Oxford Handbook of
Prescribing
for Nurses and
Allied Health
Professionals

SECOND EDITION

Edited by

Sue Beckwith

Sue Beckwith Health Care Consultancy

and

Penny Franklin

Associate Professor (Senior Lecturer)
Prescribing and Health Studies,
University of Plymouth, UK

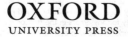

OXFORD
UNIVERSITY PRESS

OXFORD
UNIVERSITY PRESS

Great Clarendon Street, Oxford OX2 6DP.

Oxford University Press is a department of the University of Oxford.
It furthers the University's objective of excellence in research, scholarship,
and education by publishing worldwide in

Oxford New York

Auckland Cape Town Dar es Salaam Hong Kong Karachi
Kuala Lumpur Madrid Melbourne Mexico City Nairobi
New Delhi Shanghai Taipei Toronto

With offices in

Argentina Austria Brazil Chile Czech Republic France Greece
Guatemala Hungary Italy Japan Poland Portugal Singapore
South Korea Switzerland Thailand Turkey Ukraine Vietnam

Oxford is a registered trade mark of Oxford University Press
in the UK and in certain other countries

Published in the United States
by Oxford University Press Inc., New York

© Oxford University Press, 2011

British Library Cataloguing in Publication Data
Data available

Library of Congress Cataloging-in-Publication-Data
Data available

Typeset by Glyph International, Bangalore, India
Printed in Great Britain
on acid-free paper by
Ashford Colour Press Ltd., Gosport, Hampshire

ISBN 978–0–19–957581–7

10 9 8 7 6 5 4 3 2 1

Preface

This handbook gives authoritative, practical, and essential guidance on all aspects of the complex practice of non-medical prescribing. Following the style of the successful Oxford Handbooks with topic areas covering one or two pages and cross-referenced to other applicable information within the book, information is readily available to aid decision-making.

Non-medical prescribing had its inception in Julia Cumberlege's 1986 government report on neighbourhood nursing, which acknowledged that some nurses were prescribing without a legal or professional authorization[1]. The report of the Advisory Group on Nurse Prescribing (1989)[2] converted her earlier recommendations into today's prescribing mandate which was given the royal assent in 1992. Later that year the Medicinal Products: Prescription by Nurses etc. Act and the required secondary legislation were passed, enabling the selection of eight demonstration sites, and in 1994 eligible nurses (health visitors, and home/district nurses who held a community specialist practice qualification) received the then English Nursing Board (ENB) training in safe prescribing from a limited formulary.

Following successful evaluation by the Universities of Liverpool and York, a further expansion in 1996 included 60 more practices in England and two more pilot sites in Scotland. Publication of the white paper *Delivering the Future*[3] led to seven more pilot sites, and then a national roll-out to 23,000 eligible practitioners who undertook the Mode 1 course (blended learning). Students undertaking a specialist practitioner's degree completed the Mode 2 preparation (a taught module).

Gaining pace and following two favourable evaluative reports by June Crown in 1999[4,5] and the NHS Plan,[6] prescribing rights were extended to other groups of nurses as independent prescribers. By May 2001, the Nurse Prescribers Formulary and ENB training (V200) for nurses, midwives, and health visitors were extended to include four new prescribing areas:
- Minor illness
- Minor injuries
- Health promotion
- Palliative care.

1. Department of Health and Social Security (1986). *Neighbourhood nursing—a focus for care.* HMSO, London.
2. Department of Health (1989). *Report of the Advisory Group on Nurse Prescribing.* Department of Health, London.
3. Department of Health (1996). *Delivering the future.* Department of Health, London.
4. Department of Health (1998). *Review of prescribing, supply and administration of medicines. A report on the supply and administration of medicines under group protocols.* Department of Health, London.
5. Department of Health (1999). *Review of prescribing, supply and administration of medicines. Final report.* Department of Health, London.
6. Department of Health (2000). *The NHS plan: a plan for investment, a plan for reform.* Department of Health, London.

The Nurse Prescribers Extended Formulary (NPEF) included all pharmacy and general sales list (GSL) medicines and initially a list of 140 prescription-only items used for treating specific conditions in the four areas listed.

Supplementary prescribing for nurses and pharmacists was introduced in 2003 following changes within the Health and Social Care Act 2001.[7] Further amendments to legislation in May 2006 enabled nurse independent prescribers to prescribe from anywhere in the British National Formulary for any medical condition within their competence with the exception of unlicensed drugs. Following changes to legislation in 2009, Nurse Independent Prescribers can prescribe unlicensed medicines on the same basis as doctors, as long as they are competent to do so. Nurse independent prescribing includes some controlled drugs.[8] Nurses can now study for the combined qualification of Nurse Independent and Supplementary Prescriber (V300) which is recorded with the Nursing and Midwifery Council (NMC).[9]

In 2005 supplementary prescribing rights were extended to include physiotherapists, podiatrists, radiographers, and optometrists. Supplementary Prescribers are now enabled to prescribe any medicines, including controlled drugs, as part of an agreed clinical management plan (CMP).[10,11] Optometrists and pharmacists can now also prescribe as independent and supplementary prescribers.

The new standards for nurse prescribing were introduced in May 2006.[9] These standards were also adopted by the Health Professions Council.

With each extension of prescribing areas and the addition of other healthcare professionals as non-medical prescribers, the practitioners' prescribing knowledge base is constantly developing and open to challenge This handbook provides advice on all aspects of prescribing decision-making: for novice and student alike, as well as for all non-medical prescribing courses and following all the competency areas. It will act as a useful reference for newly qualified prescribers and additionally for those who are becoming more advanced in the practice.

7. *Health and Social Care Act 2001*, Chapter 15.TSO, London.

8. Department of Health (2006). *Improving patients' access to medicines: a guide to implementing nurse and pharmacist independent prescribing within the NHS in England.* Department of Health, London.

9. Nursing and Midwifery Council (2006). *Standards of proficiency for nurse and midwife prescribers.* NMC, London.

10. Department of Health (2006). *Medicines matters: a guide to the mechanisms for the prescribing, supply and administration of medicines.* Department of Health, London.

11. ▣ http://dh.gov.uk (accessed 30 November 2010).

Acknowledgements

The contents of this handbook have been peer and medically reviewed and we would like to thank our reviewers for their care and rigour.

Special thanks go to Graham Brack for being a gentlemanly critical friend. Thanks also to Caroline Hardy for her initial input to the book.

This book is dedicated to William Beckwith, Matt and Andy Franklin, and Cosmo.

We welcome constructive comments and recommendations from our readers and hope that this handbook will help towards promoting safe, effective, evidenced, and economic prescribing.

Contributors

Graham Brack, Pharmaceutical Adviser, Cornwall and Isles of Scilly PCT

Shelley Mehigan, Nurse Specialist in Contraception, Sexual Health for Berkshire East Sexual Health Services, UK

Contents

Detailed contents

Symbols and abbreviations

~	Approx
±	Plus/minus
↑	Increased
↓	Decreased
↔	Normal
1°	Primary
2°	Secondary
°	Degrees
📖	Cross reference
💾	Internet site
ABPI	Ankle brachial pressure index
ACE	Angiotensin-converting enzyme
ADE	Adverse drug effect
ADI	Adverse drug interaction
ADR	Adverse drug reaction
AIDS	Acquired immune deficiency syndrome
ASTRO-PU	Adjusted for age, sex, temporary resident originated prescribing unit
BAN	British approved name
BDA	British Diabetic Association (now Diabetes UK)
BHF	British Heart Foundation
BHS	British Hypertension Society
BMJ	*British Medical Journal*
BNF	*British National Formulary*
BTS	*British Thoracic Society*
CAMs	Complementary and alternative medicines
CAT	Critical appraisal trial
CG	Clinical governance
CHD	Coronary heart disease
CKS	Clinical Knowledge Summaries
CNS	Central nervous system
CMP	Clinical management plan
CNS	Central nervous system
COC	Combined hormonal contraceptive
COPD	Chronic obstructive pulmonary disease

CP	Community practitioner (who holds a community specialist practice qualification and who can prove that they will use prescribing in their practice).
CPD	Continuing professional development
CRAG	Clinical Resource Audit Group
CSBS	Clinical Standards Board for Scotland
CSM	Committee on Safety of Medicines
CSPHN	Community Specialist Public Health Nurse
CVA	Cerebrovascular accident (stroke)
CVD	Cardiovascular disease
DH	Department of Health
DL	Distance learning
DN	District nurse
DNA	Deoxyribonucleic acid
DVLA	Driver and Vehicle Licensing Authority
EBP	Evidence-based practice
EPACT	Electronic prescribing analysis and cost
FAQ	Frequently asked question
FSH	Follicle-stimulating hormone
GAD	Glutamic acid decarboxylase
GFR	Glomerular filtration rate
GI	Gastrointestinal
GMC	General Medical Council
GP	General practitioner
GSL	General sales list
GTN	Glyceryl trinitrate
hCG	Chorionic gonadotrophin
HDL	High-density lipoprotein
HEI	Higher education institution
HIV	Human immunodeficiency virus
HOWIS	Health of Wales Information Service
hr	hour
HRT	Hormone replacement therapy
HV	Health visitor
IDDM	Insulin-dependent diabetes mellitus
IM	Intramuscular
INR	International normalized ratio
IP	Independent prescriber
IUD	Intra-uterine device
IV	Intravenous

LA	Local anaesthetic
LDL	Low-density lipoprotein
LH	Luteinizing hormone
LSD	Lysergide
MAOI	Monoamine oxidase inhibitor
MAR	Medicines administration record
MCA	Medicines Control Agency
MDMA	3,4-Methylenedioxymetamphetamine (ecstacy)
MHRA	Medicines and Healthcare Products Regulatory Agency
MI	Myocardial infaction
ml	Millilitre
min	minute
MSU	Mid-stream urine
NCASP	National Clinical Audit Support Programme
NeLH	National Electronic Library for Health (now NHS Evidence Health Information Resources)
NHS	National Health Service
NICE	National Institute for Health and Clinical Excellence
NMC	Nursing and Midwifery Council
NMP	Non-medical prescriber
NPC	National Prescribing Centre
NPEF	Nurse Prescribers Extended Formulary
NPF	Nurse Prescribers Formulary for Community Practitioners
NSAID	Non-steroidal anti-inflammatory drug
NSF	National Service Framework
OSCE	Objective structured clinical examination
OTC	Over-the-counter
P	Pharmacy-only medicine
PACT	Prescribing analysis and cost
PASA	Purchasing and Supplies Agency
PCO	Primary care organization (now PCT)
PCT	Primary care trust
PDA	Patient decision aid
PGD	Patient-group direction
PID	Pelvic inflammatory disease
PLI	Professional liability insurance
POM	Prescription-only medicine
POP	Progesterone-only pill
PPA	Prescription Pricing Authority

PSD	Patient-specific direction
PSNC	Pharmaceutical Services Negotiating Committee
PU	Prescribing unit
PVD	Peripheral vascular disease
RCN	Royal College of Nursing
RCT	Randomized controlled trial
RHA	Regional Health Authority
RINN	Recommended international non-proprietary name
RNA	Ribonucleic acid
RTI	Renal tract infection
RTP	Return to practice
SaFF	Service financial framework
SCPHN	Specialist community public health nurse
SHA	Strategic Health Authority
SIGN	Scottish Intercollegiate Guidelines Network
SP	Supplementary prescriber
SPA	Scottish Prescribing Analysis
SPQ	Specialist Practitioner Qualification
SSRI	Selective serotonin-reuptake inhibitor
STAR-PU	Specific therapeutic group, age, sex related prescribing unit
TDM	Therapeutic drug monitoring
TENS	Transcutaneous electrical nerve stimulator
UKMI	UK Medicines Information Service
UKMIPG	UK Medicines Information Pharmacists Group
UTI	Urinary tract infection
VAT	Value-added tax
Vd	Volume of distribution
WHO	World Health Organization

Glossary

Acquired immunity
Not present at birth. Either active or passive.

Active acquired immunity
Naturally acquired immunity following exposure to an antigen within the environment or induced active immunity following deliberate exposure to an antigen, i.e. vaccination or immunization.

Adverse drug interaction (ADI)
Alteration of the drug's effects by the prior or concurrent administration of another drug (drug–drug interactions) or by food (drug–food interactions).

Adverse drug reaction (ADR)
A reaction related to the use of a specific drug (or drugs) which causes harm and/or discomfort beyond its predictable therapeutic effects, and which predictably may cause harm to the patient in the future if given in a smaller or larger dose or in the same dosage and regimen. With any ADR, treatment may warrant prevention of future reactions or alteration of the drug and dosage regimen and possible withdrawal of the product.

Audit
A systematic and official examination of a record, process, structure, environment, or account to evaluate performance.

Black triangle drugs
These are new drugs. The black triangle indicates that their safety profile is being closely monitored.

Change agent
A person skilled in the theory and implementation of planned change, who possesses well-developed leadership and management skills.

Clinical audit
Clinical audit is conducted by doctors (medical audit) and other healthcare professionals (nurses, physiotherapists, occupational therapists, speech therapists, etc.), and is the systematic critical analysis of the quality of clinical care.

Clinical management plan
The legal framework for supplementary prescribing.

Clinical supervision
This is a term used to describe a formal process of professional support and learning which enables practitioners to develop knowledge and competence, assume responsibility for their own practice, and enhance consumer protection and safety of care in complex situations.

Competent standard of care
Bolam Principle (1957): the nurse is required to act within her or his competency at all times and to exercise 'the ordinary skill of an ordinary "man" exercising that particular art', i.e. perform reasonably as practitioners trained to the same standard within the same/similar professions, within a recognized standard of competency.

Complementary and alternative medicines (CAMs)
The treatment of disease using methods other than recognized/conventional medicine.

Concordance
An informed partnership agreement which is negotiated between the prescriber and the patient.

Consent
To be valid, consent must be informed consent. Treating a patient without consent may constitute an assault and subject the nurse to damages for trespass to the person.

Constipation (difficulty in passing stools)
Stools of poor bulk, sometimes caused by a diet low in fibre, or hardness due to increased time in the intestine, or poor hydration—may be difficult to pass.

Controlled drugs
Preparations that are subject to the Misuse of Drugs Regulations 2001 and its amendments and are specified in Schedules 2 to 5.

Diabetes
Diabetes mellitus is a chronic and progressive disease which alters the body's management of carbohydrate and fat metabolism. It is divided into type 1 diabetes (previously known as insulin-dependent diabetes mellitus—IDDM) in which there is an absence of insulin, and type 2 diabetes which is caused by the body's inefficient use of endogenous insulin (insulin resistance) and/or insufficient production of insulin.

Dispensing medication
An individual who is dispensing medicine may be preparing, supplying, or administering the medication to the patient. Good practice indicates that the dispenser acts as a second checker for the prescriber. When dispensing medication always adhere to local policy.

Drug Tariff
The Drug Tariff is produced monthly as a joint compilation between the Department of Health and the NHS Business Services Authority.

Formulation
The formulation of a medicine refers to its chemical and physical composition.

Innate immunity
This is present at birth and is genetically determined. No relationship to exposure or vaccination.

Nurse Prescribers Formulary for Community Practitioners
Previously known as the Nurse Prescribers Formulary (NPF).

Nursing and Midwifery Council (NMC)
The professional regulatory body for nurses and midwives.

Overflow incontinence
The bladder overfills and urine leaks into the ureter. Symptoms include voiding small amounts of urine, hesitancy, poor flow, or post-micturition dribble. This condition may follow hysterectomy or be caused by faecal impaction, unwanted effects of a drug regimen, or prostatic hyperplasia.

PACT data
PACT (Prescribing Analysis and Cost) and SPA (Scottish Prescribing Analysis) are available as audit reports of practitioners prescribing on a quarterly (3-monthly) basis. These data provide comparisons of local and national prescribing patterns and can be broken down to indicate individual prescribing patterns.

Palliative care
Prescribing for people who require palliative care involves the active total care and suppression of symptoms for those whose disease is not responsive to curative treatments. In addition to control of pain and other symptoms, it involves a holistic approach, embracing social, psychological, and spiritual dimensions.

Passive acquired immunity
Natural passive immunity following the transfer of antibodies from another person i.e. a mother to her baby *in utero*, via the placenta, or in breastmilk, or induced passive immunity when antibodies are administered in the form of antisera to prevent or fight infection.

Patient-group directions (PGDs)
Written instructions to a specified range of health-care professionals for the sale, supply, and administration of medicines directly to groups of patients with specific defined clinical conditions who may not be individually identified before presentation for treatment. PGDs provide the legal framework for medicines to be given to groups of patients without prescriptions having to be written.

Patient-specific directions
These are written instructions from a doctor or dentist which are set out in the patient's notes (in primary care) and on the drug chart (in secondary care) to specified health-care professionals, instructing them to supply or administer medicines or appliances to a named patient. This might be a simple instruction in the patient's notes.

Pharmaid
Even BNFs which are 6–12 months old are of use for those working in developing countries. The Commonwealth Pharmaceutical Association has a scheme, Pharmaid, which dispatches older BNFs, in the month of November, to areas where they may be of use.

Public health
Public health is defined by Acheson as 'the science and art of preventing disease, prolonging life and promoting health through the organized efforts of society'.

Randomized controlled trial (RCT)
Study design where treatment, interventions, or enrolment into different study groups are assigned by random allocation. If the sample size is large enough, this design avoids bias and confounding variables.

Red flag
A system of identification for any significantly dangerous symptoms that may or may not be directly associated with the patient's presenting condition.

Social determinants of health
A person's ability to attain a standard of health and well-being is influenced by their genetic make-up and lifestyle choices.

Specific immunity
Provided by the lymphocytes, both T and B cells act as a coordinated response to specific antigens. T cells are responsible for the mediation of cell immunity, providing defence against abnormal cells and pathogens inside cells. B cells respond to antigens and pathogens in body fluids, providing humeral or antibody-mediated immunity.

Stress incontinence
An involuntary urine leak when abdominal pressure increases during physical activity (e.g. exercise or coughing). It is usually caused by muscular damage to the bladder outlet because of weakness of the pelvic floor musculature. Often precipitated by childbirth or post-menopausal oestrogen deficiency, or as a complication following prostatic surgery

Supplementary prescribing
A voluntary prescribing partnership between the independent prescriber (doctor or dentist) and a supplementary prescriber to implement an agreed patient-specific clinical management plan (CMP) with the patient's agreement.

Therapeutic range/index
The range within which plasma concentrations will be related to therapeutic effect

Urge incontinence
This is caused by instability of the detrusor muscle, or hyper-reflexia, which causes the bladder to contract at times other than intended urination. The bladder may not empty completely and a residual volume >100ml is common. The cause is unknown but it may be due to obstruction or neurological disease.

Urinary incontinence
An involuntary or inappropriate loss of urine which can be demonstrated objectively.

Vicarious liability

An employer is vicariously liable for their employee's negligent acts or omissions in the course of employment, whether authorized or not, unless the employer can show that the employee was undertaking a frolic of his own rather than the employer's business. The individual nurse still carries responsibility and, as such, is accountable for his or her actions.

Yellow card

Yellow card reporting is the reporting of adverse reactions for any drug given to patients in UK to the Medicines and Health Care Products Regulatory Agency (MHRA).

Section 1

Introduction

What is a non-medical prescriber?

Non-medical prescribing history and policy in context

Health is a devolved sphere of government and therefore policy and implementation may vary between England, Scotland, Wales, and Northern Ireland. However, the following imperatives can be applied to all countries within the UK.

Context
- Renegotiation of divisions in health-care labour.
- Changing professional boundaries.[1,2]
- Supporting the ethos of the NHS.[3]
- Expansion of health professional roles.
- Introduction of nurse-led/health-professional-led clinics.
- Supporting the nurse practitioner/health professional practitioner role.[4]

Impact on practice
- Multidisciplinary teamwork approach to care.[5–9]
- Wide range of clinical and geographical settings.
- Blurring of traditional roles and practices.

Outcome for patients
- Patient choice and convenience.[2,8,9]
- Patient-centred care.
- Structured around need.
- Appropriate, timely, effective, and cost-effective intervention.
- Giving consideration to best practice based on evidence.[10]
- Health professionals managing long-term conditions.

Caution
Practice with caution and awareness of the necessity to prescribe:
- within the limitations of competencies;
- to the required legal framework.[11–14]
📖 Seven principles of safe prescribing, p. 94.

1. Department of Health (1999). *Making a difference: strengthening the nursing, midwifery and health visiting contribution to health and healthcare.* TSO, London.
2. Department of Health (2002). *Liberating the talents: helping primary care trusts and nurses to deliver the NHS Plan.* TSO, London.
3. Department of Health (2000). *The NHS Plan: a plan for investment, a plan for reform.* TSO, London.
4. Baird, A. (2001). Diagnosis and prescribing: the impact of nurse prescribing on professional roles. *Primary Health Care*, 11, 24–6.
5. *Medicinal Products: Prescription by Nurses etc. Act* (1992). TSO, London.
6. *Health and Social Care Act* (2001), Chapter 15. TSO, London.
7. *Prescription Only Medicines (Human Use) Amendment Order* (2003). TSO, London.
8. Department of Health (2004). *Choosing health: making healthier choices easier.* TSO, London.
9. Department of Health (2008). *High quality care for all: NHS Next Stage review final report.* TSO, London. 🖳 http://www.dh.gov.uk/en/Publicationsandstatistics/Publications/PublicationsPolicyAndGuidance/DH_085825 (accessed 6 September 2009)
10. Latter, S., and Courtenay, M. (2004). Effectiveness of nurse prescribing: a review of the literature. *Journal of Clinical Nursing*, 13, 26–32.
11. Nursing and Midwifery Council (2006). *Standards of proficiency for nurse and midwife prescribers.* NMC, London.

12. Nursing and Midwifery Council (2007). *Standards of educational preparation for prescribing from the community nurse prescribers formulary for nurses and midwives without a specialist practitioner qualification (V150).* NMC, London.
13. Nursing and Midwifery Council (2008). *Code of conduct, performance and ethics.* NMC, London.
14. Health Professions Council (2008). *Standards of conduct, performance and ethics.* HPC, London.

Further reading

Department of Health (2006). *Medicines matters: a guide to mechanisms for the prescribing, supply and administration of medicines.* TSO, London.

Student non-medical prescribers and methods of training 1

Who is able to prescribe what?

For all prescribing it is essential that there is clarity regarding the prescribing regimen being used, i.e. community practitioner, nurse prescriber, nurse independent prescriber and supplementary prescriber, pharmacist independent and supplementary prescriber, or supplementary prescriber.

- Nurses, midwives, pharmacists, and optometrists can qualify and prescribe as independent and supplementary prescribers.
- Physiotherapists, podiatrists, and radiographers are able to qualify as supplementary prescribers only.
- Registered nurses who have been identified by their organization as needing to prescribe from the Community Practitioners Formulary for Nurse Prescribers (CPF) can qualify as community practitioner nurse prescribers.

Prescribing training

Training is accessed through the clinical leads of primary care organizations (PCOs) and NHS trusts or can be accessed directly via higher education institutions (HEIs). Some courses are funded by Strategic Health Authority (SHA) workforce development directorates. Each SHA has a non-medical prescribing lead. Other courses are funded directly by the employing organization or can be funded privately by the applicant.

Prescribing from the Community Practitioners Formulary for nurses with a Specialist Practice Qualification (SPQ)

Mode 1

This training, the original nurse prescribing, was available for district nurses (DNs) and health visitors (HVs), now known as specialist community public health nurses (SCPHNs), who held the specialist practice qualification.

Mode 2

This is the mode of training undertaken by students studying for a Community Specialist Practice Qualification (CSPQ)/Specialist Practitioner Qualification (SPQ) as part of a specialist practitioner degree award.[1]

- It is a taught module assessed at degree level. Assessment methods vary but examples include a written case study, a pharmacology/wider aspects of prescribing examination paper, and completed competencies in practice.
- Academic credits are awarded at degree level on successful completion of this module. You are advised to contact your organization's education coordinator and/or the HEI of your choice to discuss this further.
- Following successful completion of all aspects of the assessment the registrant will be linked to the Nursing and Midwifery Council and receive the recordable qualification of Community Practitioner Nurse Prescriber (V100).

- The successful registrant who has attained the V100 recordable qualification will then be able to prescribe from the Nurse Prescribers Formulary for Community Practitioners (CPF).

Prescribing from the Community Practitioners Formulary for nurses without a specialist practitioner qualification (V150)

This training is available at some HEIs and can be accessed in the same way as above.

Those accessing the training must be:
- a registered nurse or midwife;
- able to demonstrate to their employer their intent to practise in an area where there is an identified clinical need to prescribe from the CPF;
- able to demonstrate that such prescribing will improve care/service delivery;
- able to demonstrate to their employer competent practice in the area in which they intend to prescribe and have been working in this area for long enough to be able to demonstrate competence (usually for a minimum of 2 years);
- able to provide evidence of being able to study at a minimum of academic degree level.

Prior to accessing the programme, written confirmation is needed from:
- their employer;
- a mentor who is a community practitioner nurse prescriber, who is on their organization's live register of mentors, and who has agreed to supervise them for the duration of the programme;
- the programme lead regarding selection for the programme (this must be copied to the employer).

The training for the qualification involves:
- 10 study days that must take place in the setting of the HEI;
- a minimum of 10 days of supervised practice.

Assessment is in line with NMC standards[2] and takes the form of:
- a written applied pharmacology paper consisting of 20 multiple choice and short answer questions;
- an essay or portfolio of practice.

Successful completion of the programme will lead to the NMC recordable qualification of Community Practitioner Nurse Prescriber (V150) and the registrant will be able to prescribe from the Community Practitioners Formulary (CPF) only.

---

1. Nursing and Midwifery Council (2006). *Standards of proficiency for nurse and midwife prescribers.* NMC, London.
2. Nursing and Midwifery Council (2006). *Standards of proficiency for nurse prescribers without a Specialist Practice Qualification to prescribe from the Nurse Prescribers Formulary for Community Practitioners.* NMC, London.

Student non-medical prescribers and methods of training 2

Nurse independent and supplementary prescribing

This mode of study is open to all registered nurses and midwives who demonstrate that their ability to prescribe would enhance patient care. The students also need to demonstrate an ability to study at degree level.

- This is a taught course with 26 full days spent at university and 12 days spent in practice with a medical supervisor (a doctor).
- It is assessed at degree or masters level, usually by an examination comprising one short and one long answer paper, a portfolio, the completion of competencies in practice, and an objective structured clinical examination (OSCE). There are some variations in assessment techniques between HEIs.
- The number of academic points awarded may vary between HEIs.
- Some universities offer this course as blended learning with the addition of a distance learning component.
- On qualification and when they have recorded their qualification with their professional body (NMC) nurses and midwives attain the dual qualification of Nurse Independent and Supplementary Prescriber (V300).
- Following successful completion of this additional training and when they have recorded their qualification with the NMC, nurses and midwives who are working within their competencies may prescribe as nurse independent prescribers from anywhere in the BNF including a list of controlled drugs and both licensed and unlicensed drugs[1] from anywhere within the BNF, including a list of controlled drugs that can be found in the Drug Tariff and the BNF.[2,3] They may also prescribe within their competencies as supplementary prescribers to an agreed clinical management plan (CMP) in partnership with a doctor who is the independent prescriber. Within this agreed partnership and working within the legal parameters of the clinical management plan and within the boundaries of their competence, supplementary prescribers may prescribe any drug/medicinal product that is indicated on the clinical management plan and is within the formulary provided that they are competent to do so.[4]

Pharmacists and optometrists may also qualify as independent and supplementary prescribers.

- At the time of going to press pharmacists are not permitted to prescribe controlled drugs as independent prescribers. Optometrist independent prescribers can prescribe any licensed medicine for ocular conditions affecting the eye and surrounding tissue, but cannot prescribe any controlled drug independently.
- Supplementary prescribing by designated registered health professionals (physiotherapists, podiatrists, and radiographers) is often taught as shared learning with nurse, midwife, and pharmacist student prescribers.

- The rules for optometrist prescribers are different and are outside the scope of this handbook. However, further information can be accessed at: 🖳 http://www.orthoptics.org.uk/education/orthoptic-education.

1. 🖳 http://www.npc.co.uk/prescribers/faq.htm (accessed 1 February 2010).
2. *British National Formulary* (latest edn). British Medical Association and Royal Pharmaceutical Society of Great Britain, London.
3. Drug Tariff Online. 🖳 http://drugtariff.com/ (accessed 23 June 2010).
4. Department of Health (2006). *Medicines matters: a guide to mechanisms for the prescribing, supply and administration of medicines.* TSO, London.

Supplementary prescribing

Supplementary prescribing

The definition of supplementary prescribing (formerly known as dependent prescribing) is as follows:

A voluntary partnership between an independent prescriber (a doctor or dentist) and a supplementary prescriber to implement an agreed patient specific Clinical Management Plan (CMP) with the patient's agreement.[1]

Supplementary prescribers:

• are selected locally and must have opportunities to prescribe in the post occupied on completion of prescribing training;
• must be able to demonstrate an ability to study at level 6 (degree level);
• must be able to demonstrate 3 years post-registration clinical experience;
• are able to prescribe any medicines and controlled drugs that are listed in an agreed clinical management plan (CMP);
• are able to prescribe controlled drugs because of amendments to the Misuse of Drugs regulations 2001 and to the GMS/PMS regulations which came into effect on 14 April 2005;
• Examples of CMPs can be obtained from 🖳 www.dh.gov.uk/ PolicyAndGuidance/MedicinesPharmacyAndIndustry/Prescriptions/ SupplementaryPrescribing/fs/en.

In the case of supplementary prescribing independent prescribers:

• must be doctors or dentists;
• will discuss with supplementary prescribers which patients may benefit from supplementary prescribing and which medicines may be included in a CMP;
• should be responsible for the patient's care;
• are responsible for making the diagnosis and setting the parameters for the CMP.

The supplementary prescriber has discretion regarding the frequency, dose, and product in addition to other variables outlined within the CMP.

Supplementary prescribing training

On qualifying, physiotherapists, podiatrists, and radiographers are able to register solely as supplementary prescribers. To qualify as a supplementary prescriber a nurse, midwife, pharmacist, or optometrist also has to train as an independent prescriber.

Formularies and nurse independent prescribing

The Nurse Prescribers Extended Formulary (NPEF) ceased to exist in May 2006. Nurse independent prescibers are now able to prescribe any licensed or unlicensed medicine including some controlled drugs which are listed in the BNF and in the Drug Tariff.[2,3] Nurse independent prescribers must not prescribe unless they have assessed their patient, diagnosed the condition, and are clinically competent.[3] Nurse independent prescribers are responsible for making a diagnosis.

Changes to legislation in December 2009 enabled nurse independent prescribers to prescribe unlicensed drugs.[4] This extension means that specialist nurses running clinics where they take a history, assess the patient, and make a diagnosis could, if competent and confident, prescribe independently for their patients. Pharmacists are able to prescribe independently for the local community (e.g. controlling high blood pressure, smoking cessation, diabetes, etc.) and within an acute setting where appropriate. Independent prescribing by nurses and midwives and pharmacists is intended to support the role of doctors.[1]

Before prescribing unlicensed medicines as a nurse independent prescriber you must follow the NMC guidance which states:[4]

You may prescribe an unlicensed medication as an independent nurse prescriber providing:
- You are satisfied an alternative, licensed medication would not meet the patient's or client's needs.
- You are satisfied there is a sufficient evidence base and/or experience to demonstrate the medication's safety and efficacy for that particular patient or client.
- You are prepared to take responsibility for prescribing the un-licensed medicine and for overseeing the patient's or client's care, including monitoring and any follow up treatment.
- The patient or client agrees to the prescription in the knowledge that the medicine is unlicensed and understands the implications of this.
- The medication chosen and the reason for choosing it are documented in patient's or client's notes.

Supplementary prescribing[1]

Supplementary prescribing in partnership with a doctor or dentist independent prescriber will continue for the management of long-term conditions and for shared care. Supplementary prescribing in partnership with an independent doctor prescriber can help to support the development of the confidence of nurses, midwives, designated registered health professionals (physiotherapists, podiatrists, and radiographers), pharmacists, and optometrists as prescribers.

Patient group directions (PGDs)

PGDs are for the supply and/or administration of a medicinal product or drug. Professionals who supply or administer according to a PGD are not prescribing. There are no special training requirements for health professionals who supply and administer medicines through the use of a PGD. However, the National Prescribing Centre (NPC) suggests that those using PGDs should receive at least one day's training in their use provided at local level followed by annual updates.

The NPC have developed a competency framework to guide development and training at a local level and this can be accessed at http://www.npc.co.uk/non_medical.htm.

1. Department of Health (2006). *Medicines matters: a guide to mechanisms for the prescribing, supply and administration of medicines*. TSO, London.
2. *British National Formulary* (latest edn). British Medical Association and Royal Pharmaceutical Society of Great Britain, London.
3. Drug Tariff Online. http://drugtariff.com/ (accessed 23 June 2010).
4. Nursing and Midwifery Council (2009). http://www.nmc-uk.org/Documents/ Circulars/2010%20circulars/NMCcircular04_2010.pdf (accessed 13 August 2010).

Timeline for non-medical prescribing

1968	Medicines Act
1986	Neighbourhood Nursing: a Focus for Care
1989	First Crown Report
1992	Medicinal Products: Prescription by Nurses Act
1994	Medicinal Products: Prescription by Nurses etc. Act (Commencement No. 1)
1999	Second Crown Report (Crown Review)
2000	Consultation on Proposals to Extend Nurse Prescribing
2000	Freedom of Information Act
2001	Health and Social Care Act
2003	Amendments to the Prescription Only Medicines Order and NHS Regulation
2006	Nurse independent prescribing
2006	Introduction of Nursing and Midwifery Council standards of proficiency for nurse and midwife prescribers
2006	The Medicines for Human Use (Prescribing) (Miscellaneous Amendments) Order 2006
2006	Amendments to 1992 Medicinal Products: Prescription by Nurses Act and to medicines legislation (SI 2006/1015)
2007	Introduction of the Nursing and Midwifery Council standards of proficiency for nurse prescribers without a specialist practice qualification to prescribe from the Community Practitioners Formulary
2009	Changes to legislation enabling nurse independent prescribers to prescribe licensed and unlicensed drugs: Medicines for Human Use (Miscellaneous Amendments) (no 2) Regulations. SI 2009 3063

1968 Medicines Act

Covered the establishment of the medical agency, the manner and type of licence needed for research on medicinal products, the manufacture, import, and storage of medicines, and, of particular relevance, the manner in which medicines can be supplied and administered by health professionals.

1986 Neighbourhood Nursing: a Focus for Care

Report of the Community Nursing Review, the Cumberlege Report. Recommended limited prescribing rights for community nurses with district nurse or health visitor qualifications.

1989 First Crown Report

Report on the Advisory Group on Nurse Prescribing. Recommended nurse prescribers and other professionals as prescribers for the future enhancement of patient care.

1992 Medicinal Products: Prescription by Nurses Act
Primary legislation: royal assent to limited prescribing rights for health visitors, district nurses, and practice nurses with a health visiting or district nursing qualification.

1994 Medicinal Products Prescription by Nurses etc. Act (Commencement No. 1)
Secondary legislation enabling health visitors, district nurses, and practice nurses with a health visiting or district nursing qualification to prescribe.

1999 Second Crown Report (Crown Review)
Review of prescribing, supply, and administration of medicines. Recommended the supply and administration of medicines under group protocols for nurses and other professionals.

2000 Consultation on proposals to extend nurse prescribing
This included extending the scope of nurse prescribing, which does not require primary legislation, and also extending prescribing rights to other health professionals.

2000 Freedom of Information Act
This Act gives the public the right to view information held in the public domain by public authorities such as the NHS. This includes prescribing policies and protocols. The handling and disclosure of personal information is exempted and is regulated by the Data Protection Act 1998.

2001 Health and Social Care Act
This provided necessary legislation for the implementation of independent extended nurse prescribing. Nurses and midwives were given the rights to prescribe independently from an Extended Nurse Prescribing Formulary. It set the ground for supplementary prescribing rights to be given to other health professionals

2003 Amendments to the Prescription Only Medicines Order and NHS regulations
Allowed supplementary prescribing by suitably trained nurses, midwives, and pharmacists.

Spring 2005 Amendments to the Prescription Only Medicines Order and NHS regulations
Allowed supplementary prescribing of controlled drugs by nurses, midwives, and pharmacists in primary and secondary care. Allowed supplementary prescribing by suitably trained physiotherapists, podiatrists, and radiographers, with the exception of controlled drugs.

2006 The Medicines for Human Use (Prescribing) (Miscellaneous Amendments) Order 2006

Allowed independent non-medical prescribers (nurses, midwives, and pharmacists) to prescribe any licensed prescription-only drug within their field of competence and, for nurse/midwife prescribers only, some controlled drugs.

2006 Nurse independent prescribing

In response to the above, from May 2006, the Nurse Prescribers Extended Formulary was discontinued and qualified nurse independent prescribers (formerly known as Extended Formulary nurse prescribers) were able to prescribe any licensed medicine for any medical condition within their competence, including some controlled drugs.

2006 Prescribing from the Community Practitioners Formulary

From Spring 2006 the name of the Nurse Prescribers Formulary was changed to the Community Practitioners Formulary for Nurse Prescribers. Nurses who undertake mode 2 training as part of a community specialist practice qualification (SPQ) or as part of the V150 training are licensed with the Nursing and Midwifery Council to prescribe from this formulary only.

2006 Introduction of the Nursing and Midwifery Council standards of proficiency for nurse and midwife prescribers

These were introduced in Spring 2006.[1]

2006 Amendments to 1992 Medicinal Products Prescription by Nurses Act and to medicines legislation (SI 2006/1015)

This enabled prescribing from the Community Practitioners Formulary for suitably trained nurses and midwives without a specialist practice qualification.

2007 Introduction of Nursing and Midwifery Council standards of proficiency

These allowed nurse prescribers without a Specialist Practice Qualification to prescribe from the Community Practitioners Formulary.

December 2009 The Medicines for Human Use (Miscellaneous Amendments) (no. 2) Regulations SI 2009 3063

These changes to legislation enabled nurse independent prescribers to prescribe licensed and unlicensed drugs (NB: the regulations relating to the prescribing of controlled drugs[2] has not changed and the controlled drugs that can be prescribed are listed in the Drug Tariff[3] and the BNF[4]).

Further reading

Department of Health (2006). *Improving patients' access to medicines: a guide to implementing nurse and pharmacist independent prescribing within the NHS in England.* ⌨ http://www.dh.gov.uk/en/Publicationsandstatistics/Publications/PublicationsPolicyAndGuidance/DH_4133743.

1. ⌨ http://www.nmc-uk.org/Educators/Standards-for-education/Standards-of-proficiency-for-nurse-and-midwife-prescribers/ (accessed 1 February 2010).
2. ⌨ http://www.npc.co.uk/prescribers/faq.html (accessed 1 February 2010).
3. ⌨ http://www.ppa.org.uk (accessed 1 February 2010).
4. *British National Formulary* (latest edn). British Medical Association and Royal Pharmaceutical Society of Great Britain, London.

The legal differences between prescribing, administering, and dispensing

Administration of drugs

Administration of drugs can occur as a result of a patient-group direction (PGD) or a written patient-specific direction (PSD) of which a prescription is one example.

PGDs

Recommended by the Second Crown Report,[1] patient-group direction is legal terminology for what used to be known as group protocols.

PGDs provide written instructions to a specified range of health professionals for the sale, supply, and administration of medicines directly to groups of patients with specific defined clinical conditions who may or may not be individually identified before presentation for treatment.[2] PGDs provide the legal framework for medicines to be given to groups of patients without prescriptions having to be written.

Medication can be administered by specified health professionals under a PGD without them necessarily having to consult a prescriber, and without the patient necessarily seeing a prescriber. Responsibility for assessment to ascertain whether the patient fits the criteria within the PGD lies with the health professional.

PGDs are not designed to manage long-term/chronic conditions. Management of such conditions is best achieved by a health professional prescribing for the individual patient.

Legal framework for PGDs

- The Prescription Only Medicines (Human Use) Amendment Order 2000.[3]
- The Medicine (Pharmacy and General Sale—Exemption) Amendment Order 2000.[4]
- The Medicines (Sale and Supply) (Miscellaneous Provisions) Amendment (No 2) Regulations 2000.[5]

A senior doctor, dentist, or pharmacist who is authorized by their employing organization must provide signed authorization for a PGD. They must also have been instrumental in developing the PGD. The PGD must be ratified by the Trust or organization through governance. Individual health professionals can only administer under the authority of a PGD if it has been agreed through the governance procedures of their employing organization.

The following qualified registered health professionals can sell, supply, or administer medicines under a PGD, provided that they are named individuals and are working to the authorization of a PGD that is recognized by the governance procedures of their employing organization:

- nurses;
- midwives;
- health visitors;

- optometrists;
- pharmacists;
- chiropodists and podiatrists;
- radiographers;
- orthoptists;
- physiotherapists;
- paramedics;
- dietitians;
- occupational therapists;
- speech and language therapists;
- prosthetists.

Appropriate settings for use of PGDs
Areas where a patient has not been already identified, such as:
- minor injury clinics;
- minor illness clinics;
- first contact services;
- out-of-hours services;
- emergency situations;
- family planning clinics;
- immunization clinics.

Patient-specific directions

These are written instructions from a doctor or dentist to specified health professionals, which are set out in the patient's notes (in primary care) and on the drug chart (in secondary care), instructing them to supply or administer medicines or appliances to a named patient. This might be a simple instruction in the patient's notes or on the medicines administration record (MAR).

Dispensing medication

An individual who is dispensing medicine may be preparing, supplying, or administering the medication to the patient. Good practice indicates that the dispenser acts as a second checker for the prescriber. When dispensing medication always adhere to local policy.

1. Department of Health (1999) *Review of prescribing, supply and administration of medicines: final report*. TSO, London.
2. Department of Health (2004) *Policy and guidance: patient group directions*. ▣ http://www.dh.gov.uk/PolicyAndGuidance/EmergencyPlanning/EmergencyPreparednessArticle/fs/en?CONTENT_ID=4069610&chk=in7ZEF
3. *Prescription Only Medicines (Human Use) Amendment Order 2000*. TSO, London.
4. *Medicine (Pharmacy and General Sale—Exemption) Amendment Order 2000*. TSO, London.
5. *Medicines (Sale and Supply) (Miscellaneous Provisions) Amendment (No 2) Regulations 2000*. TSO, London.

Nursing and Midwifery Council and Health Professions Council codes

Nursing and Midwifery Council (NMC)

Background

The code Standards of Conduct, Performance and Ethics for Nurses and Midwives (4 April 2008) came into effect on 1 May 2008.[1] This document replaced the earlier UK Central Council for Nursing, Midwifery and Health Visiting Code of Conduct.

All references to 'nurses, midwives and health visitors' were replaced by 'nurses, midwives'. Since 2004 the code has contained a section outlining indemnity insurance. The main emphases for the new code of conduct are health professional accountability and placing the patient at the centre of care.

A summary of the code can be accessed at 🔲 http://www.nmc-uk.org/aArticle.aspx?ArticleID=3056

Standards of proficiency for nurse and midwife prescribers[2]

These were published in April 2006 and provide educational and practice prescribing standards for nurses and midwives. Standards are mandatory and cover both nurse and midwife independent prescribers and community practitioner nurse prescribers. The standards have also been adopted by the HPC and can be accessed at:

🔲 http://www.nmc-uk.org/aDisplayDocument.aspx?documentID=1645.

Standards of educational preparation for prescribing from the Community nurse Prescribers Formulary for nurses without a Specialist Practitioner Qualification (V150)[3] can be accessed at:

🔲 http://www.nmcuk.org/aDisplayDocument.aspx?documentID=5454

🔲 http://www.nmcuk.org/aDisplayDocument.aspx?documentID=3567.

Prescribing and the implications of delegation

The NMC (2007) has provided written standards for the administration of medicines.[4] All nurse prescribers are accountable under the law to work to these standards and they must be used in conjunction with the standards of proficiency for nurse and midwife prescribers. The NMC has produced advice on the following topics:

- accountability;
- confidentiality;
- gifts and gratuities;
- consenting;
- delegation;
- environment of care;
- alternative and complimentary medicines, and homeopathy;
- record keeping.

Further advice can be accessed at:

🔲 http://www.nmc-uk.org/aSection.aspx?SectionID=12.

The prescriber is responsible for (accountable for):
- accurate, contemporaneous, and up-to-date record keeping,[5] even if the administration is delegated;
- ensuring that the prescribed/recommended item is applied or administered as directed by the patients, their carers, the nurse him/ herself, or any other person to whom the task is delegated.

Prescribing and cooperation with others
The NMC code states that you must collaborate with those in your care by:
- listening to the people in your care and responding to their concerns and preferences;
- supporting people in caring for themselves to improve and maintain their health;
- recognizing and respecting the contribution that people make to their own care and well-being;
- arranging to meet people's language and communication needs;
- sharing with people, in a way they can understand, the information they want or need to know about their health.

Specialist community public health nurses
Specialist community public health nurses are accountable under the NMC code of conduct and, if they are prescribers, to the standards of proficiency for nurse and midwife prescribers.

NMC standards for prescribing for children
The Nursing and Midwifery Council have set specific standards related to prescribing for children. Practitioners who prescribe for children must:

. . . recognise the unique implications and developmental context of the anatomical and physiological differences between children neonates and young people.[6]

In addition they stipulate that:

Only nurses with relevant knowledge, competence and skills in nursing children should prescribe for children. This is particularly important in primary care (e.g out of hours, walk in clinics and general practice settings). Anyone prescribing for a child in these situations must be able to demonstrate competence to prescribe for children and refer to another prescriber when working outside of their area of expertise or level of competence.[4]

and:

It is the responsibility of the employer to ensure that the registrant is able to apply prescribing principles to their own area of practice.[4]

The Health Professions Council (HPC)

Background
The HPC is a regulatory body which has been set up to protect the public. It holds a register of members from the following 14 health professions:
- arts therapists;
- biomedical scientists;
- chiropodists/podiatrists;

- clinical scientists;
- dietitians;
- occupational therapists;
- operating department practitioners;
- orthoptists;
- paramedics;
- physiotherapists;
- practitioner psychologists;
- prosthetists/orthotists;
- radiographers;
- speech and language therapists.

The names of the above professions are protected by law and only individual practitioners registered with the HPC are permitted to use these titles. Publications defining the standards of proficiency and conduct for the above professions are available at:
🖳 http://www.hpc-uk.org/publications/

Health professionals who can prescribe
The following health professionals are able to prescribe as supplementary prescribers only:
- physiotherapists;
- radiographers;
- podiatrists.

These professionals share the nursing and midwifery standards of proficiency for nurse and midwife prescribers.

Pharmacists are able to prescribe as independent and supplementary prescribers and are regulated by the Royal Pharmaceutical Society of Great Britain (http://www.rpsgb.org/).

Optometrists are able to prescribe as independent and supplementary prescribers and are regulated by the General Optical Council.

NB: The specifics of prescribing for pharmacists and optometrists are not covered in this publication.

1. Nursing and Midwifery Council (2008). *Standards of conduct, performance and ethics for nurses and midwives.* NMC, London.
2. Nursing and Midwifery Council (2006). *Standards of proficiency for nurse and midwife prescribers.* NMC, London.
3. Nursing and Midwifery Council (2007). *Standards of educational preparation for prescribing from the Community Nurse Prescribers Formulary for nurses and midwives without a Specialist Practitioner Qualification (V150).* NMC, London.
4. Nursing and Midwifery Council (2007). *Standards for medicines management.* NMC, London.
5. Nursing and Midwifery Council (2009). *Record keeping: guidance for nurses and midwives.*
6. Nursing and Midwifery Council (2007). *Prescribing for children and young people.* NMC, London.

Section 2

Principles

Principles of supplementary prescribing

What is supplementary prescribing?

Supplementary prescribing is a voluntary prescribing partnership between the independent prescriber (doctor or dentist) and a supplementary prescriber, to implement an agreed patient-specific clinical management plan (CMP) with the patient's agreement.[1]

Supplementary prescribers must be clinically competent and be able to fully assess their patient and make a prescribing decision. They are accountable for any prescription that they write and for their actions and omissions when working within the framework of a clinical management plan (CMP).

Rationale for supplementary prescribing
- Maximum benefit to patients.
- Patient choice of prescriber.
- Flexible use of workforce.
- For patients with multiple health needs or multiple professional carers.
- Works well for the management of uncomplicated long term conditions.
- May not be suitable for all cases.
- The independent prescriber who is a doctor can decide in partnership with the supplementary prescriber as to suitability of implementation of a CMP.

Supplementary prescribing works well when:
- working within a team;
- a doctor is easily accessible;
- there is management of long-term conditions;
- used in a mental health setting;
- prescribing controlled drugs;
- the health professional who is a supplementary prescriber is clinically competent and the support of a doctor who is the independent prescriber increases their confidence.

Legislation
- The 1998 Crown 2 Review of Prescribing suggested widening prescribing rights to enable nurses and some allied health professionals to prescribe from patient-group directions and as dependent prescribers.
- Dependent prescribing changed to supplementary prescribing as a result of amendments to the Health and Social Care Act 2001. These amendments designated new categories of prescriber with set conditions, and supplementary prescribing for nurses and pharmacists was implemented as a result of amendments to the Prescription Only Medicines Order and changes to NHS regulations (2003).
- Supplementary prescribing was enforced for physiotherapists, podiatrists, radiographers, and optometrists in 2005.
- From 2005 nurse and pharmacist supplementary prescribers were able to prescribe controlled drugs as part of a CMP.

- In 2006 physiotherapist, podiatrist, radiographer, and optometrist supplementary prescribers were able to prescribe controlled drugs as part of a CMP.[1]

📖 Timeline for non-medical prescribing, p. 14.

Who can qualify as a supplementary prescriber?
Registered:
- nurses;
- midwives;
- pharmacists;
- optometrists;
- podiatrists;
- physiotherapists;
- radiographers.

Key principles of supplementary prescribing
- Patient safety is paramount.
- Doctor independent prescriber makes the diagnosis.
- Independent prescriber must be a doctor (or dentist).
- Voluntary partnership between doctor/dentist independent prescriber and supplementary prescriber.
- Clinical management plan needs to be agreed jointly by doctor independent prescriber/s and supplementary prescriber(s).
- Patients/carers must be informed of the plan, who will be prescribing for them, and in what role (e.g. nurses, midwives, pharmacists, and optometrists can also be independent prescribers).
- Patients/carers must give their consent.
- A supplementary prescriber must prescribe only within the parameters of an agreed CMP.
- A supplementary prescriber is accountable for actions and omissions when working within the framework of supplementary prescribing.
- The clinical management plan must be patient appropriate and patient specific.
- A supplementary prescriber should only prescribe within their competency area.
- Patient agreement is paramount.
- CMPs should refer to appropriate reputable guidelines or agreed protocols for treatment of a specific condition.
- Guidelines/protocols should be easily available to all who are prescribing within the CMP.
- Supplementary prescribing can include a team approach to prescribing with more than one independent and supplementary prescriber signed up to the plan.
- Communication between all prescribers is essential.
- Ideally, there should be shared access to patient records.
- Supports multidisciplinary care.
- The CMP needs to be relatively simple otherwise it won't happen.

1. Department of Health (2006). *Medicines matters: a guide to the mechanisms for the prescribing, supply and administration of medicines.* Department of Health, London.

Practice specific to supplementary prescribing

General principles of supplementary prescribing, as listed below, apply to prescribing in both acute and primary care. CMPs need to be set up for the patient with the patient's knowledge in advance of any prescribing and must:

- ensure that a voluntary prescribing agreement has been negotiated between the independent prescriber(s) and the supplementary prescriber(s) with the knowledge of the patient;
- prescribe only within competency area/scope of practice;
- always inform the patient/carer of prescribing actions;
- gain consent from the patient/carer;
- ensure that all parties have access to the CMP;
- communicate all prescribing decisions contemporaneously with other prescribers who are involved in the patient's care;
- where possible, use shared electronic records;
- where there is co-terminus access to records, use the template as illustrated;
- where there is no access to co-terminus records, use the template as illustrated;
- templates can be established for the treatment of specific conditions (however, these must be adapted to meet the specific needs of the individual patient).

📖 Practical examples of CMPs, p. 40

CMP templates

Template CMP 1 (blank): for teams that have full
co-terminus access to patient records

Name of patient:	Patient medication sensitivities/allergies:	
Patient identification (e.g. ID number, date of birth):		
Independent prescriber(s):	Supplementary prescriber(s)	
Condition(s) to be treated	Aim of treatment	
Medicines that may be prescribed by SP:		
Preparation Indication	Dose schedule	Specific indications for referral back to the IP
Guidelines or protocols supporting clinical management plan:		
Frequency of review and monitoring by:		
Supplementary prescriber:		
Supplementary prescriber and independent prescriber:		
Process for reporting ADRs:		
Shared record to be used by IP and SP:		
Agreed by independent prescriber(s) Date	Agreed by Date supplementary prescriber(s)	Date agreed with patient/ carer

Reproduced with permission from the Department of Health.

☒ http://www.dh.gov.uk/en/Healthcare/Medicinespharmacyandindustry/Prescriptions/
TheNon-MedicalPrescribingProgramme/Supplementaryprescribing/DH_4123030
(accessed 1 February 2010).

Template CMP 2 (blank): for teams where the SP does not have co-terminus access to the medical record

Name of patient:	Patient medication sensitivities/allergies:
Patient identification (e.g. ID number, date of birth):	
Current medication:	Medical history:
Independent prescriber(s):	Supplementary prescriber(s):
Contact details: (tel/email/address)	Contact details: (tel/email/address)
Condition(s) to be treated:	Aim of treatment:

Medicines that may be prescribed by SP:

Preparation	Indication	Dose schedule	Specific indications for referral back to the IP

Guidelines or protocols supporting clinical management plan:

Frequency of review and monitoring by:

Supplementary prescriber:

Supplementary prescriber and independent prescriber:

Process for reporting ADRs:

Shared record to be used by IP and SP:

Agreed by independent prescriber(s)	Date	Agreed by supplementary prescriber(s)	Date	Date agreed with patient/ carer

Reproduced with permission from the Department of Health.

🖳 http://www.dh.gov.uk/en/Healthcare/Medicinespharmacyandindustry/Prescriptions/
TheNon-MedicalPrescribingProgramme/Supplementaryprescribing/DH_4123030
(accessed 1 February 2010).

Supplementary prescribing within the acute sector

In the acute sector you can use either an adapted version of the hospital prescribing sheet, as long as it is line with local policy, or an FP10 (e.g. when prescribing in some outpatient clinics and some A&E departments). Ensure that the hospital pharmacy has a record of your signature.

Examples of clinical conditions where supplementary prescribing can be used in the acute setting:

- stroke;
- erythropoiesis;
- pain;
- palliative care;
- cardiology;
- oncology;
- diabetes;
- hypertension;
- chronic obstructive pulmonary disease;
- asthma;
- paediatrics;
- cystic fibrosis.

Supplementary prescribing in the primary care setting

The same general principles apply for supplementary prescribing in the primary care sector as in the acute sector.

Practice specific to prescribing in primary care

- Provide community pharmacies with a copy of your signature.
- Prescribe using FP10 independent supplementary prescriber prescription.
- Ensure that your contact number and budget code are indicated on the prescription.
- Register your entitlement with the NHS Business Services Authority (NB: if you are employed this is usually done by your organization).

Examples of clinical conditions for which supplementary prescribing can be used in the primary care setting:

- smoking cessation;
- chronic obstructive pulmonary disease;
- asthma;
- chronic eczema/skin complaints;
- hypertension;
- diabetes;
- heart failure.

Further reading

Bissell, P. Cooper, R., Guillaume L., *et al.* (2008). *An evaluation of supplementary prescribing in nursing and pharmacy. Final report for the Department of Health.* Universities of Sheffield, Nottingham, South Australia and Flinders University, Adelaide.
🖳 http://www.sheffield.ac.uk/content/1/c6/09/11/83/Supplementary_prescribing.pdf

Space for writing notes on clinical management plans

Space for your own examples of prescribing within the acute sector

Space for your own examples of prescribing within the primary care setting

Clinical management plans

What is a clinical management plan?

A clinical management plan (CMP) is an agreed defined plan of treatment for a named patient which sets the legal boundaries of the medication and the parameters of prescribing responsibility for the supplementary prescriber. The plan must be agreed as the result of a voluntary partnership between the independent doctor or dentist prescriber and the supplementary prescriber, and with the knowledge of the patient and/or carer (📖 Supplementary prescribing, p. 10).

Only qualified supplementary prescribers who hold a recordable qualification, as recognized by their regulatory body (in the case of nurses, the NMC), can prescribe as supplementary prescribers. Supplementary prescribers must only prescribe within their clinical field of competence.

A CMP:
- is the legal framework for supplementary prescribing;
- is a plan of care that relates specifically to a named patient and the specific condition(s) to be managed;
- must be in place before prescribing.

📖 Supplementary prescribing, p. 10.
📖 Practical examples of CMPs, p. 40.

What must be included on a CMP?

- The name of the patient to whom the plan relates.
- The illness or conditions which may be treated by the supplementary prescriber.
- The date on which the plan is to start.
- The date when the plan is to be reviewed by the independent prescriber.
- The date of review by the supplementary prescriber.
- The class or description of medicines or appliances which may be prescribed or administered under the plan.
- Restrictions or limitations of strength or dose of medicines which may be prescribed or administered under the plan.
- The period of administration or use of medicines or appliances which may be prescribed or administered under the plan.
- Relevant warnings about known sensitivities of the patient to medicines or appliances.
- Known difficulties that the patient has with particular medicines or appliances.
- The arrangements for notification of:
  - suspected or known reactions to any medicine which may be prescribed or administered according to the plan;
  - suspected or known adverse reactions to any other medicine taken at the same time as any medicine prescribed or administered under the plan;
  - incidents occurring with the appliance which might lead, might have led to, or has led to the death or serious deterioration of the state of health of the patient;

- circumstances in which the supplementary prescriber should refer to, or seek the advice of, the independent prescriber or prescribers who are party to the plan.
- Date for review—at least annual, and more often where needed.[1]

How can supplementary prescribing be effectively implemented into practice?
- CMPs have to be relatively simple and quick to complete.
- A plan should not duplicate information already in the shared record.

Communication
- Vital between independent prescriber(s) and supplementary prescriber(s).
- Remote partnerships work best when there are shared electronic records.
- The CMP should include national and local guidelines which must clearly identify the range of the relevant medicinal products to be used in the treatment of the patient.
- The CMP should draw attention to the relevant part of the guideline.
- Guidelines referred to need to be easily accessible.

Further reading
Department of Health (2005). *Supplementary prescribing by nurses, pharmacists, chiropodists/ podiatrists, physiotherapists and radiographers within the NHS in England.*
 🖳 www.doh.gov.uk/supplementaryprescribing
Department of Health (2006). *Medicines matters: a guide to mechanisms for the prescribing, supply and administration of medicines.* TSO, London.

1. Department of Health (2003). *Guidelines: supplementary prescribing: frequently asked questions.*
🖳 www.doh.gov.uk/supplementaryprescribing

Developing, writing, and implementing a CMP

Developing a CMP

The agreed written plan must be in place before prescribing begins. CMPs can be written on two types of template.

- The first is designed for situations where all the prescribers who are involved in the management of the case have full co-terminus access to patient records (📖 Template CMP 1, p. 41).
- The second is designed for teams and can be used where the supplementary prescriber does not have co-terminus access to the medical record (📖 Template CMP 2, p. 42).

Writing a CMP

- There are no legal restrictions on the clinical conditions which can be treated or what can be prescribed as the result of a CMP.
- All conditions which have previously (before the implementation of supplementary prescribing) been prescribed for by an independent doctor or dentist prescriber can be treated and prescribed for by a supplementary prescriber under the umbrella of an agreed CMP.
- Wherever possible, the CMP must cite national and locally agreed guidelines.
- The prescriber must (wherever possible) adhere to agreed local and national guidelines.

Essential information

When writing a CMP one should always include:

- the name of the patient;
- the condition(s) to be treated;
- class and/or description of medication(s);
- dose ranges and strengths;
- range restrictions;
- timescale over which the medication is to be given;
- reference to local and national guidelines;
- allergies and sensitivities to medication(s) or other substances;
- how to report allergies and sensitivities;
- when and why to refer back to the independent prescriber(s);
- keep the plan appropriately simple;
- write the plan in a language that everyone can understand.

What can be prescribed?

Supplementary prescribers, when working to an agreed CMP, can prescribe:

- all general sales list (GSL) medicines, pharmacy (P) medicines, appliances and devices, foods, and other borderline substances approved by the Advisory Committee on Borderline Substances;
- all prescription-only medicines for use outside their licensed indications (i.e. 'off-label' prescribing), black triangle drugs, and drugs marked 'less suitable for prescribing' in the BNF;
- unlicensed drugs.

Supplementary prescribers are advised to prescribe generically except where not clinically indicated (e.g in the case of a drug with a specific bioavailability) or when the product does not have an approved generic name.

When is supplementary prescribing best used?

- Supplementary prescribing is the most useful method for prescribing when the patient's condition requires them to be treated with unlicensed medication.
- For medication which is outside its product licence (e.g. smoking cessation products for teenagers).
- For controlled drugs which are not permitted by nurse independent prescribing.
- For complex conditions and shared care.

Practical examples of CMPs

Nurses can prescribe controlled drugs, unlicensed drugs, and drugs which are used for indications which are outside their product licence as supplementary prescribers.

Supplementary prescribing is useful in specific cases for the management of chronic conditions, palliative care, and shared nurse–doctor care.

The following examples are taken from the inpatient care of a person with diabetes, the palliative care of a person in the terminal stages of life, and public health nursing.

- **Template CMP 1:** for teams that have full co-terminus access to patient records.
- **Template CMP 2:** for teams where the SP does not have co-terminus access to the medical record.
- **Template CMP 3:** CMP for neonatal team with co-terminus access to patient records.
- **Template CMP 4:** CMP for a service user under the care of an Assertive Outreach Community Team.
- **Template CMP 5:** CMP for care of a client who wishes to stop smoking.

Template CMP 1: for teams that have full co-terminus access to patient records

Name of patient:	Patient medication sensitivities/allergies:
Mary Smith	None known

Patient identification e.g. ID number, date of birth: 20.10.35

Independent prescriber(s): Dr F Bloggs (Consultant Diabetologist)	Supplementary prescriber(s) John Jones Inpatient Diabetic Nurse Specialist

Condition(s) to be treated	Aim of treatment
Type 2 Diabetes (steroid induced)	Normoglycaemia To optimize glycaemic control thereby minimizing risk of long-term complications To support patient in self management of diabetes

Medicines that may be prescribed by SP:

Preparation	Indication	Dose schedule	Specific indications for referral back to the IP
Pre-mixed insulin 30/70 and appropriate delivery system	To achieve normal glycaemia	As indicated by clinical need (see appropriate section BNF)	Unsatisfactory blood glucose levels Significant hypoglycaemia

Guidelines or protocols supporting clinical management plan: Consult with local guidelines

NICE Guidelines for the Management of Type 2 Diabetes: Management of Blood Glucose 2002

National Service Framework for Diabetes Mellitus (DOH, 2001)

Frequency of review and monitoring by:

Supplementary prescriber: Four hourly blood sugars as inpatient. On discharge initially daily by telephone contact until stable. Continue monitoring while steroid doses are reduced.

Supplementary prescriber and independent prescriber: Monitored by GP diabetic clinic unless further outpatient clinic required.

Process for reporting ADRs: Yellow card scheme to committee of safety of medicines and in patients shared electronic records. Report to Independent prescriber and to patient's GP

Shared record to be used by IP and SP:

Patient's medical notes.

Agreed by independent prescriber(s)	Date	Agreed by supplementary prescriber(s)	Date	Date agreed with patient/carer
Dr F Bloggs	20.03.06	John Jones	20.03.06	Mary Smith 20.03.06

Template CMP 2: for teams where the SP does not have co-terminus access to the medical record

Name of Patient: Lil Ashby	**Patient medication sensitivities/allergies:** None known or reported

Patient identification e.g. ID number, date of birth: 20.10.61

Current medication: None	**Medical history:** Has a history of repeated chest infections. Patient has had two chest infections in the last six months. Patient smokes between 20 and 30 cigarettes a day.

Independent Prescriber(s): Dr Fred Bloggs Contact details: [tel/email/address] 98757428345	**Supplementary prescriber(s):** Penny Franklin Contact details: [tel/email/address] 01395 276483 pfranklin@eastenderspct.nhs.uk

Condition(s) to be treated: Nicotine dependency	**Aim of treatment:** To provide pharmaceutical support as part of a smoking cessation programme with view to supporting smoking cessation

Medicines that may be prescribed by SP:

Preparation	**Indication**	**Dose schedule**	**Specific indications for referral back to the IP**
As per East Lunghampton PCT fomulary Bupropion	Therapeutic support for smoking cessation in combination with motivational support	As per manufacturers summary of product characteristics (SPC), BNF page 248 and East Lunghampton PCT formulary pg 118	Increased adverse, common, uncommon and rare effects as indicated in summary of product characteristics: hypersensitivity reactions such as urticaria, sudden onset moderate to severe depression, sudden onset moderate to severe anxiety, chest pain, asthenia, tachycardia, increased blood pressure, confusion, anorexia, tinnitus, visual disturbance, vasodilation, syncope, seizures, moderate to severe irritability and hostility

Guidelines or protocols supporting Clinical Management Plan:
Guidance on the use of nicotine replacement therapy (NRT) and Buprorion for smoking cessation (National Institute for Health and Clinical Excellence March 2002 Prodigy guidance and patient information leaflet – smoking cessation (http://www.prodigy.nhs.uk/guidance.asp?gt= Smoking cessation)

Frequency of review and monitoring by:

Supplementary prescriber: Weekly for first four weeks as indicated by response to treatment, and then 4, 6, 8 and 12 weekly
Supplementary prescriber and independent prescriber: Annually

Process for reporting ADRs:
Supplementary prescriber to report to Independent prescriber and to record in patient's records.
Notify by CSM yellow card system if indicated.

Shared record to be used by IP and SP:
Patient's EMIS electronic records.

Agreed by independent prescriber(s)	Date	Agreed by supplementary prescriber(s)	Date	Date agreed with patient/carer
Dr F Bloggs	20.02.05	Penny Franklin	20.02.05	21.02.05

Template CMP 3: for a neonatal team with co-terminus access to patient records

Name of patient:
Molly Fairface

Date of birth:
01/01/2009

Local hospital no:
A123456

NHS no:
700123456

Birthweight:
670 grams

Current weight: *1200 grams*

Date: *02/03/2009*

Independent prescriber(s)/consultant:
Dr Iam Luvely

Supplementary prescriber(s)
ANNPs Daisy Honey; Tinker Bell; Dolly Shu

Condition(s) to be treated

Osteopaenia of prematurity

Anaemia of prematurity

Chronic lung disease (CLD)

Aim of treatment

Minimize risk of metabolic bone disease

Prevent anaemia of prematurity

Reduction in oxygen requirements

Medicines that can be prescribed by SP:

*Agreed by neonatal consultant team & BNF for Children

(Continued)

Template CMP 3 (Contd.)

Preparation	Indication	Dose schedule	Specific indications for referral back to the IP
Phosphate	Hypophosphataemia	1mmol/kg daily orally	Resistant hypophosphataemia
Chlorothiazide	Chronic lung disease	10–20mg/kg twice daily orally	Self-ventilating in air
Spironolactone	Chronic lung disease	1–2mg/kg daily orally in 2 divided doses	Self-ventilating in air

Guidelines or protocols supporting clinical management plan:

Local neonatal guidelines

British National Formulary for Children 2009

Frequency of review and monitoring by:

Supplementary prescriber	Supplementary prescriber and independent prescriber
Daily on ward rounds	Weekly, during consultant ward rounds

Process for reporting ADRs:

1 Patient hospital records

2 Parents

3 Incident reporting system local hospital NHS Trust

4 GP 5 Yellow card—BNF for children 2008

Shared record to be used by IP and SP

Dr: Iam Luvely ANNPs: Daisy Honey, Tinker Bell, & Dolly Shu

Agreed by independent prescriber(s)	Date	Agreed by supplementary prescriber(s)	Date Time	NMP/CMP information discussed with parent/s
Named consultant	02/02/09	NIPs signatures	2/3/09	Yes, with both parents, John and Mary Fairface
Dr Iam Luvely	05/02/09	1. Daisy Honey	11.00hr	
	10/02/09	2. Tinker Bell		
		3. Dolly Shu		

Template CMP 4: for a service user under the care of an Assertive Outreach Community Team

Clinical Management Plan [CMP] Version : 1   Date: xx/xx/2010

Name of Patient:
Mr Ron Test

Patient medication sensitivities/allergies:
Had dystonic reaction to depot flupentixol (xx/xx/1999). Refuses all depot anti-psychotic medication

Patient identification e.g. ID number, date of birth:
Name: Ronald Test No: xxxxxxxx NHS No: xxxxxxxx DoB: xx/xx/1979

Current medication:
Risperidone tablets 3mg at night
Lansoprazole capsules 15mg daily in the morning

Medical history:
Paranoid schizophrenia (6 admissions over past 8 years) all under section

Duodenal ulcer (diagnosed xx/xx/2000)

Independent prescriber(s) [IP]:
Dr Alan Crisp

Contact details: [tel/email/address]
xxxxxxxxxxxxx
xxx.xxx@xxxxxxx

Supplementary prescriber(s) [SP]
Steve Example xxx Assertive Outreach Team

Contact details: [tel/email/address]
xxxxxxxxxxxxxxxxxxxxxxxxx
xxxxx@xxxxxxxxx

Condition(s) to be treated:
Paranoid schizophrenia
Acute insomnia
Agitation

Aim of treatment:
Reduce breakthrough symptoms of schizophrenia
Alleviate insomnia
Reduce agitation and prevent escalation

Medicines that may be prescribed by SP:

Preparation	Indication	Dose schedule	Specific indications for referral back to the IP
Risperidone tablets	Breakthrough symptoms	Increase to 6mg daily at night	Failure to control symptoms, intolerable adverse effects or side-effects. Unable to reduce back to 3mg daily after a month. Service User's request
Aripiprazole tablets (to replace risperidone)	If service user refuses risperidone or wishes to change from risperidone	BNF 4.2.1	Failure to control symptoms, intolerable adverse effects or side-effects. Service User's request.
Zolpidem tablets	Acute insomnia	10mg at night	If needed for more than 3 weeks. Intolerable adverse effects or side-effects. Service User's request.
Lorazepam tablets	Agitation	1mg up to max. of 4mg in 24hr In divided doses. No more than 1mg every 4hr	Does not control agitation. Needed for more than 3 days. Intolerable adverse effects or side-effects. Service User's request.

(Continued)

Template CMP 4 (Contd.)

Guidelines or protocols supporting clinical management plan:

BNF 4.2.1; 4.1.1; 4.1.2. NICE (2002) Health Technology Appraisal No.43

Frequency of review and monitoring by:

Supplementary prescriber

Weekly or more frequently if required

LUNSERS* 6 monthly

PANSS† by agreement, to monitor progress of relapse prevention plan

Supplementary prescriber and independent prescriber

6 monthly or more frequently if required.

Process for reporting ADRs:

Yellow Card. Discuss with IP, GP, and pharmacy advisor before reporting. Document in patient's notes and advise GP by phone and fax.

Shared record to be used by IP and SP:

Case notes, Trust Electronic Record. Summary letters to GP, noting all changes. Copy of CMP to GP and out of hours GP service.

Agreed by independent prescriber(s):	Date	Agreed by supplementary prescriber(s):	Date	Date agreed with patient/carer
Dr Alan Crisp	12/01/08	Steve Example	12/01/08	12/01/2008

* Morrison, P., Gaskill, D., Meehan, T., Lunney, P., Lawrence, G., and Collings, P. (2000). The use of the Liverpool University neuroleptic side-effect rating scale (LUNSERS) in clinical practice. *Australia and New Zealand Journal of Mental Health Nursing*, **9**, 166–76.

† The PANSS Institute (TPI) (2006). *Positive and Negative Syndrome Scale* (www.panss.org).

Rationale for the CMP 4

This CMP (based on a real case) is for a service user under the care of an Assertive Outreach Community Team. He suffers from severe mental illness, and has been reluctant to engage with services. It illustrates how the process of developing a CMP can be user led, and helps promote concordance. The plan allows the team to deliver agreed as-required (prn) medication effectively, and help maintain the service user in the community by changing medication quickly without having to set up an appointment with the independent prescriber. This CMP acts as an advance directive for medication and, together with supportive and psychological therapies, forms part of a person-centred relapse prevention plan.

📖 Non-medical prescribing in mental health and learning disabilities, p. 218.

Template CMP 5: for care of a client who wishes to stop smoking

Name of patient:
Mrs X

Patient medication sensitivities/allergies:
None known or reported

Patient identification e.g. ID number, date of birth: 20.10.61

Current medication:
None

Medical history:
Has a history of repeated chest infections. Patient has had two chest infections in the last 6 months. Patient smokes between 20 and 30 cigarettes a day.

Independent prescriber(s):
Dr Fred Bloggs
Contact details: [tel/email/address]
98757428345

Supplementary prescriber(s):
A Prescriber
Contact details: [tel/email/address]
01234 567890/aprescribe@elunghamptonpct.nhs.uk

Condition(s) to be treated:
Nicotine dependency

Aim of treatment:
To provide pharmaceutical support as part of a smoking cessation programme with view to supporting smoking cessation

Medicines that may be prescribed by SP:

Preparation	Indication	Dose schedule	Specific indications for referral back to the IP
As per East Lunghampton PCT formulary Bupropion	Therapeutic support for smoking cessation in combination with motivational support	As per manufacturer's summary of product characteristics (SPC), BNF p.248, and East Lunghampton PCT formulary, p.118	Increased adverse, common, uncommon, and rare effects as indicated in summary of product characteristics: hypersensitivity reactions such as urticaria, sudden-onset moderate to severe depression, sudden-onset moderate to severe anxiety, chest pain, asthenia, tachycardia, increased blood pressure, confusion, anorexia, tinnitus, visual disturbance, vasodilation, syncope, seizures, moderate to severe irritability and hostility The patient no longer wishes to be involved in the supplementary prescribing partnership

Guidelines or protocols supporting clinical management plan:

NICE (2008). *Public health guidance 10. Smoking cessation services in primary care, pharmacies local authorities and work places, particularly for manual working groups, pregnant women and hard to reach communities.* NICE, London.

PRODIGY Guidance and patient information leaflets on smoking cessation.

CKS Clinical Summary. *Managing buproprion.*

🖳 http://www.cks.nhs.uk/smoking_cessation/management/quick_answers/scenario_smoking_cessation_adults#-318401

(Continued)

Template CMP 5 (Contd.)

Frequency of review and monitoring by:

Supplementary prescriber: Weekly for first 4 weeks as indicated by response to treatment, and then four-weekly in weeks 6, 8, and 12.

Supplementary prescriber and independent prescriber: Annually

Process for reporting ADRs:

Supplementary prescriber to report to independent prescriber and to record in patient's records.

Notify by CSM Yellow Card System if indicated.

Shared record to be used by IP and SP: Patient's EMIS electronic records.

Agreed by independent prescriber(s)	Date	Agreed by supplementary prescriber(s)	Date	Date agreed with patient/carer
Dr F Bloggs	20.02.05	A. Prescriber	17.10.09	21.10.09

Basic principles of pharmacology

Pharmacodynamics

Pharmacodynamics is the consideration of the effect that a drug has on the body. Body functions are mediated by control systems which depend on:
- receptors on the cell surface;
- carrier molecules;
- enzymes;
- specific macromolecules (e.g. DNA).

Once drugs reach the area of their action they either work in a specific or non-specific manner.

Specific drug action:

Interaction with receptors on the cell membrane

- A receptor, usually a protein molecule, is found on the surface of the cell or is located inside the cell in the cytoplasm.
  - drugs interact with receptors forming a drug–receptor complex.
  - a drug requires a complementary structure in order for it to interact with a receptor, i.e. lock and key model.
  - few drugs need a specific receptor and many will combine with more than one type of receptor.
  - drugs (agonists) often display an affinity for one particular receptor type.
- An agonist is a drug that has an affinity for a receptor, and once bound to that receptor it can cause a specific response. For example, morphine which binds to mu (µ) receptors in the CNS depresses the feeling of pain (📖 Opioid analgesics, p. 326).
- Drugs which bind to receptors but do not cause a response are called antagonists or receptor blockers.
  - an antagonist or receptor blocker is a drug which has an affinity for a receptor but does not cause a specific response.
  - antagonists reduce the likelihood of other drugs binding to the receptor and therefore further drug activity is blocked or reduced.
  - competitive antagonists compete with agonists for receptor sites, mitigating the action of the agonist by reducing its opportunity for action. For example, naloxone, which is used for opioid overdose, will compete with morphine for µ receptors.
  - non-competitive agonists are inactive receptors which prevent an agonist from having an affect.
- Drug–receptor binding is reversible and a drug's action reduces once it has left the receptor site.
- Partial agonists/antagonists can act on receptor sites, eliciting a smaller pharmacological response (incomplete inhibition) compared with a complete agonist/antagonist.

Interference with ion passage/channels through the cell membrane

An ion is an atom (or group of atoms) that has lost one or more electrons (cation) or gained one or more electrons (anion).

An ion passage/channel is a selective pore in the cell membrane that allows the movement of ions in and out of the cell.

Drugs which block these channels, such as the calcium blocker nifedipine, interfere with ion transport and produce an altered physiological response.

Enzyme inhibition or stimulation

An enzyme is a protein acting as a catalyst in a specific biochemical reaction. Some drugs interact with enzymes in a similar manner to the drug–receptor mechanism. ACE inhibitors and aspirin act in this way. Insulin is destroyed by proteolytic enzymes.

Incorporation into macromolecules

Some drugs are incorporated into macromolecules (larger molecules) and alter the normal functioning of that molecule.

Drugs of this type are used for cancer treatment, e.g. 5-fluorouracil which is incorporated into RNA taking the place of uracil and altering the message carried by the RNA.

Interference with the metabolic processes of micro-organisms

Some antibiotics kill the micro-organism causing infection by interfering with its metabolic processes. For example, penicillin disrupts the ability of bacteria to form cell walls.

Non-specific mechanisms

Chemical alteration of the cellular environment

Some drugs do not alter specific cell function but cause the chemical environment surrounding the cell to alter which changes the normal cellular responses. Osmotic laxatives and antacids are examples of this type of drug.

Physical alteration of the cellular environment

Drugs in this class alter the physical environment surrounding the cell, producing alterations in the normal cellular responses. Barrier preparations which protect the skin work on this principle.

Pharmacokinetics

Pharmacokinetics is the movement of drugs within the body and the way in which the body changes drugs over time. There are four basic processes:
• drug absorption;
• drug distribution;
• drug metabolism;
• drug excretion.

Drug absorption

Conveyance of the drug from the site of administration into the circulatory or lymphatic system.
• Almost all drugs require absorption into the body before they can have any affect.
• The proportion of a drug which has reached the general circulation is termed bioavailability.
• Drugs which are administered IV are said to have 100% bioavailability.
• Administration by routes other than IV leads to a decrease in bioavailability as some molecules of the drug will be lost during the absorption and distribution processes.
• Drugs administered orally are absorbed from the GI tract, carried by the hepatic portal vein to the liver.
• Metabolism of the drug may start in the liver. This is referred to as the 'first-pass effect'.

First-pass effect

The first-pass effect is the removal of a drug by the liver before it has had any therapeutic affect. This effect renders some drugs inactive and necessitates their administration by another route. GTN is an example of a drug which is rendered less active by the first-pass effect and therefore is administered by sublingual or transdermal routes.

Absorption following oral administration

Most drugs present in the gut in solution will pass through the cell membrane into the blood stream by **passive diffusion**. In this process the drug passes through the cell membrane from a stronger solution in the gut towards a weaker solution in the bloodstream (the concentration gradient). This process continues until there is an equal concentration on each side of the cell membrane. Passive diffusion is an energy-neutral process.

Some lipid-soluble drugs require **facilitated diffusion** in order to cross the cell membrane in combination with a carrier molecule. Facilitated diffusion also requires a concentration gradient and requires no energy expenditure.

Some drugs, which resemble substances occurring in the body, are absorbed against the concentration gradient and require carrier molecules and energy to be expended. This is **active transport**.

Factors affecting drug absorption from the GI tract

• Gut motility: if motility is increased less of the drug is absorbed.
• Gastric emptying: if this is increased the absorption rate of the drug is increased; if it is slowed the absorption rate of the drug is decreased.

- Surface area: the rate of drug absorption is greatest in the small intestine as it is lined with villi, which increase the overall surface area.
- Gut pH varies along the length of the gut and this changing environment may prevent optimal absorption of a drug in some areas.
- Blood flow: absorption rates ↑ in areas with good blood supply.
- Presence of food and fluid: may ↑ or ↓ drug absorption depending on the drug, e.g. absorption of tetracycline is reduced if dairy products are present in the gut.
- Antacids: these affect the pH and therefore the absorption rates.
- Drug composition: liquid preparations are absorbed faster than solid ones, and lipid-soluble preparations are absorbed faster than aqueous ones.

Absorption following parenteral administration

- Intradermal drugs diffuse slowly from the injection site into local capillaries.
- Subcutaneous drugs are absorbed faster than intradermal drugs.
- Intramuscular drugs are absorbed faster than intradermal and subcutaneous drugs.

Absorption following topical administration

- Lower rates of absorption than parenteral or oral administration.
- Rate is increased if the skin is broken or an occlusive dressing is used.
- Faster absorption in a well-vasculated area (e.g. rectum, sublingual).
- Nasal route allows local as well as systemic absorption.
- Inhalation into the lungs provides extensive absorption.
- Minimal absorption from the ear.
- Absorption from the eye depends on whether the drug is in solution or ointment.

Drug distribution

Distribution is the transportation of the drug from the site of administration to the target area. During this process the molecules of some drugs may be deposited at storage sites and other drugs may be deposited and inactivated.

Factors influencing drug distribution

- Blood flow: drug distribution is faster if the organ has a good blood supply (e.g. heart, liver) rather than being less vascular (e.g. bone).
- Plasma protein binding: in circulation drugs may either be bound to a protein, usually albumin, or 'free' and unbound. Only free drug molecules can produce an effect. As free molecules leave the circulation others are released from the protein to which they are bound to re-establish the ratio of those free to those bound.
- Displacement of one bound drug by another can have serious consequences. For example, if warfarin is displaced by tolbutamide this may precipitate haemorrhage as there is a greater amount of free warfarin in the circulation, and if tolbutamide is displaced by salicylates this may cause hypoglycaemia.
- Placental barrier: this permits the passage of poorly lipid-soluble drugs from the mother to the fetus but prohibits the passage of lipid-soluble preparations.
- Blood–brain barrier: CNS capillaries have a different structure to those elsewhere in the body and this constrains the passage of lipid-insoluble drugs.
- Storage sites: fat tissue acts as a storage facility for lipid-soluble drugs, and calcium-containing structures such as bones and teeth can accumulate drugs that bind to calcium. Drugs may accumulate in these sites and not be released until after their administration has ceased.

Drug metabolism

Metabolism is the process of modifying or altering the chemical composition of the drug, also called biotransformation.
- The pharmacological activity of the drug is removed.
- Metabolites (products of the drug's metabolism) are produced.
- Metabolites are more water soluble than the drug itself and this promotes their excretion from the body.
- Metabolic processes include oxidation, reduction, hydrolysis, and conjugation.
- Most drug metabolism occurs in the liver, catalysed by hepatic enzymes.
- Other sites for metabolism are the kidneys, intestinal mucosa, lungs, plasma, and placenta.

Certain drugs, if given repeatedly, are metabolized more rapidly in subsequent doses because of enzyme induction. This requires the drug to be given in larger and larger doses to achieve the same affect as the initial dose. This is sometimes referred to as drug tolerance, although tolerance may also be caused by changes to the drug receptors within the cells.

Factors influencing drug metabolism

- Genetic factors: enzyme systems are genetically determined and genetic variations lead to differences in metabolic reactions to medication. For example, patients genetically inheriting the possession of an atypical form of the enzyme pseudocholinesterase have a prolonged paralysis and reaction time when given the muscle relaxant suxamethonium.
- Age
  - in older people first-pass metabolism may be reduced, or there is a delayed production and elimination of metabolites resulting in increased bioavailability of the drug. Reduced doses may be indicated for older people.
  - in neonates the enzyme systems responsible for conjugation of the drug may be incompletely developed. Thus there is an increased risk of toxic effects of the drugs.
- Disease process: any alteration to body systems caused by a disease process has the potential to alter the metabolism or response to a drug. For example, liver disease reduces hepatic blood flow which slows drug metabolism, leading to an accumulation of the drug and eventually toxicity.
- Mental and emotional factors: confusion, depression, amnesia, stress, and many other mental illness may reduce a patient's capabilities and motivation, which can result in inability to follow a medication regime correctly.
- Ethnicity: the metabolism of drugs varies from one ethnic group to another. It is also important to remember that different cultures have different health beliefs and practices.

Table 4.1 Some common interactions between drugs and foods or herbs[1-5]

Food or herb	Drug	Reaction	Reason
Grapefruit juice	Simvastatin Atorvastatin	Headache, muscle weakness	Reduced metabolism and elimination
Grapefruit juice	Nifedipine	Hypotension, tachycardia and flushing	
Barbecued meat	Diazepam	Dose ↑ to obtain the therapeutic effect	Accelerates the action of enzymes in the gut and liver
St John's wort	Antidepressants	Mild serotonin syndrome	Inhibits enzymes clearing SSRIs
Liquorice	Corticosteroids	Fluid retention Hypertension Hypokalaemia	Decreased renal clearance
Liquorice 100–200g/day	Antihypertensives	Fluid retention Hypertension Hypokalaemia	Retention of corticosteroid hormones
Ginko and ginseng	NSAIDs	Bleeding	Interference with clotting
Garlic, ginko, ginger, feverfew, cranberry juice	Warfarin	Bleeding	Platelet dysfunction
St John's wort, ginseng, camomile, brewed green tea	Warfarin	Clotting	Drug inactivated
Evening primrose oil	Antipsychotics	Possible ↑ risk of siezures	Possible additive effect

1. Dresser, G., Bailey, D.G., Leake, B.F., et al. (2000) Fruit juices inhibit organic anion transporting polypeptide-mediated drug uptake to decrease the oral availability of fexofenadine. *Clinical Pharmacology and Therapeutics*, **71**, 11–20.
2. Fugh-Berman, A. (2000). Herb–drug interactions. *Lancet*, **355**, 134–8.
3. Karch, A. (2000). *Focus on nursing pharmacology* (2nd edn). Lippincott, Philadelphia, PA.
4. Sørenson, J. (2002). Herb–drug, food–drug, nutrient–drug and drug–drug interactions: mechanisms involved and their medical implications. *Journal of Alternative and Complementary Medicine*, **8**, 293–308.
5. Stockley, I. (1999). *Drug interactions* (5th edn). Blackwell, Oxford.

Drug excretion

Excretion is the elimination of drugs and their metabolites from the body. Most drugs and metabolites of drugs are excreted through the kidneys. Factors affecting the rate of excretion of drugs and metabolites through the kidneys are:
- presence of kidney disease;
- altered renal blood flow;
- pH of urine;
- concentration of drug in plasma;
- molecular weight of the drug.

Other routes of excretion

Bile
- Some drugs and metabolites are secreted from the liver into the bile and then via the common bile duct to the duodenum.
- Some drugs may be reabsorbed from the terminal ileum and then return to the liver. This is termed enterohepatic recycling and may extend the duration of action of the drug.
- Drugs eventually pass to the large intestine and are eliminated in the faeces.

Lungs
- Pulmonary excretion accounts for small amounts of alcohol and anaesthetic gases.

Breastmilk
- Small amounts of a drug may pass from the capillaries surrounding the milk-producing glands and be ingested by a suckling infant who may be unable to metabolize and excrete the drug.

📖 Prescribing for special groups, pp. 197–224.

Perspiration, saliva and tears
- Some lipid-soluble drugs may be passively excreted via these routes.

Half-life of a drug

This is the time taken for the concentration of a drug in the blood to fall to 50% (half) of its original value.
- Many standard dose calculations are based on this value.
- It allows a dose to be calculated which produces a stable plasma concentration and is below the toxic value and above the minimum effective level.

Loading dose

This is a dose which is larger than the normal dose and allows a plasma steady state to be reached quickly. A maintenance dose is given subsequently. A loading dose is useful for antibiotic therapy or digoxin.

Calculation of loading dose

The loading dose (LD) is calculated as follows:

$$LD = Vd \times Cp$$

where Vd is volume of distribution and Cp is plasma concentration of the drug.

Therapeutic drug monitoring (TDM)

Regular plasma levels of a drug with a narrow therapeutic index are taken in order to ensure that it is used effectively.

- Drugs such as digoxin, lithium, and phenytoin are monitored in this way.
- It is also used as a tool to check patient concordance with a regime.

Therapeutic index

The therapeutic index is the ratio of a drug's toxic dose to its minimally effective dose.

Volume distribution (Vd)

This is the estimated amount of a drug left in the bloodstream after absorption and distribution is complete.

- Vd has to be an estimate because we can only measure the drug concentration in the bloodstream.
- Drugs are distributed unevenly between various body fluids and tissues according to their physical and chemical properties. High lipid solubility allows a drug to cross membranes. High tissue protein-binding properties leaves less of the drug in the plasma. For example, gentamicin has good water solubility and poor lipid solubility and therefore it stays mainly in body fluids and blood.
- A low Vd indicates that the drug is mainly confined to blood and body water, as with gentamicin.
- A high Vd indicates that the drug has overflowed into the tissues.

Calculation of volume distribution

The volume distrbution is calculated as follows:

$$Vd = X/Cp$$

where X is the total amount of drug in the body and Cp is the plasma concentration of the drug.

Uses of volume distribution

- If a drug is highly distributed to the tissues the first few doses are not apparent in the bloodstream.
- The use of a loading dose is indicated to enable the dose to be present in both the tissue and the bloodstream. This is important if the site of action of the dose is in tissue (e.g. digoxin).
- Vd can be used to help calculate the dose needed to achieve critical plasma concentration.

Prescribing for the extremes of life

Both the very old and very young have problems with excretion and breakdown of drugs.

Neonates

Neonates (newborns) have a deficient hepatic enzyme system, resulting in incomplete metabolism of drugs and raised levels of toxicity. Neonates also have increased water-to-fat ratio for the first 28 days after their birth and therefore need higher doses of some drugs (e.g. aminoglycosides). It is beyond the scope of this handbook to give guidance on prescribing for the very young, and specialist advice is required.

Older people

Healthy older people often have a degree of renal impairment which delays drug excretion through the kidneys, thus increasing the duration of action of a preparation. However, a further rapid reduction in renal clearance in older people suffering from an acute illness will exacerbate this process. Liver function may also be impaired, resulting in delayed drug metabolism (📖 Prescribing for older people, p. 198).

Potential and unwanted effects

Drug effects

The effect that a drug (or drugs) has on the body:
• can be beneficial;
• can be harmful—adverse drug effects (ADEs).

Adverse drug reactions (ADRs) and adverse drug interactions (ADIs):
• cause 2–6% of admissions to hospital;
• cause 0.24–2.9% deaths of hospital inpatients;[1]
• are between the 4th and 6th leading cause of deaths;[2]
• can affect the quality of life;
• can be costly;
• can copy symptoms of disease;
• can affect concordance.

📖 Basic principles of pharmacology, pp. 53–64.
📖 Adverse drug reactions (ADRs), p. 68.

Adverse drug reaction

Definition
A reaction related to the use of a specific drug or drugs which causes harm and/or discomfort beyond its predictable therapeutic effects, and which predictably may cause harm to the patient in the future if given in a smaller or larger dose or in the same dosage and regimen. With any ADR, treatment may warrant prevention of future reactions or alteration of the drug and dosage regimen and possible withdrawal of the product. The study of adverse drug reactions is known as pharmacovigilance.

Classification
• Mild: treatment is not necessary and medical attention is short term.
• Moderate: there is a required change in the treatment (e.g. where the same drug can be continued but at a reduced dose). Treatment might require the patient to be hospitalized for a significant time.
• Severe: there is a possibility of death. The drug will need to be stopped and the reaction treated.
• Lethal: a direct or indirect response to the reaction causes death.[3]

Causes
• The pharmacological or physiological actions of the drug (often common and predictable).
• The patient's response to the drug (often rare, idiosyncratic, unavoidable, and unpredictable).
• Prescribing error or inappropriate prescribing.

When making prescribing decisions remember:
• Any drug has the potential for adverse drug reactions and interactions (some more than others).
• As part of baseline prescribing assessment when prescribing more than one drug, always consider risk versus benefit for the patient in

partnership with the patient and, if prescribing as a supplementary prescriber, with the independent prescriber.
- Special precautions and contraindications are indicated in Appendix 1 of the British National Formulary (BNF).[4]
- Always document an adverse drug reaction in the patient's notes/computerized records.

The National Patient Safety Agency

The National Patient Safety Agency (NPSA) was established in 2001. It was commissioned by the Department of Health as a result of the Chief Medical Officer's Report *An organisation with a memory* which made the following recommendations:[5]
- unified mechanisms for reporting and analysis when things go wrong;
- a more open culture, in which errors or service failures can be reported and discussed;
- mechanisms for ensuring that, where lessons are identified, the necessary changes are put into practice;
- a much wider appreciation of the value of the system approach in preventing, analysing and learning from errors.

Further reading

Lee, A. (2006). *Adverse drug reactions* (2nd edn). Pharmaceutical Press, London.
National Audit Office and Department of Health (2005) *A safer place for patients: learning to improve patient safety*. TSO, London.
Pirmohamed, M., James. S., Meakin, S., *et al.* (2004). Adverse drug reactions as cause of admission to hospital: prospective analysis of 18820 patients. *British Medical Journal*, **329**, 15–19.
World Health Organization (1966). *International drug monitoring: the role of the hospital*. WHO, Geneva.

1. Kelly, J. (2000). *Adverse drug effects: a nursing concern*. London, Whurr.
2. Lazarou, J., Pomeranz, B.H., Corey, B. (1998). Incidence of adverse drug reactions in hospitalized patients: a meta-analysis of prospective studies. *JAMA*, **279**, 1200–5.
3. MERCK Manuals Online Medical Library: Adverse Drug Reactions. http://www.merck.com/mmpe/sec20/ch305/ch305a.html (accessed 4 October 2009)
4. *British National Formulary* (latest edn). British Medical Association and Royal Pharmaceutical Society of Great Britain, London.
5. Department of Health (2000) *An organisation with a memory. Report of an expert group on learning from adverse events in the NHS*. TSO, London.

Adverse drug reactions (ADRs)

Drug reactions

The reaction the body has to a drug:

- can carry clinical significance and cause a noticeable effect;
- may not be clinically significant;
- can be beneficial (levodopa/carbidopa in Parkinson's disease);
- can be harmful (ADR);
- may be more common in older people as a result of changes in pharmacokinetics and pharmacodynamics, polypharmacy, and polymorbidity.

British National Formulary classification of the frequency of side effects

- Very common: >1 in 10.
- Common: 1 in 100 to 1 in 10.
- Uncommon: 1 in 1000 to 1 in 100.
- Rare: 1 in 10 000 to 1 in 1000.
- Very rare: <1 in 10 000.

Some patients will experience side effects when they first start to take a drug but these may abate with time. If prescribing drugs with known adverse side effects, but which have been considered to be of benefit to the patient, inform patients of known side effects and urge them to persevere (e.g. combined contraceptive pill).

Minimizing ADRs

- Identify patients who are taking potentially interacting drugs.
- Only use a drug where there is good indication and where benefit exceeds risk.
- Always ask if the patient is taking other medications, including drugs and herbal medicines, products purchased over the counter, homely remedies.
- Identify high-risk groups, including older people, children, pregnant and breastfeeding women, and patients with polymorbidity or subject to polypharmacy. Only use for these special groups if a full risk–benefit assessment has been completed.
- Always ask about allergy and previous ADRs.
- Use as few concurrent drugs as possible.
- Gradually titrate to greatest therapeutic effect.
- Start with the lowest effective dose and when appropriate reduce dose.

📖 Basic principles of pharmacology, pp. 53–64.
📖 Classification of adverse drug effects and drug interactions, p. 72.

Monitoring adverse drug reactions

Yellow card reporting of adverse reactions for any drug given to patients in UK to the MHRA at:
Medicines and Healthcare Products Regulatory Agency (MHRA)
Committee on Safety of Medicines (CSM) Freepost
London SW8 5BR, UK.[1]
Online reporting to MHRA: 🖥 medicines.mhra.gov.uk
Tel: freephone 0808 100 3352, 10.00 to 14.00 Mondays to Fridays.

Report suspected ADRs to any drug, including those self-medicated by the patient. Also report reactions to blood products, vaccines, radiographic contrast media, and herbal products.
• Can report drugs of any age.
• Can be used by all prescribers.
• Confidential.
• No blame attached.

The Medicines and Healthcare Regulatory Agency, which incorporates the Commission on Human Medicines, monitors the safety of marketed drugs, advising the government on the licensing of medicines and their safety. The MHRA publishes regular drug safety bulletins.
🖥 http://www.mhra.gov.uk/Publications/Safetyguidance/CurrentProblems inPharmacovigilance/index.htm

Report
• Black triangle drugs: these are new drugs. The black triangle (▼) indicates that their safety profile is being closely monitored.
• Serious reactions with established drugs, e.g. those that have been on the market for more than 2 years.
• All ADRs in children.
• All ADRs for complementary and unlicensed medicines.
• Record in patient's notes.

Post-marketing surveillance[2]
• Detects risks in a target population after the drug has been marketed.
• Establishes efficacy for the population in general.
• Establishes cost effectiveness.
• Identifies therapeutic benefits which were not previously predicted.
• Interprofessional cooperation between all prescribers, pharmacists, and patients/carers can help to avoid ADRs.
📖 Seven principles of safe prescribing, p. 94.

Further reading
Edwards, I. and Aronson, J.K. (2000). Adverse drug reactions: definitions, diagnosis and management. *Lancet*, **356**, 1255–9.
Grahame-Smith, D and Aronson, J.K. (eds) (2002). *Oxford Textbook of Clinical Pharmacology and Drug Therapy* (3rd edn). Oxford University Press, Oxford.
Kelly, J. (2000). *Adverse drug effects: a nursing concern*. Whurr, London.
Pirmohamed, M., Breckenridge, A.M., Kitleringham, N.R., et al. (1998). Adverse drug reactions *British Medical Journal*, **316**, 1295–8.

1. 🖥 http://www.mhra.gov.uk/Publications/Safetyguidance/CurrentProblemsinPharmacovigilance/index.htm (accessed 2 February 2010).
2. *British National Formulary* (latest edn). British Medical Association and Royal Pharmaceutical Society of Great Britain, London.

Adverse drug interactions (ADIs)

Definition
Alteration of the drug's effects by the prior or concurrent administration of another drug (drug–drug interactions) or by food (drug–food interactions).[1]
📖 Basic principles of pharmacology, pp. 53–64.

Drug interactions
Modification of the effect of one drug by the administration of another or with several different drugs. Drug interactions can be:
- beneficial;
- harmful (ADIs);
- may affect normal body processes;
- effects can oppose each other or be additive (synergistic)—the combined effect of two drugs.

📖 Basic principles of pharmacology, pp. 53–64.
📖 Adverse drug reactions (ADRs), p. 68.
📖 Drug effects, p. 66.

Types of interaction
- Pharmacokinetic: drug absorption, distribution, metabolism, and excretion.
- Pharmacodynamic: antagonism of one drug at the receptor site changes the effect of the drug.
📖 Basic principles of pharmacology, pp. 53–64.
- Interactions can occur between one drug (or group of drugs) and another drug (or group of drugs):
  - during absorption, distribution, metabolism, and excretion
  - as a result of competition at the site of action.
- They can be additive and potentiate an effect, or antagonistic and block an effect.

Serious interactions can occur as a result of inhibition or induction of metabolic enzymes by one drug (or drugs), leading to an increase or decrease in plasma concentrations of another drug (or drugs).[2]

A list of likely drug–drug and drug–food interactions can be found in Appendix 1 of the BNF.[3]

📖 Classification of adverse drug effects and drug interactions, p. 72.

1. Merck (2007) 🖳 http://www.merck.com/mrkshared/mmanual/section22/sec22.jsp (accessed 2 February 2010).
2. McGavock, H. (2005). *How drugs work: basic pharmacology for healthcare professionals* (2nd edn). Radcliffe Medical Press, Oxford.
3. *British National Formulary* (latest edn). British Medical Association and Royal Pharmaceutical Society of Great Britain, London.

Classification of adverse drug effects and drug interactions[1,2]

Refer to Appendix 1 in the current BNF.

Type A effects: augmented

Aetiology
- Dose related.
- Usually relate to the pharmacology of the drug.
- Are responsible for at least 80% of adverse drug effects.
- Can be of therapeutic benefit.
- Can cause toxicity or decreased therapeutic benefit.
- Can be harmful for the patient.

Actions to prevent/minimize effects
- Take a thorough past and current medical history including past or current drug interactions, sensitivities, and allergies.
- Take a thorough history of current medication.
- Ask about any medication purchased over or 'under' the counter.
- Record prescribing actions in shared medical notes and in patient's hand-held records.
- Start with the lowest effective dose (dose reduction may resolve the problem).
- Gradually titrate dose to greatest therapeutic effect.
- Where applicable, administer drug only to required site of action (e.g. inhaled corticosteroids).
- Target drug to treat specific condition (e.g. organism-specific anti-microbials.
- Use National Prescribing Centre (NPC) prescribing pyramid[3] to complete holistic prescribing assessment.

Examples of interactions that might lead to adverse drug effects
- Concomitant use of antihypertensives leading to hypotension.
- Concurrent administration of drugs to maximize effects.
- NSAIDs and opioid analgesics for pain control.
- β-antagonist and diuretic for hypertension.

Type B effects: bizarre

Aetiology
- Rare
- Unpredictable
- Unrelated to dose
- Idiosyncratic
- Hard to prevent in the first instance
- Relatively high morbidity and mortality.

Actions to prevent/minimize effects
- As for type A effects.
- Ask about family history of allergies, sensitivities, and reactions.
- Ask about any other drugs the patient might be taking including drugs purchased over and 'under' the counter.

Examples Anaphylactic immunological reaction to a specific antibiotic; myositis, myalgia, myopathy with statins.

Type C: chronic effects
Aetiology
• Result from long-term drug usage.
• Usually associated with treatment for chronic disease.

Actions to prevent/minimize effects
As for type A and type B effects.

Examples Tolerance to nicotine; osteoporosis with steroids.

Type D: delayed effects
Aetiology
Can occur many years after therapy has stopped.

Actions to prevent/minimize effects
As for type A and B effects and:
• monitoring, audit;
• clinical research;
• longitudinal post-marketing surveillance.

Examples Vaginal cancer following stilboestrol.

Type E: end-of-use effects
Aetiology
Occur as a result of abrupt cessation of some therapies (e.g. systemic anabolic steroids) and withdrawal from some antidepressants.

Type F: effect failure
Aetiology
Failure of drug to achieve therapeutic effect.

Actions to prevent/minimize effects
Give adequate information and advice as to how to take, when to take, and precautionary measures.

Examples Inadequate dose of contraceptive when used with rifampicin.

Further reading
McGavock, H. (2005). *How drugs work: basic pharmacology for healthcare professionals* (2nd edn). Radcliffe Medical Press, Oxford.
Stockley's *Drug Interactions*.
🖥 https://www.medicinescomplete.com/mc/stockley/current/login.htm?uri=http%3A%2F%2Fwww.medicinescomplete.com%2Fmc%2Fstockley%2Fcurrent%2Findex.htm (accessed 27 September 2009).

1. Kelly, J. (2000) *Adverse drug effects a nursing concern*. Whurr, London.
2. Rawlins, M.D. and Thompson, J.W. (1977). *Pathogenesis of adverse drug reactions*. In: *Textbook of adverse drug reactions* (ed. D.M. Davies). Oxford University Press, Oxford.
3. National Prescribing Centre (1999). *Signposts for prescribing nurses: general principles of good prescribing*. National Prescribing Centre, Liverpool.

Therapeutic range/index

This is the range within which plasma concentrations are related to therapeutic effect. Concentrations below this range have little therapeutic effect. Toxicity is related to increasing concentration and may occur within the therapeutic range of a drug or in concentrations above this range. Special care needs to be taken with certain drugs that have a narrow therapeutic range; where the plasma concentration is higher than the therapeutic range, severe adverse drug reactions can occur.

Drugs with a narrow therapeutic range/index
- Methotrexate.
- Digoxin.
- Warfarin.
- Lithium.
- Theophylline.
- Phenytoin.
- Valproate.

Plasma protein binding
Most drugs bind to plasma protein and are transported around the body in this way. A drug which is bound to plasma protein is not available for the body for use. It is the free drug which exerts its effect. The concentration of the free drug rises when the drug is displaced from the plasma protein. Some drugs, such as phenytoin and other anti-epileptic drugs, can be highly plasma protein bound (>90%). If phenytoin is displaced from its plasma protein binding by other drugs, its plasma concentration will increase without a change in total concentration. Toxicity can occur with rapid displacement.

Steady state
This is a constant state of balance between the metabolism and elimination of a drug from the body and the absorption of a drug into the body to replace that which is metabolized and eliminated.

Half-life
This is the time taken for the plasma concentration of a drug to fall by half. It is important to understand half-life when considering the potential toxic effects of drugs on the body.
- It is used to predict the rate of accumulation of a drug in the body.
- It can be used to predict the length of time a drug takes to be eliminated from the body.
- It takes approximately five half-lives to achieve steady state and as long again for a drug to be eliminated from the body.
  Some drugs have a very long half-life, e.g. digoxin (40hr).

Toxicity
- This refers to any adverse reaction by the body to the administration of drugs for therapeutic purposes, regardless of dosage or amount.
- Displacement of digoxin from plasma protein can, and does, lead to toxicity.
- Digoxin takes 160–200hr to leave the body; this can cause problems in states of toxicity.

📖 Basic principles of pharmacology, pp. 53–64.

Special precautions

Drugs of bioequivalence act on the body with the same strength and similar bioavailability at the same dosage, although they may be different formulations or chemical compounds. When prescribing most drugs the prescriber is encouraged to use the non-proprietary title (name) of the drug as this supports the prescribing of any suitable product of bioequivalence, so that if one drug is not available, another brand can be dispensed. However, note that it is important to prescribe some drugs by brand name rather than by generic name.

📖 Drug effects, p. 66.
📖 Adverse drug reactions (ADRs), p. 68.

Managing adverse drug effects (in the event of toxicity)

- If the patient is having difficulty breathing or is not breathing, maintain airway, assess all vital signs, and provide life support.
- Take a history of events and make a record.
- Keep evidence.
- Reduce or stop dose.

Where to get up-to-date information 1

Review of prescribing websites

🖳 *Pharmaceutical Journal: www.pharmj.com*

This is the electronic version of the *Pharmaceutical Journal*. Subscription is free and it provides an excellent source of evidence-based information, including continuing professional development (CPD) with a pharmacist-based slant. The website links to *Clinical Evidence* (BMJ Publishing Group). This publication has up-to-date reviews of clinical evidence related to prescribing. It is useful for systematic reviews of up-to-date randomized control trials and clinical comparison of drugs and their clinical application.

🖳 *Clinical Knowledge Summaries: http://www.cks.nhs.uk/home*

This site provides patient, nurse, and doctor information for a wide range of disease management. There are brief updates which inform practice. The site provides information leaflets with patient-friendly diagrams, as well as details of self-help groups, patient groups, and similar organizations. There is also an up-to-date Cochrane review, podcasts, and drug safety updates.

🖳 *Association of the British Pharmaceutical Industry: www.abpi.org.uk*

This site contains useful information pertaining to the drug industry, its code of conduct, and vital statistics. The site includes some patient information produced by drug companies and summaries of product characteristics.

🖳 *Prescriber/escriber: http://www.prescriber.co.uk/view/0/index.html*

The online electronic journal *Prescriber* is free to health professionals who register online and covers peer-reviewed articles relating to primary care, therapeutics, and prescribing-related issues. Good for research articles about pharmacology, pharmacokinetics, and pharmacodynamics. The site links to NICE guidelines and the National Service Frameworks (NSFs) and also has medical humour. Once registered to the site, readers can also elect to receive SMS alerts to their mobile phones.

🖳 *National Prescribing Centre (NPC): www.npc.co.uk*

Links to sites related to clinical governance, knowledge and skills framework, standards, and competencies related to prescribing. This site provides authoritative and up-to-date information on all aspects of medical and non-medical prescribing. The site also produces MeReC bulletins. http://www.npci.org.uk/ is a virtual interactive learning resource for all prescribers it also provides a blog relating to up to date prescribing news. At the time of going to press it is anticipated that NPC will integrate with NICE from April 2011.

▣ Medicines and Health Care Regulatory Agency: www.mhra.gov.uk.
This excellent site is devoted to protecting the public, maintaining and regulating standards for the pharmaceutical industry, and prescribing. It provides comprehensive information on drug safety and medical device alerts, information on how products are licensed, and information related to prescribing and public health.

▣ National Electronic Library for Health (NeLH): www.nelh.nhs.uk
Links via Athens or NHS log in to all major academic and information sites for prescribing, including BNF, the Cochrane database, *Clinical Evidence*, and *Drugs and Therapeutics Bulletin*.

▣ Scottish Intercollegiate Guidelines Network (SIGN): www.sign.ac.uk
This site is the Scottish equivalent of NICE. It links with NICE to work in partnership to provide evidence-based guidelines for standardized treatment for disease management. Good reliable source of evidence-based information.

▣ UKMIPG-UK Medicines Information Pharmacists Group: www.ukmi. nhs.uk
This site is a source of up-to-date online information for pharmacists working in primary care. Useful links to National Electronic Library for Medicines (NHS NeLM) (www.nelm.nhs.uk), other up-to-date sources of guidance and information, and specialist advice services.

▣ Medicines: www.medicines.org.uk
The official site for the electronic medicines compendium. It provides a summary of product characteristics for drugs and a search engine for information regarding specific medicines.

Where to get up-to-date information 2

Other sources of electronic information

▣ *Free Medical Journals.com: www.freemedicaljournals.com*
This site provides access to useful free online journals.

▣ *Chemist and Druggist: www.dotpharmacy.com*
Useful for self-testing for continuing professional development (CPD).

▣ *Drug and Therapeutics Bulletin: www.which.net/health/dtb*
Up-to-date information regarding common drugs.

▣ *Hospital Pharmacist: www.pharmj.com/backissues.html*
Has lots of information about medicines management. Good access to free electronic journals related to prescribing. Useful updates from *Pharmaceutical Journal* online.

▣ *Bandolier: http://www.medicine.ox.ac.uk/bandolier/*
Rich source for evidence-based pharmacology and prescribing.

▣ *British Medical Journal (BMJ): www.bmj.com*
Access to evidence-based medicine, news, and reviews.

▣ *British National Formulary: www.bnf.org/*
Provides an online up-to-date BNF if you subscribe to the site. It has lots of links to useful sites related to prescribing.

▣ *NPC Plus: www.keele.ac.uk/schools/pharm/npcplus*
NPC Plus is a partnership programme within the Faculty of Health at Keele University. This site offers links to other sites with prescribing information and case studies, e.g. the NPC Medicines Partnership Programme. Membership gives access to advice, CPD, promoting training and education for all non-medical prescribers.

▣ *Association of Nurse Prescribers: www.anp.org.uk*
Membership gives access to advice, CPD, promoting research, training, and education for all non-medical prescribers.

Other sites you have found useful:

Where to get up-to-date information 3

See also 📖 Additional prescribing information available in the BNF, p. 472, and 📖 Advice and support; p. 466

National guidelines[1]

The National Institute for Health and Clinical Excellence (NICE) provides up-to-date technology appraisals, which are nationally recognized guidelines that adhere to best clinical evidence and which recommend best practice and cost-effective prescribing. Technology appraisals are updated every 5 years.

Nationally recognized guidelines are also produced by:
- 🖵 The British Thoracic society (BTS) www.brit-thoracic.org.uk
- 🖵 The British Hypertension Society (BHS): www.bhsoc.org
- 🖵 The British Diabetic Association (BDA): www.diabetes.org.uk
- 🖵 The British Heart Foundation (BHF): www.bhf.org.uk
- 🖵 Scottish Intercollegiate Guidelines Network (SIGN): www.sign.ac.uk

NHS Clinical Knowledge Summaries (🖵 www.cks.nhs.uk) provides a nationally recognized knowledge source for independent and supplementary prescribers in primary and secondary care.
All sites were accessed on 4 October 2009.

Local guidelines

Locally produced NHS formularies provide evidence-based guidelines and protocols for prescribing medications and appliances. They also advise on locally accepted practice and safe and cost-effective prescribing.

Guidelines are exactly what they say, and in supplementary prescribing, in agreement with the independent prescriber and the patient, can be tailored to meet the needs of the individual patient. However, whenever possible, it is best practice for the prescriber who is working for the NHS to follow the guidelines as indicated both nationally and within the local NHS formulary.

PACT data

PACT (Prescribing Analysis and Cost) and SPA (Scottish Prescribing Analysis) are available as audit reports of practitioners prescribing on a quarterly (3-monthly) basis. These data provide comparisons between local and national prescribing patterns and can be broken down to indicate individual prescribing patterns.
📖 Audit, p. 428.
📖 Approaches to audit, p. 434.

The Drug Tariff

This is available online as the electronic Drug Tariff
🖵 http://www.nhsbsa.nhs.uk/924.aspx (accessed 4 October 2009).
The Drug Tariff is a joint compilation between the Department of Health and the Prescription Pricing Authority[1] (now renamed the Business Services Authority).

Useful information obtainable from the Drug Tariff
- The basic price of named drugs, appliances, and chemical reagents.
- Endorsements including pack sizes.
- Whether the prescription is in pharmacopoeial or generic form.
- Brand name and name of manufacturer or wholesaler from whom the drug was purchased.
- Quantity supplied (if at variance with quantity ordered).
- Pharmacists' professional payments fees.
- Commonly used pack sizes.
- Advice on domiciliary oxygen service.
- Advice to care homes.
- Borderline substances.
- The dental prescribing formulary.
- The Community Practitioners Formulary for Nurse Prescribers.
- Drugs and other substances not to be prescribed under the NHS pharmaceutical services (blacklisted drugs).
- Drugs to be prescribed in certain circumstances under the NHS pharmaceutical services.
- A list of controlled drugs.
- National out-of-hours formulary.

The Drug Tariff is obtainable online from 🖳 www.drugtariff.com (accessed 3 February 2010).

1. Department of Health (latest edition). *Drug tariff*. TSO, London.
🖳 www.ppu.org.uk

Holistic assessment

In contrast with the medical model of assessment which seeks to identify a problem from symptoms, investigations, and physical examination,
and then make a curative response. A holistic assessment by non-medical
prescribers takes into account the physical, emotional, psychological, and
environmental or social aspects of the symptoms and feelings presented
by the patient, their family, or carers. Notions of well-being, quality of life,
and the values and aspirations of the individual are also considered.

The non-reductive holistic account of health derives from exploration
of what it is to be a person and the acceptance that persons are partly
defined by their aspirations and goals, and this extends to their notions of
illness and well-being.

There is a fundamental difference between the biomedical model which
decides if a person is ill by examination and requires no input from the
patient and the holistic account of ill health which includes the patient's
own view of the matter.

Helen Close[1] suggests that the prescriber may find it useful to adapt
a seven-point holistic assessment model from Twycross and Black,[2]
originally used in the treatment of nausea and vomiting but applicable to
more general use:

1. Evaluation of the history given by the patient
- Time and onset of symptoms.
- Physical, emotional, and social effects of the symptoms.
- Past and current medical history, current prescribed medication
  including over-the-counter (OTC), and 'borrowed medication' and
  homely remedies.
- Any known allergies.
- Any red flag symptoms, e.g. bleeding, obstruction?

2. Record the severity of the symptoms
- How often are they experienced?
- Does the patient regard the symptoms as serious?

3. Correct reversible causes
- Before treating the symptoms identify any causes which can be
  eliminated.

4. Non-drug treatments
- Are there actions which can be taken to avoid the symptoms?

5. If needed prescribe and start a drug treatment
- Move to point 5 only when points 3 and 4 have failed to relieve the
  symptoms.

6. Check route of administration
- Optimize the effect of treatment by using the most suitable route of
  administration, e.g a non-oral route if vomiting prevents absorption.

7. Re-evaluate

- If there are no improvements in symptoms recommence at point 1 and reconsider.

📖 Using the medical model for clinical or physical examination, p. 178.
📖 History-taking, p. 174.
📖 Using models of consultation for prescribing, p. 184.
📖 Concordance, p. 84.

1. Close, H. (2003). Nausea and vomiting in terminally ill patients: towards a holistic approach. *Nurse Prescribing*, **1**, 22–6.
2. Twycross, R. and Black, I. (1998). Nausea and vomiting in advanced cancer care. *European Journal of Palliative Care*, **5**, 39–45. 🖥 http://www.npc.co.uk/nurse_prescribing/

Concordance

What is concordance?

Initially defined by the Medicines Partnership in 2003, concordance was a new approach to prescribing and taking medicines based on an informed partnership agreement between the prescriber and the patient.

- Based on mutual negotiated agreement regarding illness and treatment.
- Taking into account previous experience, patient health beliefs, skills, and wishes.
- With the aim to support adherence to treatment.[1]

There is now a greater emphasis on shared decision-making based on the patient's understanding of and involvement in their treatment with a view to supporting adherence to the recommendations and advice given by the prescriber.[2]

Why do we need concordance?

- The cost of prescribed drugs is ~10% of NHS expenditure.
- Patients with long-term conditions only take between a third and half of the drugs they have been prescribed.
- Non-adherence to taking medicines costs the health service an estimated £100 million per year.[2]

Concordance between prescriber and patient is essential:

- to promote safe prescribing;
- reduce adverse drug reactions;
- to reduce cost and waste for the NHS.

Adherence

If achieved, concordance promotes and improves the patient's adherence, i.e whether they take their medication as prescribed and agreed

Holistic assessment and prescribing concordance

A holistic assessment will support concordance and promote harmony.

To establish concordance

Remember that patients have the right to refuse treatment/ prescribing.

Respect the patient

- Involve the patient as an active partner.
- Work in collaboration with the patient to gain a negotiated agreement as to how to proceed.
- Give the appropriate amount and type of information to the patient at the right place and at the right time to meet patient needs and appropriate to their level of understanding.
- Make the consultation patient-specific.
- Facilitate patient options and choice.
- Listen to and respect the health beliefs of the patient.
- Use consultation style to break the information into smaller pieces and to check that the patient understands.
- Explain the mode of action of the drug to the patient.
- Tell the patient what to expect.

- Consider and respect the patient's lifestyle, culture, and ethnic background.
- Consider disability, language barriers, and learning disabilities.
- Take the patient's concerns seriously.
- Allow the patient to disagree and take a suboptimal treatment or no treatment.

Communicate
- Speak the patient's language.
- Avoid medical jargon.
- Communicate decisions verbally and in writing.
- Signpost information into a logical sequence.
- Summarize.
- Use patient information leaflets.
- Use pictures/diagrams.
- Look at the patient when talking and listening, not at the computer.
- Observe the patient's body language.
- Explain medical tests/terms.

Mutual decision-making
- Involves a dialogue between yourself and the patient.
- What does the patient want?
- What does he/she think/feel?
- Draw up an agreed plan.
- Discuss choices and limitations of choice.
- Consider the options, benefits to the patient, drawbacks to therapy, and limitations of agreement.
- Can agree to disagree.
- Concordance should be empowering for the patient.

Ask
- What is the patient's initial knowledge base?
- What else do they want/need to know?
- What do they already understand?
- What don't they understand?

Contract with patient—give clear instructions
- Explain how to seek help (safety netting).
- Is the patient happy with the plan?
- Does he/she know what to do?
- When does the plan start?

Aids to concordance
- Large-print leaflets.
- Audio and audiovisual tapes.
- Braille.
- Language interpreters.
- NHS Direct.

Causes of non-adherence
- Lack of patient understanding.
- Lack of patient participation.
- Lack of patient empowerment.

- Unwanted/unpleasant side effects.
- Medication taken over a long period, e.g. chronic disease.
- Cost of medication to patient.

📖 Seven principles of safe prescribing, p. 94.

Further reading

Anon. (2003). Time to mobilise expert patients' skills. *Pharmaceutical Journal*, **270**, 743–4.

Heath, I. (2003). A wolf in sheep's clothing: a critical look at the ethics of drug taking. *British Medical Journal*, **327**, 856–8.

1. Britten, N. and Stevenson, F. (2002). Concordance—not just another word for compliance. *Prescriber*, **13**, 13–14.
2. National Institute for Health and Clinical Excellence (2009). Medicines adherence involving patients in decisions about prescribed medicines and supporting adherence.
🖳 http://www.nice.org.uk/nicemedia/pdf/CG76NICEGuideline.pdf (accessed 4 October 2010).

Safe prescribing

Safe prescribing

Accountability

Accountability covers four distinct areas:
- **personal**—liable under civil legislation to protect others from harm;
- **criminal**—may be called to account should harm result from their actions;
- **professional**—required to adhere to a standards relating to their scope of practice working to a code of professional conduct;
- **contractual**—must work within their job description as agreed by their employer.

Prescribers are called to account for their practice and in order to practice safely they must have:
- satisfactorily completed a recordable and recognized educational programme;
- maintained and updated prescribing knowledge and recorded any additional competencies;
- prescribed within their competency and the scope of their practice;
- agreed and followed a clinical management plan when undertaking supplementary prescribing. 📖 What is a clinical management plan?, p. 36.

Legal consent may be considered as:
- active—the patient is participating;
- oral—verbal confirmation has been obtained from the participating patient;
- written—the patient has signed a document stating that they have consented.

To be valid, consent must be informed, which requires the patient to be aware of:
- the reasons for the prescribed medication;
- the process for taking the prescribed medication;
- risks involved in the use of the prescribed medication;
- the demonstrated efficacy of the prescribed medication;
- any alternatives to the prescribed medication.

📖 NMC and HPC codes, p. 20
📖 Legal differences between prescribing, administering, and dispensing, p. 18

Gaining consent

- Prescribers must consider the patient's understanding and capacity to accept or decline treatment.
- If the patient is legally considered as unable to consent, the prescriber must act within their own competence and for the patient's good (beneficence). 📖 NMC and HPC codes, p. 20.

Prescribers must:
- document all prescribing decisions and actions;
- prescribe within the legal framework for independent prescribing and supplementary prescribing;

- understand that they are legally responsible for prescriptions they write, including acts and omissions;
- adhere to trust/organization policy;
- adhere to code of conduct;[1]
- do no harm to the patient;
- keep up to date with prescribing competencies[2] and provide evidence of these through appraisal processes;
- only prescribe within their competency area;
- be aware that they are still accountable when delegating to others;[3]
- be aware that they cannot prescribe for a patient whom they have not themselves assessed;
- understand the potential for drug abuse and misuse;
- keep clear contemporaneous records;
- maintain good lines of communication;
- undertake clinical supervision from another prescriber.

Principles

- Follow the principles of prescribing as set out by the National Prescribing Centre (NPC).[2]
- Use the prescribing pyramid as a model for prescribing.
- Work as part of a team.
- Understand the pressures that will be placed on you as a prescriber.

📖 Seven principles of safe prescribing, p. 94.

1. Nursing and Midwifery Council (2008) Code of professional conduct, performance and ethics. 🖥 http://www.nmc-uk.org
2. Nursing and Midwifery Council (2006) Standards of proficiency for nurse and midwife prescribers. 🖥 http://www.nmc-uk.org
3. Nursing and Midwifery Council (2007). Guidance for the administration of medicines. NMC, London.
4. NPC. 🖥 www.npc.co.uk. (accessed 23.11.2010).

Practice

Practising legally

- Non-medical independent prescribers can prescribe licensed and unlicensed drugs from anywhere in the British National Formulary (BNF), including some controlled drugs, provided that they are clinically competent to do so.
- Community practitioner nurse prescribers prescribe only from the Community Practitioners Formulary (CPF).
- Supplementary prescribers must work in partnership with an independent prescriber (who is a medical doctor) and the patient/carer. Prescribing decisions are documented in the CMP and where possible a copy of this plan is given to the patient.
- Always consult the formulary prior to prescribing.

📖 The legal differences between prescribing, administration, and dispensing, p. 18.
📖 Prescribing and the law, p. 134.

The practice of assessment

- Only prescribe if you have assessed the patient yourself.
- Complete a holistic assessment.
- Follow a structured model of assessment.
- Consider the patient's past medical history.
- Ask about the patient's current health status.
- Take a thorough medication history.
- Ask about other medication bought over or under the counter, including herbal and family homely remedies and borrowed medications.
- Ask about allergies and sensitivities.

The practice of concordance

- Always consider side effects, cautions, contraindications, and interactions.
- Inform the patient of potential side effects, how, when, and how often to take the medication, the dose, and what to do if he/she has an unfavourable reaction.
- Explain the rationale for prescribing to the patient.
- Gain full and informed consent.

📖 Holistic assessment, p. 82
📖 Concordance, p. 84.

Practice safely

- Check that the patient can read the label on the medication.
- Explain how to obtain medicines.
- Advise the patient to keep medicines out of reach of children and animals.
- Advise the patient not to share their medication with others.
- Be aware of the public health implications of your prescribing.

Further reading

Courtenay, M. and Butler, M. (2002). *Essential nurse prescribing*. Greenwich Medical Media, London.

Courtenay, M. and Griffiths, M. (2010). *Independent and supplementary prescribing: an essential guide*. Cambridge University Press, Cambridge.

Health Professions Council (2006). *Standards for education and training*. ▣ http://www.hpc-uk.org/aboutregistration/medicinesandprescribing/ (accessed 3 February 2010).

Health Professions Council. ▣ www.hpc-uk.org (accessed 3 February 2010).

Nursing and Midwifery Council (2006). *Standards of nursing and proficiency for nurse and midwife prescribers*. NMC, London.

Scottish Executive Health Department (2006). *Non-medical prescribing*. ▣ http://www.scotland.gov.uk/Publications/2006/08/23133351/0 (accessed 3 February 2010).

Responsibility

As well as being accountable to others for their prescribing actions and decisions, prescribers are also responsible for their own decision-making and actions.[1]

Responsibility and safety

- Have a clear rationale for prescribing.
- Consider alternatives to prescribing.
- Have a sound knowledge of the therapeutics of any medication you prescribe.
- Give written information to the patient.
- Consider patients who may have special needs.
- Gain concordance between the patient and prescriber.
- Be aware of the needs of patients for whom English is not their first language.
- Prescribe with caution for people from special groups, e.g. those with renal and hepatic disorders, children, older people, pregnancy, and breastfeeding.
- Review the patient on a regular basis.
- Maintain awareness of limitations of and changes to formularies.
- Be aware of your own limitations in practice.
- Maintain contemporaneous shared record-keeping.
- Establish and maintain clear communication with other professionals who are involved in the patient's treatment.
- Report adverse drug reactions using the Yellow Card Scheme.
- Recognize, analyse, and learn from critical incidents and significant events.
- Understand the requirements of clinical governance.
- Keep up to date with new information.

Responsibility and continuing professional development

In the 21st century a trusting assumption of professional responsibility is not enough, and professional bodies and the public now require evidence and 'objective assurance'.[2] In response to the Report from the Shipman Inquiry the NMC produced guidance relating to continuing professional development (CPD) for nurse and midwife prescribers.[3]

Maintain CPD in line with requirements of professional bodies

- Identify CPD needs at appraisal.
- Gain employer's support to enable you to meet CPD needs.
- Keep your prescribing portfolio up to date.
- Network with other prescribers.
- Develop leadership skills.
- Understand the roles of others.
- Perform audit.
- Share good practice.

📖 NMC and HPC codes, p. 20.

Remember to record: failure to record actions is unsafe practice and constitutes negligence.

📖 Record-keeping, p. 192.

1. Nursing and Midwifery Council (2006). *Standards of proficiency for nurse and midwife prescribers.* 🖥 http://www.nmc-uk.org (accessed 3 February 2010).
2. *Trust, assurance and safety—the regulation of health professionals in the 21st Century* (2007). TSO, London.
3. Nursing and Midwifery Council (2008). *Guidance for continuing professional development for nurses and midwives.* 🖥 http://www.nmc-uk.org/aArticle.aspx?ArticleID=3265 (accessed 11 October 2009).

Seven principles of safe prescribing

Prescribing a product or medicine is a complex process which involves far more than writing a prescription and has considerable impact on the patient, colleagues, and the NHS in general. The National Prescribing Centre have a model: the prescribing pyramid which gives a useful framework for prescribing considerations.

The prescribing pyramid

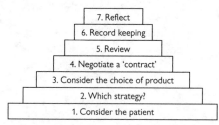

Fig. 6.1 The prescribing pyramid. Reproduced with kind permission of the National Prescribing Centre from *Nurse Prescribing Bulletin* (1999), **1**(1). NPC Liverpool

1. Examine the holistic needs of the patient
- Is a prescription really necessary?
- A thorough needs assessment may show that a non-drug therapy is indicated.
- A full medical and social history should be taken, along with an holistic assessment (📖 Holistic assessment, p. 82) before prescribing.
- The mnemonic 2-WHAM[1] may prove a helpful aide-memoire:
  W Who is it for?
  W What are the symptoms?
  H How long have the symptoms been present?
  A Any action taken so far?
  M Any other medication taken?

When taking a drug history include:
- Any prescribed items.
- OTC medications.
- Home remedies (home-made medicines handed down over generations, e.g. an infusion of the plant feverfew for migraine).
- Alternative therapies such as homeopathic and herbal remedies.
- Any prescribed items 'borrowed' from another person.
- Any known allergies.
- Medications purchased over the internet.
- Complementary or alternative medicines;
- Products described as 'natural remedies' (e.g. ginseng).

2. Consider the appropriate strategy

- Is the diagnosis established?
- Is a GP referral indicated?
- Is a prescription needed at all?
- Is patient expectation a factor in your decision?
- A prescription should only be given when it is genuinely needed. Patients may want prescriptions for reasons other than treatment, e.g.:
  - to legitimize the sick role;
  - to gain attention;
  - because a friend recommended it;
  - because a family member or friend would like the product.

3. Consider the product of choice

The use of the mnemonic EASE may be helpful.

   E How effective is the product?
   A Is it appropriate?
   S How safe is it?
   E Is the prescription cost effective?

- To ensure that the product is appropriate, familiarize yourself with the relevant section of the formulary.
- Critically appraise the evidence to assess a product's effectiveness.
- Check the BNF for any ADRs, contraindications, special precautions, or drug interactions.
- Consider dose, formulation, and the duration of treatment with regard to the individual patient.
- Does the patient fall within a particular group requiring specialist knowledge and consideration, e.g. the extremes of life?

  📖 Cost-effective prescribing, p. 438
  📖 Adverse drug reactions (ADRs), p. 68

4. Negotiating a contract

Shared decision-making between the patient and the health-care professional is known as concordance.

- The patient has a central role in the decision-making process.
- The patient needs to understand:
  - what the prescription is for;
  - how long it will take to work;
  - how to take the product;
  - how long to take it;
  - at what dose to take it;
  - any possible side effects;
  - how and whom to contact if they have concerns.

  📖 Concordance, p. 84.

5. Reviewing the patient

Regular review will determine whether the prescribed item(s) are effective, safe, and acceptable.

6. Keeping records

The NMC has guidelines regarding record-keeping.[2]

📖 Record-keeping, p. 192.

7. Reflecting on your prescribing

Reviewing and reflecting your prescribing decisions will help improve your practice and knowledge base.

📖 Repeat prescriptions, p. 122
📖 Non-medical prescribing history and policy in context, p. 4
📖 Concordance, p. 84
📖 Safe prescribing, p. 88

NB: for any given therapeutic intervention, the potential benefits of the intervention must be balanced against safety concerns.

1. Hayes, A. (1997). Sale of medications in pharmacies: protocols. Where now? *Pharmaceutical Journal*, **259**, 60–8.
2. Nursing and Midwifery Council (2001). *Guidelines for records and record keeping*. NMC, London.

Reason to use EASE

Information Centre statistics[1] show that 842.5 million items were prescribed in 2008, a rise of 5.8% compared with 2007. The net costs of prescribed items for the UK were £8325.5 million, a fall of 0.6% compared with 2007. It is the responsibility of the prescriber to consider the cost and efficacy of any and all items prescribed in order to optimize expenditure and minimize waste.

Information regarding the costs of prescribable items can be obtained from the Drug Tariff which is published monthly on behalf of the Secretary of State and is obtainable from the Stationery Office.

In addition prescribers can reduce their prescribing budget by adopting the following procedures.

- Consider, when appropriate, recommendation of an OTC product. If the patient pays for their prescriptions, this may save them money and will have no impact on the NHS budget.
- Always prescribe using the generic name of the product. The only exception is where there may be bioavaiabilty problems. In these cases the BNF recommends that patients always receive the same brand, and therefore the items should be prescribed using the brand name.

1. 🖳 www.ic.nhs.uk (accessed 9 September 2009).

Controlled drugs (CDs)

Detailed advice on writing a prescription for CDs is contained in the current BNF and you can also refer to *Guidance on prescribing: controlled drugs and drug dependence.*[1]

Non-medical prescribers (NMPs) prescribe controlled drugs according to current legislation and must ensure that they maintain up-to-date knowledge. All NMPs must be aware of who the accountable officer is in their trust or organization. The Health Act 2006 created the new role of accountable officer for controlled drugs.[2]

• Each NHS trust, primary care trust, foundation trust, and independent hospital must appoint an accountable officer for CDs.
• The accountable officer is charged with specified responsibilities in relation to the safe, appropriate, and effective management and use of CDs.
• The definition of safe and effective management of CDs includes destruction and disposal.
• A list of accountable officers for controlled drugs is held by
• The Care Quality Commission and is accessible at http://www.carequalitycommision.org.uk/serviceproviderinformation/controlleddrugs/acc
• NMPs must be aware of the audit requirements and the local procedures for prescribing of CDs.
• NMPs must *not* prescribe a CD for themselves, and only prescribe a CD for someone close to them if:
  • no other person with the legal right to prescribe is available
  • the treatment is immediately necessary to:
    ○ save life;
    ○ avoid significant deterioration in the patient/client's health;
    ○ alleviate otherwise uncontrollable pain.
• An NMP must be able to justify their actions and must have documented their relationship and the emergency circumstances that necessitated their prescription of a controlled drug for someone close to them.

Record-keeping[1]

From 1 February 2008, the regulations require the following information to be recorded in the Controlled Drug Register (CDR), under the following specified headings, when CDs are obtained:
• date supply obtained;
• name and address from whom obtained (e.g. wholesaler, pharmacy);
• quantity obtained.

When CDs are supplied to patients (in response to prescriptions) or to practitioners (in response to requisitions), the regulations require information to be recorded in the CDR, under the following specified headings:
• date supplied;
• name and address of person or firm supplied;
• detail of authority to possess—prescriber or licence-holder's details;
• quantity, name, form, and strength of the CD supplied.

The Department of Health notes that the following information *may* (not must) be recorded in the CD register:

- running balances;
- prescriber identification number (i.e. the six-digit private doctor code or the NHS prescriber code) and/or the professional registration number of the prescriber where known, and also the name and professional registration number of the health-care professional supplying the CD.

When electronic registers and electronic prescribing for CDs are in widespread use and subject to parliamentary approval, the government will mandate the inclusion of running balances and prescriber and sup-plier identification.

From February 2008 and as specified in the amended Misuse of Drugs Regulations 2001, it is a requirement to record the following informa-tion in relation to the identity of the person collecting a schedule 2 CD supplied on prescription.

- Whether the person who collected the drug was:
  - the patient;
  - the patient's representative;
  - a health-care professional acting on behalf of the patient.
- If the person who collected the drug was a health-care professional acting on behalf of the patient, that person's name and address should be recorded.
- Whether evidence of identity was provided by the person collecting the drug.
- If the person who collected the drug was the patient or their representative, whether evidence of identity was requested (annotated in the yes/no columns). As a matter of good practice a note as to why the dispenser did not ask may be included but this is not mandatory.

Further reading

National Prescribing Centre (2007). *A guide to good practice in the management of controlled drugs in primary care (England)*. NPC, Liverpool.

1. Department of Health (2007). *Safer management of controlled drugs (CDs): changes to record keeping requirements guidance (for England only), revised 2008*. TSO, London. ▣ http://www.dh.gov. uk/publications (accessed 9 September 2009).

2. ▣ http://www.opsi.gov.uk/si/si2006/20063148.htm (accessed 10 October 2009).

Safe storage of controlled drugs

The Care Quality Commission[1] offer the following advice on the safe storage and disposal of CDs.

Storage

Schedule 2 controlled drugs are subject to the safe custody requirements set out in the Misuse of Drugs (Safe Custody) Regulations 1973, amended 2007.[2] They state that CDs must be stored in a locked receptacle, usually in an appropriate controlled drug cabinet or approved safe, which can be opened by a person in possession of the controlled drug or a person authorized by that person.

Destruction

The person carrying out the destruction of schedule 2 controlled drugs must be appropriately authorized and witnessed by a person authorized to do so.

📖 Prescribing for public health, p. 205

1. Care Quality Commission (2009). *The safer management of controlled drugs. Annual Report 2008*. 🖳 http://www.cqc.org.uk/db/documents/Thesafermanagementofcontrolleddrugs Annualreport2008.pdf (accessed 10 October 2009).
2. Department of Health (2007). *Guidance on the destruction of controlled drugs: new role for accountable officers*. TSO, London.

Working as a non-medical prescriber for out-of-hours services

The principles relating to non-medical prescribing apply to any prescribing context.

- Always take a thorough history and conduct a full prescribing assessment.
- Only prescribe within your field of competence.
- Adhere to policy.
- Adhere to NMC standards for record-keeping.
- Communicate your prescribing actions and decisions to patients, doctor, and carers.
- Remember to review the patient and your prescribing decision.

The NMC have produced guidance regarding remote assessment and prescribing. This guidance can be accessed at:
 http://www.nmc-uk.org/aArticle.aspx?ArticleID=3460 (accessed 2 March 2010).

Numeracy and drug calculations 1

It is imperative that, as a prescriber, you are able to perform drug calculations competently. If you struggle in this area, you must seek help before prescribing. Never prescribe unless you are sure that the calculation is correct. If in doubt, check it with another colleague and only ever prescribe if you are sure that the calculation is correct.

SI units are units of measurement, e.g. grams, milligrams, micrograms, millilitres, or litres. When calculating drug doses, make sure that you are aware of the SI unit that is being used (e.g. grams or milligrams).

Table 6.1 Equivalence of weight and volume

Units of measurement (SI units) for weight	Units of measurement (SI units) for volume
1000 micrograms = 1 milligram and 1000 milligrams = 1 gram	1000 microlitres = 1 millilitre and 1000 millilitres = 1 litre

Why do we need to know?

Drug calculation is a critical area when managing medicines and is open to error. All health professionals who are dispensing, supplying, or administering drugs will need to perform drug calculations to a greater or lesser extent. Registered professionals are accountable and responsible for their decisions and actions, and cannot rely on others to check the accuracy of their calculations.

Main areas of error when calculating drug dosages

- Moving the decimal point in the wrong direction when converting dosages to the same units of measurement (SI units), for example grams to milligrams or litres to millilitres.
- Miscalculating the quantities of tablets/dressings etc. to be administered over a period of time.
- Miscalculating the time interval between doses.
- Miscalculating the volume of drug in solution.
- Miscalculating the rate of administration (IV fluid).

Calculating drug dosages

For a dose that is in a solution, ensure that the dosage of the drug is at the same level of the SI unit as the solution that it is in. If it is not, convert it so that it is.

> *Example*
> 0.005 grams in 10 millilitres is better expressed as 5 milligrams in 10 millilitres (5mg in 10mL).

Remember that a microgram is smaller than a milligram and a milligram is larger than a microgram but smaller than a gram:

1000 micrograms = 1 milligram
1000 milligrams = 1 gram
1,000,000 micrograms = 1gram

To convert from a smaller unit to a larger unit, divide by multiples of a 1000. Therefore to convert micrograms to milligrams divide by 1000:

1000 micrograms/1000 = 1 milligram.

To convert milligrams to grams divide by 1000:

1000 milligrams/1000 = 1 gram.

A simple way of doing this is to move the decimal point three places to the left. For example,

300mg/1000 = 0.3g

300mg/1000 = 0.3g

To convert from a larger unit to a smaller unit, multiply by multiples of 1000. Therefore to convert grams to milligrams, multiply by 1000:

1 gram × 1000 = 1000 milligrams

A simple way of doing this is to move the decimal point three places to the right, for example

0.005 g

0.005g is better expressed as 5mg.

Numeracy and drug calculations 2

Calculating the volume of drug that needs to be administered in solution

The dose of the drug that needs to be given is divided by the dose of the drug that is in the volume. This is then multiplied by the volume of the solution that contains the drug.

Example

To administer 10mg of sintomycin (made-up name) that comes in a stock amount of 40mg in 80mL:

- 10mg of a drug is to be given;
- the stock amount of the drug in the solution is 40mg in 80mL;
- a simple way of expressing this is as follows:

> What you want (the dose of the drug to be given)
> × the stock volume you have
> _____
> What you have (the dose of the drug you have)

- This can be expressed as:

   (10mg × 80mL)/20mL = 40mg.

Calculating the number of tablets to be administered over a period of time

Prescribe in the form that is most acceptable for the patient as this will support adherence. For example, a 1g tablet might be more acceptable for the patient to take than two 500mg tablets, or an oral solution might be more acceptable for a patient who has difficulty in swallowing.

Calculating the number of tablets to be given in 24 hours

You will need to be aware of the time interval between the doses, e.g. to be given 4 hourly. You will also need to be aware of the dose of the drug to be given and of the stock dose of the drug. To calculate the total number of tablets needed to be prescribed over a given time period:

- identify the dose of the tablet that is required to be given;
- identify the stock dose of the tablet (what dose does it come in?);
- identify the total number of tablets to be given in the time period;
- identify the time interval between dosages;
- identify the number of times that you need to give the dose.

Example 1
- If a tablet is to be given no less than 4 hourly for a maximum period of 24 hours then you must divide the required time period for the total dose to have been given (in this case 24 hours) by the time interval between doses (in this case not less than every 4 hours):

    $24/4 = 6$

- Therefore the tablet needs to be given six times a day with an interval of not less than 4 hours between administrations.

Example 2
- 5mg of antopotin (made-up name) to be given every 4 hours for 24 hours.
- Stock dose (the dose in which the tablets are supplied) of antopotin is 2.5mg.
- Required single dose of 5mg divided by the stock dose of 2.5mg is two tablets in a single dose.
- To give 5mg for each dose you will need to give 2 × 2.5mg. Therefore administer two tablets every 4 hours.
- To calculate the number of times that the dose needs to be given in 24 hours divide the total number of hours by the minimum dose frequency, e.g. 24/4 = 6 (administer six doses in 24 hours).
- To work out the total dose, multiply the dose given at each single administration by the dose frequency (how many times the dose is given in 24 hours): 5mg × 6 times in 24 hours. Thus the total dose in 24 hours is 30mg.
- To work out the number of tablets to be prescribed for a 24 hour period, multiply the number of tablets to be given at each dose by the number of times to be given in 24 hours. For example, 2 tablets (at each single administration) × 6 (times a day) = 12 tablets to be prescribed for a 24 hour period.

Calculating the total number of tablets to be given for a period longer than 24 hours

Multiply the number of tablets to be given over a 24 hour period by the number of days that the tablets are to be given for.

Example

12 tablets to be given in 24 hours (1 day). Therefore
no. to be prescribed for 5 days = 12 × 5 = 60 tablets.

Calculating the administration of intravenous fluid

Giving sets are commonly designed to administer fluid at either 20 drops/mL or 60 drops/mL (as a microdrip). To calculate the number of drops to be given per minute:

    rate (drops/min) = volume (drops)/time (min).

For example, 1000mL is to be given over 10 hours and the giving set delivers 20 drops/mL. Since we want a rate in drops per minute, we must convert the time to minutes:

10 hours = 10 × 60 = 600 minutes.

We must also convert the volume to drops if we have 1000mL and there are 20 drops/mL:

1000 × 20 drops = 20000 drops in total

Therefore:

rate = volume (drops)/time (min) = 20000/600 = 33.3 drops/min.

NB: this is not practical to administer, so you would need to make it into a whole number by rounding it up to 34.

Percentage weight per volume

Percentage weight per volume (%w/v) is a way of describing the percentage mass (weight) of the drug in an ointment. It is expressed as the number of grams per 100mL.

Example

An ointment containing 8%w/v = 8g of the drug in the ointment base. When dissolving 8g of the drug in 200mL, to work out how many grams per millilitre divide the weight by the volume of the ointment or solution:

8/200 = 0.04g/mL.

Then to obtain the percentage multiply by 100:

0.04g × 100 = 4%.

Further reading

Chernecky, C., Butler, S., Graham, P., and Infortuna, H. (2002). *Drug calculations and drug administration*. W.B. Saunders, Philadelphia, PA.
Coben, D., and Atere-Roberts, E. (2005). *Calculations for nursing and healthcare* (2nd edn). Palgrave Macmillan, Basingstoke.
Nursing and Midwifery Council (2006). *Standards of proficiency for nurse and midwife prescribers*. NMC, London.

Consideration of product choice

Generic prescribing

- The BNF directs all prescribers to use the generic name of a product when prescribing, rather than the brand name.
- Since 1997 wound care products and appliances can be prescribed by brand name as it was proving very time consuming and confusing to refer to 'vapour permeable adhesive film dressing', for instance, when OpSite® or Tegaderm® was required.
- Brand names are those given to a particular version of a product by an individual manufacturer.
- Some products are only marketed by one manufacturer. However, the generic name should still be used when prescribing.
- Other products are only produced in their generic forms.
- Patients should be told that items will be prescribed generically and that although the packaging may differ the content is the same as they have had before.
- Conversely, a branded product may be dispensed instead of the generic one prescribed if the branded product is cheaper. PACT data will still record the prescriber as having prescribed generically. See 🖥 www.nhsbsa.nhs.uk/3230.aspx (accessed 4 February 2011).
- Patients can be reassured that both branded and generic items conform to the licensing requirements of the Medicines Control Agency (part of the MHRA) and are equally safe.
- UKMiCentral offer drug comparison charts online (🖥 www.ukmicentral.nhs.uk).
- Products imported from the European Union may prove to be less expensive, resulting in the patient receiving a product with packaging not labelled in English. Reassurance can be given that the same licensing standards apply and instructions in English are included in the package.
- Since 2000 the free market for the supply and sale of generic products has been regulated by the Department of Health, which imposes a maximum price.
- Some patients need to be kept on branded anti-epileptic and lithium products because these products have a narrow therapeutic margin and can be toxic if the prescribed dose is exceeded.

Suitability of formulation

Definition
The formulation of a medicine refers to its chemical and physical composition. This includes the chemical compositions of both the active ingredients and the excipients which stabilize the active ingredients or modify their release.

It is important to select the appropriate formulation to suit the desired therapeutic outcome and the physical condition, abilities, and psychological inclination of your patient.

Formulations
- Tablets (including dispersible and dissolvable)
- Liquid
- Gums and lozenges
- Patches
- Topical—creams, lotions, emollients, patches, etc.
- Rectal preparations
- Parenteral—IV, IM, ID, SC, IT
- Mouthwashes
- Gargles
- Paint/varnish
- For inhalation
- Drops—eye, ear, and nasal.

Considerations

Excipients
- May be responsible for some ADRs. For example, some penicillins and warfarin contain sodium as do some indigestion remedies and analgesics. Patients with incipient heart failure who take any of these may find the sodium content sufficient to precipitate fluid retention and breathlessness.
- Excipients may vary from one branded product to another, and this could have an effect on the bioavailability of the active ingredients. For example, with some anti-epileptic and lithium preparations, changing from one branded product to another or to a generic product can result in loss of control of the patient's condition.
- Oral preparations that do not contain fructose, sucrose, or glucose are described as 'sugar free' as are those containing hydrogenated glucose syrup, mannitol, malitol, sorbitol, or xylitol as there is evidence that these do not cause dental caries. This is an important consideration when prescribing for children.

Oral medications
- Tablets and capsules should be swallowed with a glass of water and the patient should sit erect and remain so for the following 30min. This is in order to prevent prolonged contact between a potentially corrosive substance, the medication (bisulphates, aspirin, iron and potassium salts), and the lining of the mouth and oesophagus.

- When prescribing an oral preparation it is important to be aware of potential interactions between drugs, food, and herbs.
- Not only can food affect a drug's bioavailability and alter the therapeutic outcome, but drugs can have an adverse impact on a patient's nutritional status.
- Foods and herbs may also counteract the action of a drug. For example, fexofenadine (non-sedating antihistamine) loses effect if taken with orange, apple, or grapefruit juice, the activity of ciclosporin is reduced by St John's wort, and the metabolism of warfarin is inhibited by grapefruit juice.
- Drugs and food may bind together, leading to their retention in the intestine (e.g. digoxin).
- Administration with food can be beneficial for some preparations (e.g. nifedipine) as it prevents a sudden onset of action of the drug.
- Some drugs (e.g. bisulphates or tetracycline) will not be absorbed if given with food.
- The timing of administration of enteral or oral medication is imperative. For example, iron relies on gastric acidity in order to be absorbed which may be too low if:
  - administered between meals in older people;
  - administered to those with HIV/AIDS and also those taking antacids and H2-receptor agonists.
- Conversely, ampicillin and some antivirals for HIV/AIDS (didanosine, indinavir) are destroyed by stomach acid and therefore should not be taken within 2 hours of meals or enteral feeds.
- Changing from a tablet to a liquid preparation of the same medication often requires a reduction of dose.

📖 Where to get up-to-date information, p. 462.

📖 Basic principles of pharmacology, pp. 53–64.
See also the relevant section of the latest version of the BNF.

How to obtain prescription pads

At the time of going to press FP10P prescription forms are preprinted by Astron. Orders for a new prescriber's prescription forms should not be placed more than 42 days prior to the date that the individual is scheduled to begin prescribing. Allow 6 working days between notifying changes to the NHS Business Services Authority and ordering prescriptions. Pads are normally delivered to the address of the person who orders them. Any prescriber who works for more than one employer or in more than one setting must either have separate prescription pads for each organization or use FP10SS prescriptions printed with the correct organization details in the prescriber details area of the form.

What appears on the prescription

The top of the prescribing area will be overprinted to identify the type of prescriber, for example:

NURSE INDEPENDENT/SUPPLEMENTARY PRESCRIBER

or

PHARMACIST INDEPENDENT/SUPPLEMENTARY PRESCRIBER.

The address box will be overprinted to identify:

- the nurse or pharmacist independent prescriber;
- the organization on whose behalf they are prescribing.

For those nurse or pharmacist independent prescribers who are directly employed by a PCT or prescribing through a community practitioner nurse prescribing contract, there is a space for the relevant practice number to be added for each patient for whom they prescribe (Astron printed prescriptions only). If the prescription is printed by a GP system, the practice code will be printed in the relevant place.

How do non-medical prescribers prescribe for hospital inpatients or outpatients?

There are three methods by which they can prescribe.

- Hospital in-patient prescription form or sheet—this is used for in-patients and discharge supplies only as a prescription charge is not levied for inpatients.
- Internal hospital prescription form—used for outpatients but only in cases where the hospital pharmacy will dispense the prescription as a prescription charge may be payable unless the patient is exempt from charges. (NB: internal hospital forms cannot be accepted for dispensing by community pharmacies).
- The prescriber may also use a prescription form which will be dispensed by the community pharmacist.

Who can write a prescription

- NMPs can only prescribe within their area of competency.
- NMPs can only prescribe for a patient whom they have assessed.
- They must use the prescription pad which has been issued to them.
- Repeat prescriptions may only be issued under DoH guidelines.
- 📖 Repeat prescriptions, p. 122.

Writing a prescription 1

Always use indelible ink, preferably black, unless directed otherwise. If possible use a computer-printed prescription.

- Write legibly.
- Date the prescription.
- Give the full name, address, and postcode of the patient for whom you are prescribing.
- Where possible give the patient's NHS number.
- Sign the prescription and date it.
- It is preferable to include the age and date of birth of the patient.
- It is a legal requirement to state the age of a child under 12 years when prescribing a POM.
- Any directions should be in English and not abbreviated.
- Where there is more than one item on a form, a line should be inserted between each item for clarity.
- Unused space in the prescription area of the form should be blocked out with, for example, a diagonal line (to prevent subsequent fraudulent addition of extra items).
- The BNF recommends avoidance of the unnecessary use of decimal points (e.g. 3mg not 3.0mg).
- Quantities of 1g or more should be written as 1g etc., and quantities of less than 1g should be written as 500mg not 0.5g.
- If the decimal point is unavoidable, a zero should be put in front (e.g. 0.5ml not .5ml).
- The decimal point may be used when expressing a range (e.g. 0.5 to 1g).
- The units micrograms and nanograms should not be abbreviated.
- Use the term millilitre (ml or mL) not cubic centimetre (cc or cm^3).
- On *hospital prescriptions only*, the name of the nurse or pharmacist independent prescriber should be printed or hand-written in the box provided to ensure that the dispensing pharmacist is aware of whom to contact if he/she has a query.

Principal legal requirements

The prescription must be:

- signed;
- dated;
- indelibly written and include:
  - the patient's name and address;
  - the case, form, and strength of the preparation;
  - the total quantity of the preparation, or number of dose units in both words and figures;
  - the dose;
  - if issued by a dentist, the words 'for dental treatment only'.

📖 Prescribing and the law, p. 134.

	Age Two	**Name (including first names) and address**	
	D.o.B 21/5/97	Joanna Bloggs 14 Any Road Fulchester Northshire XS34 4LP	**1. Patient details:** • Full name (surname and first name) • Full address • Age and date of birth
Pharmacy Stamp			

Dispenser's Endorsement	**Number of days' treatment** N.B. ensure dose is stated	**NP**	**Pricing** *Office*

Pack and Quantity	Paracetamol sugar free oral suspension, 120 mg/5ml One 5ml spoonful to be taken every four to six hours, as required to relieve pain. Max. 4 doses in 24 hours. <u>Supply 100ml</u> Aqueous cream Apply to the affected areas four times a day and use to wash instead of soap. <u>Supply 500g</u>	2. **Details of the item(s) to be supplied:** (a) **Name, form,** and **strength** of the item(s): • Use **generic** name, except for dressings and appliances or when clinically inappropriate • Do not use abbreviations (b) **Dose** and **frequency** of dose (c) Directions of how to use the item(s) • Always write **full** directions in English • Do not use abbreviations (d) Quantity to be supplied • Specify and appropriate amount to meet the patient's need while avoiding waste • Generally this should be for no more than one calendar month • Where possible prescribe the pack size specified in the NPF under each preparation – do not use the term 'OP' • Consider patient packs/special containers where appropriate

Signature of Nurse	*Date*	3. **Signature** of prescriber and date.

For *Dispenser* No. of Presens on form [ ]	Please complete patient's Practice details PATIENTS PRACTICE CODE .... NURSE CONTACT TEL. NO.	4. **Practice Code** – Code for the practice where the patient is registered. 5. **Nurse's contact telephone number** The pharmacist must be able to contact the nurse if there is a problem with the prescription.
NHS		

Writing a prescription 2

For prescribing in **primary care** and in the **community**, the prescription should contain:
- the name of the prescribed item;
- the formulation;
- the strength (if any);
- the dosage;
- the frequency with which the medication is to be taken;
- the quantity to be dispensed, which should reflect the patient's needs (normally the pack size as indicated in the BNF);
- full directions on how to use the items e.g.rectally or orally.

The name of the prescribed item should reflect the description in the *NHS Dictionary of Medicines and Devices* (NHS dm+d), the NHS standard for naming medicines and devices (🖳 www.dmd.nhs.uk). Use the generic name except for appliances and dressings.

For prescribing in **secondary care**, in hospitals, prescriptions for in-patients should contain:
- the name of the prescribed item;
- the formulation;
- the strength (if any);
- the dosage;
- the frequency.

Where a defined length of treatment is required, this should be stated.

The requirements for **outpatients** and **discharge prescriptions** are the same as those for primary/community care, whilst recognizing local policies on, for example, the length of treatment provided for outpatients and patients who are being discharged.

Computer-generated prescription

- A computer-generated prescription must include the date of issue, the patient's second name, forename(s) as initials, and their address.
- It may print their title and date of birth.
- The age of children under 12 years and adults over 60 must be printed in the box available.
- The age of children less than 5 years should be printed in years and months.
- The prescriber's name, surgery address, telephone contact number, forename(s), and reference number should be included.

See latest version of the BNF for more guidance.

Further information

Royal Pharmaceutical Society of Great Britain. *Clinical governance framework for pharmacist prescribers and organisations commissioning or participating in pharmacist prescribing (GB wide).*
🖳 http://www.rpsgb.org/pdfs/clincgovframeworkpharm.pdf (accessed 5 May 2010).
Advice regarding prescribing in Scotland:
🖳 http://www.scotland.gov.uk/Publications/2006/08/23133351/17 (accessed 5 May 2010).
Advice regarding prescribing in Northern Ireland:
🖳 http://www.dhsspsni.gov.uk/best_practice_guidance.pdf (accessed 7 May 2010).
Advice regarding prescribing in Wales:
🖳 www.wales.nhs.uk/sites3/docopen.cfm?orgid=371&id=85949 (accessed 7 May 2010).

Security and safety of the prescription pad

- The prescription pad/form is the property of the local health board or NHS trust.
- It is the responsibility of the prescriber to ensure security of the pad or form at all times.
- Take the same care of the prescription pad as you would your cheque book.
- Under no circumstances should a blank prescription pad or form be pre-signed.
- The prescription pad or form should only be produced when needed, and should never be left unattended or visible.
- When not in use, prescription pads/forms should be stored in a lockable drawer in a filing cabinet or in a secure box.
- When travelling between patients or venues the prescription pad or form should not be visible and must be locked in the car boot within a bag.
- The bag and prescription pad or form must always be removed from the car at the end of the working day.
- Some prescribers take only a few prescriptions out with them rather than risking the whole pad.
- It is helpful to record the numbers of prescription pads as you receive them.

What to do if a prescriber:
- terminates their employment;
- moves to another job which involves prescribing;
- commences maternity leave;
- commences a secondment;
- commences long term sick leave or a sabbatical.

Return prescription pads and any loose forms to the line manager whose responsibility it is to complete the appropriate forms and return or destroy the prescription pads or forms subject to local guidelines.

What to do if a prescription pad or form is lost or believed to be stolen
- Prescribers must be aware of their local guidelines which may vary (complete Box 7.1).
- The prescriber must immediately report the loss or suspected theft to their line manager.
- Either the prescriber or their manager will report the loss/theft to the police.
- You are advised to notify local pharmacists and may be requested to complete future prescriptions in a distinctively coloured ink to enable detection of any forgeries.

Box 7.1 Local procedure for reporting lost or stolen prescription pads

Name of person to contact:

Telephone/email contact address:

Review

Repeat prescriptions

Approximately 75% of prescriptions are dispensed as repeat prescriptions.[1]

Repeat prescriptions are convenient for patients and prescribers, but care must be taken to avoid either waste and over-prescribing, or detection of adverse or dangerous patient reactions.

The guidance for repeat dispensing,[2] issued in a joint document by the NHS, BMA, and PSNC in 2009, notes that two-thirds of primary care prescriptions are repeat prescriptions. The Medicines Management newsletter[3] offers guidance on the optimal repeat prescribing times of 28 or 56 days for individual patients. A further newsletter suggests that, where the drugs are expensive and the patient may not tolerate the medication, a duration of less than 28 days may be suitable for a patient's initial prescription (see later).

The NPC issued the first Service Improvement Guide (SIG), focusing on repeat prescriptions, in 2005. This can be accessed at http://www.npc.co.uk

Luker and Austin[4] conducted a review of repeat prescriptions at two of the nurse prescribing pilot sites and found that many patients were receiving repeat prescriptions of items in the CPF which had originally been prescribed by doctors. Many of the products were no longer indicated and considerable savings were realized.

Therefore it is important to have a system in place which identifies products that a nurse would not usually wish to prescribe repeatedly, and it is recommended that 'nurses should be mindful of any protocols already in place'.[5]

28-day prescriptions

28-day prescriptions were seen as more appropriate for:
- first prescriptions and until the dose and regimen are established;
- patients in residential and nursing homes;
- vulnerable patients on complex drug regimens;
- those likely to be admitted to hospital;
- terminally ill patients receiving palliative care support;
- drugs liable to abuse;
- all antidepressants;
- patients requiring dressings;
- all controlled drugs (except under exceptional circumstances);
- other 'hospital-driven' high-cost drugs, e.g. antipsychotics and drugs for dementia.

56-day prescribing

56-day prescribing is recommended as appropriate for patients on a stable medication regime, who express a preference for 56-day prescribing, or those who would be financially disadvantaged or inconvenienced by 28-day prescribing.

Computer-generated prescriptions

Most repeat prescriptions are computer-generated and guidelines are issued by the NHS regarding computer-generated prescriptions.[6] It is important that you are aware of your local practices regarding the number of repeat prescriptions allowed before a review of the patient or a review date. A medication review comprises appraisal of:

- the continued effectiveness and need for the drug;
- the appropriateness of the dose and presentation;
- the patient's understanding of the treatment;
- monitoring, tests, examinations, and follow-up;
- checks for side effects, drug interactions, and contraindications;
- any discontinuing item(s);
- appropriate frequency of requests;
- all prescriptions are for the same length of time;
- any OTC or home-made remedies taken are recorded.

📖 Over-the-counter (OTC) drugs, p. 422

1. Anon. (2003). Repeat dispensing products due to take off in Scotland. Prescribing and Medicines Management, 1 Jan/Feb, 2003.
2. 🖥 www.nhsemployers.org/publications (accessed 5 May 2010).
3. Medicines Management newsletter (2009). Guidance to prescribers on optimal duration of repeat prescriptions, Vol. 4, Issue 2. 🖥 http://www.sheffield.nhs.uk/professionals/resources/mmnewsletterjun09.pdf (accessed 1 September 2009).
4. Luker, K. and Austin, L. (1997). Nurse prescribing: study findings and GP's views. Prescriber, **8**, 31–4.
5. NHS Executive HQ (1997). Nurse prescribing guidance (April). NHS Executive, Leeds.
6. 🖥 http://www.connectingforhealth.nhs.uk/

Problems with repeat medication

The key potential problems with repeat medication are:
- unnecessary therapy;
- ineffective therapy;
- absent or inadequate routine monitoring;
- inappropriate choice of therapy type, dose, or dosing schedule;
- non-concordance with therapy;
- polypharmacy.

Good practice for repeat prescriptions systems[1]
- Written explanation of the process for repeat prescriptions for the patient or their carer.
- Designated personnel with responsibility to ensure the patient recall and regular medication review does take place.
- Agreed policy with the practice on the length of medication supply on a repeat prescription.
- Authorization check made every time a repeat prescription is signed.
- Practice staff to be given training on elements of good practice with regards to patient concordance.
- Records kept up to date.

📖 Seven principles of safe prescribing, p. 94.
📖 Suitability of formulation, p. 110.

1. Adapted from Keele University, Department of Medicines Management (2000). *Seizing the opportunities. Report of the Walsall GP/Practice Pharmacy project.* Cited in *Medicines and older people.* 🖥 http://www.wales.nhs.uk/sites3/Documents/439/NSF%20for%20Older%20People%20-%2 0Medicines%20and%20Older%20People.pdf

Medication reviews

Definition
A medication review is:
> *A structured critical examination of a patient's medication with the objective of reaching an agreement with the patient about treatment optimizing the impact of medicines, minimizing the number of medication-related problems and reducing waste.*[1]

Principles
All patients should have the chance to raise questions and highlight problems about their medicines. A medication review should improve or optimize impact of treatment for an individual patient. The review:
- should be undertaken in a systematic way;
- should be undertaken by a competent person;
- any changes resulting from the review should be agreed with the patient and documented in the patient's notes;
- the impact of any changes should be monitored.

Who can undertake a review?
- A doctor
- A practice or specialist nurse
- A pharmacist
- A suitably trained pharmacy support technician
- A qualified non-medical prescriber.

Which groups are at greatest risk of medication-related problems?
- Older people and those prescribed four or more medicines.
  - Polypharmacy is a risk factor for adverse drug reactions and for re-admissions of patients discharged from hospital. 📖 Prescribing for older people, p. 198.
- Those recently discharged from hospital.
  - Changes in medication after discharge may be intentional, but unintentional discrepancies in medication can occur. These include patients or the GP practice restarting medicines that were stopped in hospital, and duplication of treatment (e.g. a medicine being prescribed by both its generic and branded names).
- Older people in care homes.
  - A study of pharmacist-conducted medication reviews of all medicines showed that modifications to treatment were needed for half the medicines prescribed.[1,2] The most frequent recommendation (47%) was to stop medication, and in two-thirds of these cases there was no stated indication for the medicine being prescribed.[3–5] Longer-term follow-up showed that the number of medicines prescribed for older people can be reduced with no adverse impact on morbidity or mortality.[6]
- Patients with special psychiatric needs.

- Patients prescribed high-risk medication.
  - Those prescribed medications that require special monitoring (e.g. warfarin), with a wide range of side effects (e.g. NSAIDs) or with a narrow therapeutic range (e.g. digoxin).

It may also be necessary to review those who have been indicated as having medicines-related problems identified through routine monitoring or assessment.

1. Duggan, C., Feldman, R., Hough, J., and Bates, I. (1998). Reducing adverse prescribing discrepancies following hospital discharge. *International Journal of Pharmacy Practice*, **6**, 77–82.
2. Duffin, J., Norwood, J., and Blenkinsopp, A. (1998). An investigation into medication changes initiated in general practice after patients are discharged from hospital. *Pharmaceutical Journal*, **261**(Suppl.), R32.
3. Furniss, L., Craig, S.K.L., Scobie, S., Cooke, J., and Burns, A. (1998). Medication reviews in nursing homes: documenting and classifying the activities of a pharmacist. *Pharmaceutical Journal*, **261**, 320–3.
4. Furniss, L., Craig, S.K.L., and Burns, A. (1998). Medication use in nursing homes for elderly people. *International Journal of Geriatric Psychiatry*, **13**, 433–9.
5. Klepping, G. (2000). Medication review in elderly care homes. *Primary Care Pharmacy*, **1**, 105–8.
6. Furniss, L., Burns, A., Craig, S.K.L., Scobie, S., Cooke, J., and Faragher, B. (2000). Effects of a pharmacist's medication review in nursing homes: randomised controlled trial. *British Journal of Psychiatry*, **176**, 563–7.

Medication reviews for older people

Format of a detailed medication review

Reviews covering the following core areas may take place in the surgery, an older person's home, or a day-care facility (Box 8.1). They may involve the patient, family members, and/or carers, and should include an explanation of the review's purpose and reasons why it is important.

The review should include the following.

- A listing of all medicines being taken including:
  - prescribed medicines;
  - OTC products;
  - herbal medicines;
  - homeopathic remedies;
  - medicines shared with others;
  - home remedies;
  - supplements.
- Comparison of the list of medicines used with those prescribed.
- The patient/carer perceptions of the purpose of medicines taken, including any misconceptions (a Danish study[1] showed that 40% of older people did not know the purpose of their medication).
- The patient/carer perceptions of the frequency, amount and method of taking the medicines including any misconceptions.
- Use of 'prescribing appropriateness indicators',[2] e.g. the indication of the use of the drug in the BNF.
- Any side effects noted, including social side effects which restrict people's lives.
- Review of any monitoring tests, e.g. HbA1c for diabetes and INR for patients taking anticoagulants.
- 📖 Holistic assessment, p. 82

Types of questions which might be asked of a patient or carer during a medicines review[1]

- How long have you been taking/using this medicine/product?
- Is the medicine in its original container?
- Why do you take the medicine? What is its purpose?
- How often do you take it?
- Do you have a routine for taking it?
- Have you had any side effects from the medicine?
- Do you have any allergies to medicines?
- Do you buy or do you take any medicines which are not prescribed but have been bought from the chemist, shops, or supermarkets?
- Has anyone—a friend, neighbour, or family member—lent you or suggested that you should take some of their prescribed medicines, home remedies, or vitamin or herbal products?
- Do you take any other forms of medication?

Possible action following a review

- Patients/carers may need access to a prescriber or pharmacist to clear up any misconceptions.
- Provision of support items, e.g. reminder charts, multi-compartment aids, modified containers, large-print labels.[3]
- Examine current diagnosis/order investigations or additional monitoring and rationalize treatment according to clinical condition.

Box 8.1 Milestones for medicines management for older people[4]

Date	Action
2002	All people over 75 years should normally have their medication reviewed at least once a year and for those taking four or more medicines (polypharmacy) every 6 months. All hospitals to have a one-stop dispensing/dispensing for discharge scheme and, where appropriate, self-administration schemes for older people.
2004	Every PCT will have schemes in place to enable older people to get more help from their pharmacists.

---

1. Barat, I., Andreason, F., and Damsgaard, E.M. (2001). Drug therapy in the elderly. What doctors believe and patients actually do. *British Journal of Clinical Pharmacology*, **51**, 615–22.
2. Cantrill, J.A., Sibbald, C., and Buetow, S. (1998). Indicators of the appropriateness of long-term prescribing in general practice in the United Kingdom: consensus development, face and content validity, feasibility and reliability. *Quality in Health Care*, **7**, 130–5.
3. Raynor, D.K., Nicolson, M., Nunney, J., *et al.* (2000). The development and evaluation of an extended adherence support programme by community pharmacists for elderly patients at home. *International Journal of Pharmacy*, **8**, 157–64.
4. Department of Health (2001). *National Service Framework for Older People*. Department of Health, London.

Reflective practice

Why reflect?

Reflection in action and on action is now recognized as an essential tool to support safe and effective care delivery for all aspects of health care.[1] Reflective practice is essential in supporting the analytical rationale for safe, effective, and appropriate prescribing.[2] Reflection links prescribing to continual professional development and to lifelong learning.

Reflection can be considered as a process critical to improving patient care, and the process of critical reflection can be used to move practice forward. Written reflections can form part of a portfolio of prescribing practice which the prescriber may be called upon to provide to their professional body as evidence of continuing professional development and of safe and up-to-date practice. Reflection on prescribing should be considered an essential part of structured clinical supervision.

Models of reflection

There are several different models for reflection.[3] Choice of model of reflection depends on the individual prescriber's experience. The key models are listed below. It is essential that the reflector chooses a model which will best suit both their individual style and the subject matter on which they are reflecting. Some reflectors choose not to apply a model but prefer to reflect 'freestyle'.

Examples

- The What? model of structured reflection[4]
- Kolb's model[5]
- The Gibbs Reflective Cycle (Fig. 8.1):[6]
  - description (what happened?)
  - feelings (what was I thinking and feeling?)
  - evaluation (what was good about the experience?)
  - analysis (what sense can I make of the experience?)
  - conclusion (what else could I have done?)
  - action plan (what would I do if it happened again?).

Reflecting on individual prescribing practice

PACT (prescribing analysis and cost) data,[7] as issued by the Prescription Services, NHS Business Services Authority (formerly the Prescription Pricing Authority) can be useful for reflecting on group and individual prescribing practice. Reflective analysis of prescribing practice can be brought to clinical supervision and key reflective questions can be applied.

Audit in organizations in services other than primary care is done through a variety of instruments, and more detail can be found in Chapter 14.

📖 Approaches to audit, p. 434.

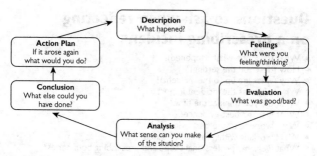

Fig. 8.1 The Gibbs Reflective Cycle. Adapted from Gibbs.[6]

Further reading

Health Professions Council (2008). *Standards of conduct, performance and ethics.* HPC, London.

Nursing and Midwifery Council (2006). *Standards of proficiency for nurse and midwife prescribers.* NMC, London.

Nursing and Midwifery Council (2008). *Standards of conduct, performance and ethics for nurses and midwives.* NMC, London.

1. Schon, C. (1987). *Educating the reflective practitioners: how professionals think in action.* Temple Smith, London.

2. National Prescribing Centre (1999). Signposts for prescribing nurses: general principles of good prescribing. *Prescribing Nurse Bulletin,* **1**(10).

3. Atkins, S. and Murphy, K. (1993). Reflection: a review of the literature. *Journal of Advanced Nursing,* **18**, 1188–92.

4. Driscoll, J. (2000). *Practising clinical supervision: a reflective approach.* Ballière Tindall, London.

5. Kolb, D. (1984). *Experiential learning: experience as a source of learning and development.* Prentice Hall, Englewood Cliffs, NJ.

6. Gibbs, G. (1988). *Learning by doing: a guide to teaching and learning methods.* Oxford Polytechnic, Oxford.

7. *British National Formulary* (latest edn) British Medical Association and the Royal Pharmaceutical Society for Great Britain, London.

Questions to ask when reflecting on a prescribing incident

- What (describe what happened)?
- How (describe the setting)?
- Why (what led up to the incident)?
- Why (why was the incident important)?
- What did you think at the time?
- What was the best evidence?
- Was I working to the best evidence?
- Was I working within my competence?
- What were my professional scope and prescribing boundaries?
- Was I working within my contractual obligations?
- Was I working within my professional code of conduct?
- To whom was I accountable?
- What were my responsibilities?
- What did I think after the incident?
- How did I feel during and after the incident?
- What was good about the incident?
- What was bad about the incident?
- How could the incident have occurred differently?
- What knowledge and skills did I use during the incident?
- What else could I have done?
- What more did I need to know?
- How could I have found the answers?
- What could I have done differently at the time?
- What would I do differently next time?
- Was anybody harmed or treated badly as a result of this incident?
- If harm occurred, what do I now need to do about it?
- Having reflected on the above, what action do I now need to take?
- How will my reflection affect my actions next time?
- Do I have recommendations for future changes to practice?

Remember when reflecting always to reflect on your practice in light of the latest and best evidence.

Prescribing and the law

Categories of the legal system
- Criminal law—this relates to crimes against the state. Criminal law can be broken if a patient is deliberately harmed, or if his/her property is stolen.
- Civil law —this relates to legal proceedings that fall outside criminal law. Examples of civil law include:
  - tort (delict in Scotland) (e.g. damage that occurs as a result of negligence);
  - breach of contract.

Negligence
Practical examples of negligence:
- giving the wrong drug to a patient;
- not doing something for a patient to alleviate suffering.

To avoid negligence when prescribing:
- check the drug;
- check the patient;
- question orders;
- follow principles of prescribing;
- keep up to date;
- seek supervision.

To succeed in a claim for negligence
The patient must demonstrate that:
- the nurse owed them a duty of care;
- there was a breach of the duty of care;
- harm occurred as a result of that breach.

The standard of proof is on the 'balance of probabilities' rather than 'beyond reasonable doubt'.

Vicarious liability
An employer is vicariously liable for his/her employee's negligent acts or omissions in the course of employment, whether authorized or not, unless the employer can show that the employee was undertaking 'a frolic of his own'[1] rather than the employer's business. The individual prescriber still carries responsibility and, as such, is accountable for his/her actions.[2]

Prescribers need to ensure that the prescribing role is clearly stated in their job description.

Competent standard of care
According to the Bolam principle,[3] the nurse/health professional is required to act within his/her competency at all times and to exercise 'the ordinary skill of an ordinary "man" exercising that particular art', i.e. to perform reasonably as practitioners trained to the same standard within the same or similar professions, within a recognized standard of competency.

Prescribing practice must be in accordance with a responsible body of opinion, even if the practice of other prescribers differs. This also means that if prescriber actions are based on best and widely accepted medical evidence and they can justify their actions in the light of this evidence, they can make a prescribing decision that might differ from that of other prescribers. A non-medical prescriber must have a strong rationale for doing so and is always fully accountable for his/her actions.

Consent

To be valid, consent must be informed. Treating a patient without consent may constitute an assault and subject the patient to damages for trespass to the person. In the case of children, the court can overrule the wishes of the parent.[7]

Consent prescribing and the implications of parental responsibility

Consent for treatment of a child can be given by a person with parental responsibility for that child.

Definition

Parental responsibility covers all the rights, duties, and powers a parent has over a child and includes the right to consent to treatment. Rights include the right to consent to treatment up until the child's 18th birthday.

Parental responsibility may be conferred automatically, i.e. a mother has this right conferred by law (Children Act 1989) on the birth of her child, or it may be acquired by operation of the law, e.g. a person who is appointed as the child's guardian or a local authority by obtaining a care order (Children Act 1989).[5]

Children under 16

Children under the age of 16 can give consent if it can be proved that they have a competent level of understanding. In Scotland, this is laid down in statute law.[6] In England and Wales, it is expressed in the Fraser ruling.[7] The age of consent for medical treatment in England and Wales is 16.[7]

📖 Legal differences between prescribing, administering, and dispensing, p. 18.
📖 Safe prescribing, p. 88.
📖 Prescribing for children, p. 212.

1. 🖳 http://www.jstor.org/pss/1112332 (accessed 2 February 2010).
2. Nursing and Midwifery Council. (2008). *Standards of conduct, performance and ethics for nurses and midwives*. NMC, London.
3. *Bolam v Friern* HMC [1957] 1 WLR 582. Quoted in Dimond, B. (2002). *Legal aspects of nursing* (3rd edn). Prentice-Hall, London.
4. *Family Law Reform Act* 1969, section 8(1). TSO, London.
5. *Children Act* 1989. TSO, London.
6. *Age of Legal Capacity (Scotland) Act* 1991, section 2(4). 🖳 www.opsi.gov.uk/ACTS/acts1991.
7. Fraser LJ in *Gillick v West Norfolk and Wisbech Area Health Authority* and another [1985] 3 All ER 402 at 413.

Mental Capacity Act

The Mental Capacity Act (2005)[1] covers England and Wales and came into force in 2007. It is underpinned by a set of five key principles.

- A presumption of capacity:
  - this means that every adult has the right to make his/her own decisions and must be assumed to have capacity to do so unless it is proved otherwise.
- The right for individuals to be supported to make their own decisions:
  - people must be given all appropriate help before anyone concludes that they cannot make their own decisions.
- Individuals must retain the right to make what might be seen as eccentric or unwise decisions.
- Best interests:
  - anything done for or on behalf of people without capacity must be in their best interests.
- Least restrictive intervention:
  - anything done for or on behalf of people without capacity should be the least restrictive of their basic rights and freedoms.

Lacking capacity

The last two points of the Mental Capacity Act refers to those who lack capacity. For the purpose of the Act this refers to a person who:

lacks capacity to make a particular decision or take a particular action for themselves at the time the decision or action needs to be taken.[2]

This statement acknowledges that a lack of capacity may not be permanent, and that an ability to make minor decisions such as 'what to eat or wear'[2] need not imply an ability to make complex decisions regarding financial matters. Further, it accepts that people are individuals and that their capacity must be judged on their ability rather than any diagnosis or assumption.

Who will be legally required to act in accordance with this Act?

- An attorney under a Lasting Power of Attorney (LPA).
- A deputy appointed by the new Court of Protection.
- A person acting as an Independent Mental Capacity Advocate.
- A person carrying out research approved in accordance with the Act.
- A person acting in a professional capacity for/in relation to a person who lacks capacity or being paid for acts for/in relation to a person who lacks capacity.

This will include a variety of health and social care staff acting in their professional capacity, for example:

- doctors;
- dentists;
- nurses;

- therapists;
- radiologists;
- paramedics and ambulance crews;
- housing workers;
- social workers;
- care managers.

Differences in the law in Scotland and Northern Ireland

Adults with Incapacity (Scotland) Act 2000[3]

This Act sets out in law a range of options to help people aged 16 or over who lack the capacity to make some or all decisions for themselves and allows others to make decisions on their behalf. In addition the Act enables those who fear a diminution in their capacity to make arrangements for specific others to make decisions and manage their affairs.

The Office of the Public Guardian in Scotland provides advice and guidance to the general public and is responsible for supervising the people appointed under the Act.

Northern Ireland

At the time of going to press there is no equivalent law in Northern Ireland, and the Bamford Review of Mental Health and Learning Disability is considering the effect of the current law on people with mental health needs or a learning disability.[4]

NMC guidance on the Mental Health Act

The NMC has worked with the Care Services Improvement Partnership to produce two publications:

- Mental Health: New Ways of Working for Everyone.
- New Ways of Working with You.

These give information for users and carers and can be downloaded from the website of the National Institute for Mental Health in England (NIMHE).[5]

1. ⊞ http://www.mentalhealth.org.uk/information/mental-health-a-z/mental-capacity/mental-capacity-act-2005/#Safeguards (accessed 2 February 2010).
2. ⊞ http://www.rmhldni.gov.uk/ (accessed 2 February 2010).
3. ⊞ http://www.nmc-uk.org/Nurses-and-midwives/safeguarding/Scotland (accessed 25 November 2010).
4. ⊞ http://www.dca.gov.uk/menincap/legis.htm (accessed 2 February 2010).
5. ⊞ http://www.dh.gov.uk/en/publicationsandstatistics/publications (accessed 25 November 2010).

Ethics

Health-care ethics are rooted in moral philosophy which tries to formulate sound arguments justifying our decisions and practices.

What is philosophy?

[Philosophy] is something… intermediate between theology and science. Like theology it consists of speculation on matters, as to which definite knowledge has so far been unascertainable, but like science it appeals to human reason, rather than to (for example) divine authority…Between theology and science is a No Man's Land…this No Man's Land is Philosophy.[1]

Some of the vocabulary of philosophy

Epistemology

The concept of what constitutes knowledge. Asking questions such as:
- How can we differentiate knowledge from belief?
- Can sense or reason or intuition provide knowledge?
- Can we distinguish different types of knowledge, e.g. practical, theoretical, moral aesthetic etc?

Ontology

Considers questions such as:
- Does the world exist independent of human thought?
- Is existence inseparable from thought?
- What is it to be a person?
- Does a person have free will?
- What is the nature of time?

Moral reasoning

Justifies decisions and practice on the following grounds.
- Deontology:
  - justification on the grounds of a moral duty to do good. (*deon* is Greek for duty);
  - maintains that the concept of obligation or a right to something is independent of the concept of good (i.e. some actions are right because they are intrinsically right);
  - Immanuel Kant (1734–1804) was a proponent of deontology;
  - the notions of beneficence and non-maleficence are deontological theories (see NMC code of conduct).
- Consequentialism:
  - judgement is based on the amount of good generated by an action;
  - utilitarianism, founded by Hume, Bentham, and Mill in the 18th century, is the most prominent consequentialist theory. It maintains that the moral rightness of an action is determined by its good consequences, where goods might be the amount of pleasure, health, friendship, or knowledge the action generates (see Table 8.1).

1. Russell, B. (1946). *History of Western Philosophy*. Allen and Unwin, London.

Table 8.1 Examples of theoretical deontological and consequentialist decisions

(Remember that our practice is governed by both ethical and legal decisions.)

Moral problem	Deontological argument (judged on duty)	Consequentialist argument (judged on outcome)
Telling the truth	Have a duty always to tell the truth regardless of the outcome; therefore it is morally right to tell the truth.	It depends on the outcome of truth telling, it may cause harm and if it does it would be morally wrong.
Euthanasia	Life is sacred and therefore it is morally wrong to take it.	If it stops pain and suffering it would be a morally right act.
Informed consent	This is morally right as it respects autonomy.	It could be morally wrong, as it might frighten the patient and stop them having a life saving procedure.
Abortion	Life is sacred and to take it is morally wrong.	If it prevents suffering, it is morally right.

Four principles which supply a framework for biomedical ethics

Autonomy

From the Greek *autos* (self) and *nomos* (rule or govern), it now encompasses such meanings as: self-governance, liberty, rights, privacy, and individual choice. Respect for autonomy is regarded as a duty and therefore is justified under the theory of deontology.

An autonomous act has to have intentionality. It has to be done with understanding of the issues. and without influences that control or determine the action.[1]

Non-maleficence

It is morally wrong to inflict evil or harm. Harm can be an injury that is physical, emotional, or financial.

Beneficence

This is the capacity of promoting and achieving good. It can be applied to individuals or to society as a whole.

Justice

This encompasses notions of fairness and equity. It requires a system of universal rules and principles to ensure that verifiable and transparent decisions are made. It also includes concepts of respect for autonomy, objectivity, and impartiality.

Four additional independent principles

These are justified on the basis of the preceding four principles:
• promise keeping;
• truthfulness;
• privacy;
• confidentiality.

Consent (Table 8.2)

There are two distinct meanings of consent within the field of health care.
• An autonomous action by the patient that authorizes the professional to involve the patient in research or to initiate a medical plan or intervention.
• Within the term of social rules of consent, it is used within institutions where it is legally necessary to obtain valid consent before proceeding with any therapeutic procedures or research.

Elements of informed consent
• Full disclosure.
• Understanding— the individual patient's needs, knowledge of the purpose and nature of the intervention, any likely effects or risks, and the likelihood of success and any alternatives.
• Voluntariness.
• Competence.
• Consent.

NB: You can treat without consent in an emergency where the patient is unconscious and/or the treatment cannot be safely delayed.

Table 8.2 Issues regarding consent

Issue	Advice	
When the practitioner has the right to treat	Adults with a lack of capacity to decide for themselves	
	Patients who are unable to consent or refuse medical treatment	
	People with long-term mental disability or temporary lack of capacity	
	Those who pass the best interest test	
Best interest test	Is it a case of necessity to save a life?	
	Will the action ensure an improvement in the patient's condition?	
	Will the action prevent deterioration in the patient's condition?	
	In many cases it is not only lawful to treat but it is a doctor's duty to do so.	
	See NMC code of conduct[2]	
Who can consent if the patient is unable to do so?	Relatives?	No (consult only to ascertain if there is a living will)
	Doctor?	Yes if the best interest test is passed
	Court of law? No	
A person's competency to consent	Needs to be comprehending and retaining information	
	Needs to believe the information	
	Needs to be able to weigh up the information	
Overriding refusal for consent.	Lack of capacity—non-competence or undue influence	
	Change in circumstances at the time consent was given or withheld	

For more advice regarding consent see NMC Code of Conduct, part 3, p. 5.[2]

1. Department of Health (2001). *Twelve key points on consent: the law in England*. Department of Health, London.
2. Nursing and Midwifery Council (2008). *The NMC code of professional conduct: standards of conduct, performance and ethics*. NMC, London.

Rights

What is a right?
- An implied permission to follow a course of action.
- Restriction of what others may do.
- Creation of obligations to observe the right.

How do we enforce a right?
- Justified coercion.
- Resistance.
- Compensation.
- Punishment.

What is a natural right?
- An obligation that is held by all (universal), e.g. the right to life.
- An obligation that is grounded in the nature of being a person, e.g. the right to respect of human dignity.

What is a negative right?
- The right to prohibit another from interference in your life, e.g. the right not to violated by theft or fraud.
- It can be respected by doing nothing at all.

Ethical, moral, and clinical decisions are complex. Using a 'decision tree' (Fig. 8.2) can be helpful.

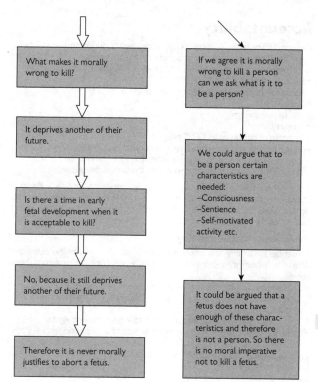

Fig. 8.2 Example of a decision tree.

Accountability

Accountability is the professionally recognized term for responsibility for something to someone. All practioners are personally accountable for their practice regardless of whether they are following the directions or advice of others.[1]

Prescribers are accountable for all aspects of:

- assessment;
- decision-making;
- prescribing;
- recommendation of an OTC product;
- ensuring that the prescribed/recommended item is applied or administered as directed by the patient, his/her carers, the nurse him/herself, or any other person to whom the task is delegated.

Since accountability is an integral part of professional practice, the prescriber has to be accountable, i.e. be able to give an explanation of actions or omissions, to him/herself, to the profession through the NMC, to the patient, and to society as a whole.

Professional accountability

Prescribers are fully accountable for their actions and for the actions of others to whom they delegate. As such the prescriber must satisfy themselves:

- that the person to whom they delegate can carry out instructions;
- that the outcome of the task that has been delegated meets the required standards;
- that they supervise and support those to whom they delegate.[2]

The NMC advice sheet outlining the standards for professional accountability can be found at: 🖳 http://www.nmc-uk.org/aArticle.aspx?ArticleID=3056 (accessed 16 October 2009).
📖 Responsibility, p. 92

NMC standards of proficiency

The NMC has standards of proficiency for nurse and midwife prescribers (2006)[3] and standards for the administration of medicines (2008).[4] These standards can be extrapolated to other registered health professionals.

Under the NMC 2006 standards the prescriber is accountable for the delegation of the dispensing, supply, or administration of medicines, and must assure themselves that the person to whom they have delegated the above is competent to do so. According to the NMC (2008, section 4, p. 4)[4] any registrant when administering medicines:

- *must be certain of the identity of the patient to whom the medicine is to be administered;*
- *must check that the patient is not allergic to the medicine before administering it;*
- *must know the therapeutic uses of the medicine to be administered and its normal dosage, side effects, precautions, and contraindications;*
- *must be aware of the patient's plan of care (care plan/pathway);*
- *must check that the prescription or the label on medicine dispensed is clearly written and unambiguous;*

- *must check the expiry date (where it exists) of the medicine to be administered;*
- *must have considered the dosage and patient's weight where appropriate;*
- *must have considered the method of administration, route, and timing;*
- *must administer or withhold in the context of the patient's condition (e.g. digoxin should not usually be given if pulse below 60) and coexisting therapies (e.g. physiotherapy);*
- *must contact the prescriber or another authorized prescriber without delay if contraindications to the prescribed medicine are discovered:*
  - *where the patient develops a reaction to the medicine;*
  - *where assessment of the patient indicates that the medicine is no longer suitable.*
- *must make a clear, accurate, and immediate record of all medicine administered, intentionally withheld, or refused by the patient, ensuring the signature is clear and legible.*

NB: it is also your responsibility to ensure that a record(s) is made when delegating the task of administering medicine.

Further, if a nurse fails to follow these standards, it is possible that the NMC will consider disciplinary action under its code of conduct (NMC 2008, Section 3, p. 47):[4]

> *When considering allegations of misconduct arising from errors in the administration of medicines, the NMC takes great care to distinguish between those cases where the error was the result of reckless or incompetent practice and/or was concealed, and those that resulted from other causes, such as serious pressure of work, and where there was immediate, honest disclosure in the patient's interest. The NMC recognises the prerogative of managers to take local disciplinary action where it is considered to be necessary but urges that they also consider each incident in its particular context and similarly discriminate between the two categories described above.*

1. NMC (2008). *Standards of conduct, performance and ethics for nurses and midwives.* NMC, London.
2. NMC (2008) Accountability advice sheet. ▣ http://www.nmc-uk.org/
aArticle.aspx?ArticleID=3056 (accessed 16 October 2009).
3. NMC (2006). *Standards of proficiency for nurse and midwife prescribers.* NMC, London.
4. NMC (2008). *Standards for medicines management.* NMC, London.

Indemnity

Indemnity is the legal term for protection. Prescribers may be shielded from the consequences of a court case regarding actions or omissions if indemnity for those actions and omissions exist.

Liability

Liability is the legal term for responsibility and is used to identify who was responsible for any harm which occurs as a result of clinical practice.

Criminal liability

- The Medicines Act 1968 describes exactly the permitted actions that can be taken by identified clinicians when prescribing.
- The Act also sets out penalties for any breaches of the strict wording of the legislation.
- Any such breach is a criminal offence.

Civil liability

- If a patient is harmed by a medication error, they may sue for negligence and ask a court to compensate them for the harm.
- The court will decide who is responsible by asking:
  - *Was there a duty of care?* Yes, if a nurse prescribes or administers a medication to a patient.
  - *Was the standard of care the same as a reasonable nurse would have provided?* An expert witness will be called to see if the standard of care was sufficient.
  - *Was the harm a direct result of the failure in delivery of a sufficient standard of care?* This is the most difficult part for the patient to prove as they must demonstrate that the injury was as a direct result of the failure in the standard of care and was not caused by the underlying condition being treated.

Protection for prescribers regarding accountability, responsibility, and liability

Vicarious liability

Vicarious liability may be explained as legal protection provided to employed staff working within agreed protocols or established and agreed methods by their employer, who is insured to cover claims.

The prescriber is protected from being sued for harming a patient because the law requires the employer to take legal responsibility for any acts or omissions on the part of the employee. The self-employed need to obtain personal insurance cover.

If you are working for a different practice, perhaps as part of an influenza immunization campaign, you need to check that you are still covered and you have a responsibility to inform your patients if you do not have indemnity insurance.

See also NMC code of conduct (2008): http://www.nmc-uk.org/aArticle.aspx?ArticleID=3056 (accessed 16.October 2009).

Professional indemnity
- If a prescriber takes action outside agreed protocols or procedures, the employer may argue that vicarious liability does not apply.
- The prescriber will require professional indemnity insurance cover which will provide legal advice, representation, and, if appropriate, compensation.
- The main professional organizations (RCN, RMN, Unison, CDNA, and CPHVA), for example, provide indemnity as part of their membership fee. (The RCN indemnifies current members for up to £3 million for each claim.)

Patient-group directions (PGDs)

History
Following questioning of the legality of group protocol practice,[1] a recommendation was made that protocols should offer practitioners the minimum of discretion and, in order to remain within the law, be patient specific. The government set out guidelines for the development of these protocols, to be called patient-group directions (PGDs).[2] The legal concerns were addressed by the Department of Health in a statutory instrument.[3]

Definition
Written instructions for the supply and administration of a named medicine to groups of individuals who may not be individually identified prior to presentation for treatment.

Further reading
Department of Health (2006). Medicines matters: a guide to the mechanisms for the prescribing, supply and administration of medicines. ☑ http://www.dh.gov.uk/en/Publicationsandstatistics/Publications/PublicationsPolicyAndGuidance/DH064325. (accessed 15 June 2009).

Griffith, R. (2005). A nurse prescriber's guide to the legal implications of parental responsibility. Nurse Prescribing, **3**(3).

Nursing and Midwifery Council (2004). *Code of professional conduct*. TSO, London

Nursing and Midwifery Council (2002). *Guidelines for the administration of medicines*. NMC, London.

Russell, B. (1939). *A History of Western Philosophy*. Allen and Unwin, London.

1. Department of Health (1998). *Report on the supply and administration of medicines under group protocols (Crown Part 1)*. TSO, London.
2. Department of Health (2000). *Patient group directions (England only)*. Health Service Circular HSC2000/026 (9 August 2000). Department of Health, Leeds.
3. Department of Health (2001). *Twelve key points on consent: the law and England*. ☑ www.doh.gov.uk/consent (accessed 3 May 2005).

Data Protection Act

Purpose

The purpose of the Data Protection Act 1998[1] is to ensure fair and lawful access to and processing of data. Personal data are both electronically and manually stored data which, in the case of prescribing, relate to the individual (patient or client).

Eight principles have been put into place by the Act to ensure that information is handled properly.

Eight principles

The eight principles of the Act state that data must be:

- fairly and lawfully processed;
- processed for limited purposes;
- adequate, relevant, and not excessive;
- accurate;
- not kept for longer than is necessary;
- processed in line with your rights;
- secure;
- not transferred to countries without adequate protection.

The Act covers personal data which are held in both electronic format and manually if the data are held within a structured filing system which is relevant to the subject (patient/client).

The Department of Health recommends that GP records are kept for a minimum of 10 years and hospital records are kept for a minimum of 8 years following the end of any treatment, or the patient's death if he/she died whilst receiving treatment. At the end of that specified time, the health records would remain at the NHS trust or, in the case of GP health records, transferred to the relevant primary care trust/health authority who will then make a decision as to whether to retain or destroy the records.[2,3]

If a patient moves abroad, they can make a request for their medical records under the Data Protection Act. Those with proof of parental responsibility can request to access children's medical records. The legal age to give consent to medical treatment is 16. However, if a child is deemed as having the capacity to make an informed decision, consent must first be obtained from that child before confidential information is shared.

📖 Record keeping, p. 192.

1. *Data Protection Act* 1998. TSO, London.
2. Department of Health (2006). *Records management: NHS code of practice*. Department of Health, London.
3. *The Human Rights Act* 1998. TSO, London.

Access to medical records

Patients have the right to obtain copies of their medical records under the Data Protection Act 1998.[1] The records should be presented to the patient in a format that they will understand.

Legal exceptions to the right to access records
Exceptions include:
- where health professionals believe that the ability to access their records may seriously harm the patient or another person;
- information regarding other people—this may be removed from the records;
- access to records on behalf of a third party—this requires the subject's consent or power of attorney.

Records can be requested informally or formally. Formal application must be in writing and entitles applicants to a response within no more than 40 days after the application has been made. The applicant will need to provide signed proof of identity. There is usually a charge, ranging between £10 and £50, when requesting access to records.

If access to medical records is refused, the applicant can appeal through the Information Commissioner's office (UK tel. 01625 545745). Complaints about the service can be made through the health service ombudsman (www.ombudsman.org.uk).

Human Rights Act 1998
The rights of the individual are protected under the Human Rights Act 1998,[2] and they can apply to access to information, confidentiality, and the protection of family and private life. Prescribers have a duty of care to ensure that any records which they maintain with regard to individual patients are confidential.[3] On rare occasions the prescriber may be called upon by the courts to disclose information which may be strongly in the interest of the public or which may support the proceedings of the prescriber's regulatory body or with the patient's specific consent for teaching or research purposes.

📖 Prescribing and the law, p. 134.

Further reading

BBC Action Network (2005). How to access your medical records. ⌨ http://www.bbc.co.uk/dna/actionnetwork/A1181657.

Department of Health (2003). *Guidance for access to health records requests under the Data Protection Act 1998.* Department of Health, London.

Mullan, K. (2003). Supplementary prescribing and access to medical records. 2: Access rights of patients and others. *Pharmaceutical Journal*, **271**, 24–6.

1. *Data Protection Act* 1998. TSO, London.
2. ⌨ www.legislation.gov.uk/ukpga/1998/42/contents (accessed 26.11.2010).
3. NMC (2008). *Standards of conduct, performance and ethics for nurses and midwives.* NMC, London.

Understanding research papers

Questions to ask when considering the evidence
- How many in subjects are in the trial?
- What are you measuring?
- What measurement tools are being used?
- Is the study quantitative?
- Is the study qualitative?
- Is it a combination of both?
- How are data analysed?

Why do we need evidence?
- Governance and quality assurance.
- Complex treatment regimens.
- To stop geographical variations in treatment.
- Challenge the established versus effective.
- Expert patients.
- Critical appraisal.
- Resource allocation.

📖 What is evidence-based prescribing (EBP)? p. 442.

Weighing up the evidence/points to consider
- Who told me about it?
- Cost versus risk benefit?

Questions to ask when evaluating the evidence
- Was it a qualitative or quantitative piece of research?
- What was the research question?
- Who sponsored the trial?
- What kind if trial was it—randomized/double blind?
- How does the drug in question/intervention compare with other agents/interventions?
- How many participants were there?
- Was the trial population reflective of future potential user population?
- Is the methodology clear and logical?
- Did the results produce relevant outcome measurements?
- Did the researchers produce justifiable interpretation of results? If it was a drug trial was there an intention-to-treat analysis?
- Were the conclusions valid in that they reflected the results?
- Was the trial outcome relevant to the age group in the trial?
- How many participants were there in trials before the product was marketed?
- Are there reports of post-marketing surveillance?

Desirable attributes for research trials
- They should be valid.
- Suitable research methods should be employed.
- They should be cost effective.
- They should be reproducible and reliable.

- They should represent the best interests of both patient and professionals.
- They should be clinically applicable.
- They should be clinically flexible.
- They should be clear.
- They should be well documented.
- There should be a clear schedule for review.
- Recommendations for sensible audit and/or monitoring should be in place.

Best evidence for National Service Frameworks (NSFs)

Gold standard—randomized control trials (RCTs) and systematic reviews.

Typology of supporting evidence for evidence-based practice (EBP) as used by NSFs

- A1: systematic reviews which contain at least one RCT (e.g. systematic reviews from Cochrane or Centre for Reviews and Dissemination).
- A2: other systematic and high-quality reviews which synthesize
- references (e.g. meta-analysis).
- B1: individualized RCTs.
- B2: individual non-randomized experimental/interventional studies.
- B3: individual well-designed non-experimental studies which are controlled statistically, if appropriate. Includes studies using case control, longitudinal, cohort, matched pairs, or cross-sectional random sample methodologies, well-designed qualitative studies, and well-designed analytical studies including secondary analysis.
- C1: descriptive and other research or evaluation not in B.
- C2: case studies and examples of good practice.
- D: summary review articles and discussions of relevant literature and conference proceedings not otherwise classified.

Evidence from expert opinion

- P: professional opinion based on clinical evidence or reports of committees.
- U: user opinion.
- C: carer opinion.

Clinical trials

- In phase I trials, researchers test an experimental drug or treatment in a small group of people (20–80) for the first time to evaluate its safety, determine a safe dosage range, and identify side effects.
- In phase II trials, the experimental study drug or treatment is given to a larger group of people (100–300) to see if it is effective and to further evaluate its safety.
- In phase III trials, the experimental study drug or treatment is given to large groups of people (1000–3000) to confirm its effectiveness, monitor side effects, compare it with commonly used treatments, and collect information that will allow it to be used safely.
- In phase IV trials, post-marketing studies delineate additional information including the drug's risks, benefits, and optimal use.

Research design terms are explained in Table 8.3.

Some evidence-based guidelines
- NICE (National Institute for Health and Clinical Excellence)
- SIGN (Scottish Intercollegiate Guidelines Network)
- BHS (British Hypertension Society)
- BDS (British Diabetes Society).

Why use guidelines?
- Avoids prescribing from habit
- Guides new staff
- Improves patient confidence
- United front
- Time saving
- Governance
- Standardized practice
- New therapies
- Educational tools
- Familiarity with best practice.

Points to consider when implementing guidelines
- Workload and practice implications?
- Resources?
- The need to improve skill?
- Implications for patient?
- Computer support?
- Dissemination?
- Local policy/formularies and protocols.

Table 8.3 Explanation of research design terms

Research term	Explanation	Flaws in study design
RCT	Study design where treatment, interventions, or enrolment into different study groups are assigned by random allocation If the sample size is large enough, this design avoids bias and confounding variables	No power calculation for group sizes lower than 20 No blinding of outcome measurement
Systematic review	An approach based on a strategy, which has clear inclusion and exclusion criteria. Aims to detect biases, random errors, unsupported claims in the methodology, interpretation of results, and content	No explicit assessment of validity of included study Studies combined inappropriately
Descriptive study	Describes the distribution of variables within a group	Can be subjective
Experimental study	Allocation or assignment is under the control of the investigator	Unblinded
Intervention study	Observation of the effect of an intervention	Unblinded
Case study	Focuses on the situation, dynamics, and complexity of a single case, or compares a small number of cases	Inclusion/exclusion criteria need to be stated, justified, and adhered to
Qualitative study	Research which is carried out in the real world and is analysed in non-statistical ways	Analysis and interpretation procedures are often unclear Interpretations not explicitly based on data

Further reading

Bero, L., Grilli, R., Grimshaw, J.M., *et al.* (1998). Getting research findings into practice: closing the gap between research and practice: an overview of systematic reviews of interventions to promote the implementation of research findings. *British Medical Journal*, **317**, 465–8.

Crombie, I.K. (1996). *The pocket guide to critical appraisal*. BMJ Books, London.

Greenhalgh, T. (1997). Assessing the methodological qualities of published papers. *British Medical Journal*, **315**, 305–8.

Grol, R., Dalhuijsen, J., Thomas, S., Veld, C., Rutten, G., and Mokkink, H. (1998). Attributes of clinical guidelines that influence the use of guidelines in general practice. *British Medical Journal*, **317**, 858–61.

Walsh, K. and Ham, C. (1997). *Acting on the evidence: progress in the NHS*. NHS Confederation www.jr2.ox.ac.uk/bandolier.

Reviewing guidelines

Oxman *et al.* (2006)[1] found at least 24 different instruments available for assessing the quality of clinical practice guidelines. They made the following suggestions.
- The World Health Organization (WHO) should develop processes to ensure that routine internal and external reviews of guidelines are undertaken.
- Use of a checklist, such as the AGREE instrument.[2]
- Checklists require adaptation and testing to ensure suitability for the broad range of recommendations that WHO produces for:
  - public health;
  - health policy.
- Any checklist includes questions about equity and other items that are particularly important for WHO guidelines.
- Regular monitoring of guidelines should be carried out by reviewers familiar with the topic (e.g. Cochrane review groups).
- Independent periodic review of guidelines by experts not involved in their development.
- Members of review panels should rotate, serving for predetermined fixed periods.
- Recommendations may need to be specifically adapted to particular settings:
  - implemented only in specific settings;
  - their impact assessed only in specific settings.

Evaluating evidence

Systematic reviews of evidence are aimed at showing:
- the relationship of an intervention to particular outcomes;
- the explicit process for translating the evidence provided into recommendations.

Evidence can include:
- information that is appropriate for answering questions about an the effectiveness of an intervention;
- the generalizability and applicability of effectiveness data (i.e. the extent to which available effectiveness data are thought to apply to additional populations and settings);
- other effects of the intervention (i.e. side effects):
  - important outcomes of the intervention not already included in the assessment of effectiveness;
  - harms or benefits, intended or unintended;
  - health or non-health outcomes.
- the economic impact of the intervention;
- barriers that have been observed when implementing interventions.

Briss et al.[3] suggested the following procedure for obtaining and evaluating evidence and translating that evidence into recommendations:
- form a multidisciplinary development teams (e.g. a task force);
- develop a conceptual approach to organizing, grouping, and selecting the interventions;
- select the interventions to be evaluated;
- search for and retrieve evidence (e.g. systematic review);
- assess the quality and summarize the body of evidence of effectiveness;
- translate evidence of effectiveness into recommendations;
- consider evidence other than effectiveness;
- identify and summarize research gaps and withheld data.

1. Oxman, A.D., Schünemann, H.J., and Fretheim, A. (2006). Improving the use of research evidence in guideline development. 16: Evaluation. *Health Research Policy and Systems*, **4**(28).
2. AGREE Collaboration (2003). Development and validation of an international appraisal instrument for assessing the quality of clinical practice guidelines: the AGREE project. *Quality and Safety in Health Care*, **12**, 18–23
3. Briss, P.A., Zaza, S., Pappaioanou, M., et al. (2000). Developing an evidence based guide to community preventive services—methods. *Am J Prev Med* **18**(15).

Reviewing the data

One approach to review is the following seven-step analysis procedure which is synthesized[1] from those outlined by Clancy,[2] Egger et al.,[3] and Greenhalgh et al.[4]

Step 1. The research question
Focus the research through the use of a specific research question(s).

Step 2. Eligibility criteria
Eligibility, quality criteria and data retrieval forms can be based on information from ▣ http://www.policyhub.gov.uk. These include:
• the studies population;
• the locality of the research.

NB: Care needs to be taken when evaluating research from different cultures. Pang et al.[5] have shown that cultural influences produce changes in role interpretation and practice.

Step 3. Location of studies
Studies should include details of:
• the databases searched;
• the time frame and search terms used.

Step 4. Select studies
Select literature published within the time frame and meeting the inclusion criteria.

Step 5. Assess study quality
Evaluate the quality of each study using the criteria outlined in Box 8.2. Note the characteristics of each study, the methodological quality, the results, and any concealment of information.

Step 6. Extract data
• Screen by title, abstract, and finally full text, excluding papers at each stage.
• Read closely and make a critical analysis of the research quality (Box 8.2).
• Add articles identified from reference lists which meet the inclusion criteria.
• A data extraction form can be generated for each study, recording:
  • study citation;
  • philosophical stance;
  • research method;
  • quality appraisal;
  • inclusion and exclusion criteria;
  • setting for the study;
  • intervention and process if applicable;
  • intervention outcome if applicable;
  • procedure and process;
  • procedure outcome if applicable;
  • main finding and subsidiary findings.

Step 7. Analyse and present results

Citations of methodological quality and results from each study can be tabulated and a log kept of all excluded studies.

Box 8.2 An approach to quality evaluation

- Are the aims and objectives of the study clearly stated?
- Was a clear and answerable question asked?
- Is there clarity in exposition of a theoretical framework?
- Is there a clear description and justification of the methods, settings, and participants chosen?
- Is there sufficient information to assess the data collection process?
- Is there rigour in documentation and process?
- Is there a clear ethical basis?
- Are possible sources of bias acknowledged?
- Is the researcher's perspective acknowledged?
- Is analytical precision demonstrated?
- Are any deviant cases included and discussed?
- Are the conclusions justified by the findings?
- Is applicability and representativeness discussed?

1. Beckwith, S., Dickinson, A., and Kendall S. (2010). What the papers say. Exploring understanding of the term nursing assessment: a mixed-method review of the literature. *World Views on Evidence Based Nursing*, **7**(2), 98–110.

2. Clancy, M. J. (2002). Overview of research designs. *Emergency Medicine Journal*, **19**, 546–9.

3. Egger, M., Smith, G.D., and Altman, D. (2001). *Systematic reviews in health care: meta-analysis in context*. BMJ Publishing, London

4. Greenhalgh, T., Roberts, G., McFarlane, F., Bate, P., Kyriakidou, O., and Peacock, R. (2005). Story lines of research in diffusion of innovation: a meta-narrative approach to systematic review. *Social Science and Medicine*, **61**, 417–30.

5. Pang, M.C.S., Wong, T.K.S., Wang, C.S., et al. (2004). Towards a Chinese definition of nursing. *Journal of Advanced Nursing*, **46**, 657–70.

Risk management

Definition of risk
Risk is the likelihood, high or low, that somebody or something will be harmed by a hazard multiplied by the severity of the potential harm.[1]

The NHS Executive has emphasized the importance of developing holistic approaches to risk management and has noted the difficulty in differentiating between 'clinical' and 'non-clinical' risk management. A move has been made away from a concentration on litigation towards a broader focus on adverse events.

The scale of the problem
The annual scale of adverse events within the NHS has been summarized by the Department of Health[1] as follows.
- 400 people die or are seriously injured in adverse events involving medical devices.
- Almost 10 000 people are reported to have experienced serious adverse reactions to drugs.
- Around 1150 people who have been in recent contact with mental health services commit suicide.
- Almost 28 000 written complaints are made about aspects of clinical treatment in hospitals.
- The NHS pays out about £400 million a year in settlement of clinical negligence claims, and has a potential liability of about £2.4 billion for existing and expected claims.
- Hospital-acquired infections, of which about 15% may be avoidable, are estimated to cost the NHS nearly £1 billion.

The Department of Health[1] further stressed the need for the NHS to learn from mistakes identified in order that they are not repeated and listed the following processes for doing this:
- local, regional, and national incident reporting schemes;
- national studies in specific areas of care, e.g. confidential enquiries;
- systems for complaints and litigation designed to investigate/respond to specific instances of poor-quality care;
- periodic external studies and reviews, e.g. the Audit Commission's value for money studies;
- health and public health statistics;
- internal and external incident inquiries;
- clinical governance where clear clinical risk strategies are developed.

It was noted that the 40-year-old guidance on reporting adverse incidents lacked both a standardized reporting system and a standard definition of what should be reported.[1]

Definition of risk management
Risk management involves the systematic identification, analysis, and assessment of all hazards associated with an activity so that effective measures can be established to control the risks.[2]

The organizational culture required to minimize risk

The following organizational characteristics needed to minimize risks have been identified.[3]

- A reporting culture:
  - people are prepared to report their errors/near-misses;
  - data are properly analysed and fed back to staff showing the action that is being taken.
- A just culture:
  - an atmosphere of trust in which people are encouraged to provide safety-related information;
  - clearly drawn lines between acceptable and unacceptable behaviour where blame may be fairly apportioned for the latter.
- a flexible culture:
  - respects the skills and abilities of 'front-line' staff;
  - allows control to pass to those with expertise working in the field.
- a learning culture:
  - willingness and competence to draw the appropriate conclusions from its safety information system;
  - ability and willingness to make changes and implement major reforms where necessary.

Further reading

Walshe, K (2001). The development of clinical risk management. In C. Vincent (ed.), *Clinical risk management: enhancing patient safety*. BMJ Books, London.

1. Department of Health (2000). *An organisation with a memory. Report of an expert group on learning from adverse events in the NHS*. TSO, London.
2. NPCi (2009). *Managing risk in medicines management*. ⬚ http://www.npci.org.uk/ medicines_management/safety/mmrisk/library/5mg_risk.php (accessed 21 October 2009).
3. Reason, J. (1997). *Managing the risks of organisational accidents*. Ashgate, Aldershot.

Learning from incidents

Barriers to organizational learning[1-3]

- Focusing on the immediate event rather than on the root causes of the incident.
- Identifying one superficial cause to the exclusion of other less obvious but essential lessons.
- Rigidity of traditional patterns of behaviour or core beliefs, values, or assumptions, i.e. 'It has always been done that way';
  - challenging these entrenched beliefs may lead to resistance.
- Lack of corporate responsibility.
- Ineffective communication.
- An incremental approach to issues of risk—attempting to resolve problems with small adjustments rather than effecting fundamental change.
- Misplaced organizational or individual pride may lead to dismissal of external sources of censure.
- Human alliances such as profession or department lead people to:
  - overlook the mistakes of members of their team;
  - act defensively against ideas from outside the team.
- Scapegoating/blaming individuals may allow avoidance of addressing more fundamental organizational deficiencies.
- Difficulties in understanding complex events, often compounded by changes among key personnel within organizations/teams.
- Unwillingness to learn from negative events.
- Contradictory imperatives, e.g. open communication versus confidentiality.
- Work levels with high stress and poor job satisfaction can engender resistance to change and apathy.
- Inability to recognize/prioritize the financial costs of failure results in the loss of a powerful incentive for organizational change.

Patient decision aids (PDAs)

Definition

> Patient decision aids are intended to prepare patients to participate with their health care professionals in making deliberated, personalised choices about health care options. They supplement counselling by providing information on options. The aim is that patients are better able to judge the value of the benefits versus the harms.[4]

Patient decision aids (PDAs) are different from informed consent materials. The NPCi produce PDAs based on the best available evidence. However, they stress that their use is not a substitute for discussion with a 'suitably skilled health professional'.

One approach to risk management

Risk management can be described as using a stepped approach.
- Step 1: risk assessment—understanding the problem.
- Step 2: identification of solutions to the problem or control measures.

1. Smith, D. and Elliot, D. (2000) *Moving beyond denial: exploring the barriers to learning from crisis.* Centre for Risk and Crisis Management, University of Sheffield.
2. Firth-Cozens, J. (2000). Teams, culture and managing risk. In Vincent C. (ed.), *Clinical risk management.* BMJ Books, London
3. Wason, P.C (1960). On the failure to eliminate hypotheses in a conceptual task. *Quarterly Journal of Experimental Psychology,* **12**, 129–40.
4. O'Connor, A. and Edwards, A. (2001) The role of decision aids in promoting evidence based patient choice. In Edwards, A. and Elwyn, E. (eds) *Evidence based patient choice: inevitable or impossible?* Oxford University Press, Oxford.

Practice

Working as a non-medical prescriber

Working as a prescriber

Accountability

- You are accountable for all prescribing acts and omissions.
- You are personally accountable for each prescription you write.
- Keep up to date with competencies.
- Work only within your competencies, your professional scope of practice, and the remit of your job description.
- Only prescribe if you have assessed the patient.
- Resist the pressure to prescribe on behalf of other colleagues.
- Seek regular clinical supervision with a medical prescribing mentor.
- Do not prescribe unless there is a prescribing policy in place.

Questions to answer prior to and on qualifying

- Who is identified as the prescribing lead from within your organization?
- Is there a policy for prescribing (this is often included within the policy for medication management)?
- Is prescribing written clearly within your job description?
- Will you be covered by your employers under vicarious liability? (Remember that you may also be personally liable.)
- What is the mechanism for continual professional development?
- Are your prescribing needs addressed through the human resources review mechanism, can you discuss your CPD needs at appraisal?
- How are you going to keep up to date?
- Are you a member of a professional body which supports/informs your prescribing?
- How are you going to prove that you are keeping your competencies sharp?
- Are there other prescribers with whom you can seek supervision/ network?
- Have you informed your medical colleagues of your ability to prescribe?
- Do your patients know that you prescribe?
- Have you negotiated a mechanism and local working agreement to prescribe?
- Do you have appropriate professional liability insurance (PLI) which covers you as a non-medical prescriber?

On qualifying

- Notify the organization's prescribing lead of your qualification.
- Ensure that prescription pads are ordered or that there is a clear mechanism enabling you to prescribe.
- Provide the prescribing lead with a specimen of your signature.
- Provide local pharmacies with specimens of your signature (primary care).
- Provide hospital pharmacies with specimens of your signature (secondary care).

Prescribing from the BNF

- Prescribe within the limitations of your competency. You can prescribe unlicensed drugs as a nurse or pharmacist independent prescriber. However, if the drugs are unlicensed you must have a strong rationale for prescribing.
- You can prescribe a limited range of controlled drugs if you are a nurse independent prescriber. These are listed in the Drug Tariff[1] and the BNF.[2]
- You are not able to prescribe controlled drugs as a pharmacist or optometrist independent prescriber.[3]
- Keep up to date with changes to the BNF which is updated twice yearly.
- Keep up to date with developments in prescribing practice.
- Keep up to date with changes to prescribers' remit.
- Access the Department of Health FAQs and latest updates on http://www.dh.gov.uk/en/Healthcare/Medicinespharmacyandindustry/Prescriptions/TheNon-MedicalPrescribingProgramme/index.htm (accessed 28 April 2010).
- Maintain your portfolio of prescribing practice.

Questions to ask before prescribing

- Have you informed your colleagues of your new role?
- Have you informed your patients/clients of your new role?
- How have you informed the above?
- How has this information been received?
- Is the software in place to support your prescribing?
- Do your employers have electronic systems that 'talk to each other'?
- Are there recognized templates for CMPs?
- Are templates for CMPs adaptable to the needs of individual patients?
- Do you have prescription pads with your identifier on them (primary care)?
- Do you have drug charts that have been amended to include the signature of the nurse prescriber?
- Does the pharmacy have a sample of your signature?
- Do you have access to shared electronic records?
- Does your patient have patient-held records?
- Do you have internet access?
- Do you have access to key prescribing websites?
- Are you going to be using mechanisms for electronic prescribing?
- How secure are the above?

Prescribing legally from the British National Formulary

- Legal classification of medicines: the classification can relate to the pack size that is being sold.
- Prescription-only medicines (POMs) can only be supplied and dispensed if a prescription is issued by a legally qualified prescriber or under a patient-group direction.[1]
- Pharmacy only/over-the-counter (P) medicines: products that are for sale supervised by a registered pharmacist.
- General sales list products: available from shops other than pharmacies, such as petrol stations and supermarkets.
- Over-the-counter medicines (OTCs): a colloquial term for medicines which can be purchased without the need for a prescription or on advice from a pharmacist.

Prescribing legally from the BNF

- Prescribe only within your competency area.
- Prescribe only within your professional standards.
- Be clear of what you are able to prescribe following your legal parameters as either a non-medical independent prescriber or a supplementary prescriber.
- The drugs and appliances must be listed within the BNF.
- Write prescriptions only for the route or form as indicated by the BNF.
- Understand drug licensing and what you are qualified to do.

Drug licensing and non-medical prescribing

- All non-medical independent prescribers must prescribe only within their field of competence:
  - licensed and unlicensed drugs;
  - drugs that have a product licence for a particular indication but are used for another indication that is not described within their product licence/summary of product characteristics (off-label prescribing);
  - nurse independent prescribers but not pharmacist independent prescribers can prescribe some controlled drugs for specific indications (as listed in the Drug Tariff[2]).
- Supplementary prescribers can prescribe any drug(s) listed in the BNF provided that they are competent to do so and that they are working within the boundaries of a negotiated patient-specific clinical management plan.
- Community practitioner nurse and midwife prescribers:
  - can prescribe only within their field of competence;
  - can only prescribe drugs and appliances that are listed in the Nurse Prescribers Formulary for Community Practitioners (CPF).[3]
- Nurse and pharmacist independent prescribers can prescribe any appliance and dressings listed in Part IX of the Drug Tariff.

- Nurses and pharmacists who are independent and supplementary prescribers, and who are prescribing in secondary care are not restricted to prescribing appliances/dressings from Part IX of the Drug Tariff, but should take into account local formulary policies and the implications for primary care. (NB: the Drug Tariff restrictions only apply to prescribing in primary care or community care, if employed by a trust, when NHS WP10 prescriptions are written.)
- Pharmacist Independent Prescribers can prescribe only within their field of competence:
  - licensed and unlicensed drugs;
  - drugs that have a product licence for a particular indication but that are used for another indication that is not described within their product licence (off-label).
- As supplementary prescribers, pharmacists can prescribe any drug(s) listed in the BNF provided that they are competent to do so and that they are working within the boundaries of a negotiated patient-specific clinical management plan.
- Physiotherapist, podiatrists, and radiographers can prescribe as supplementary prescribers:
  - only within their scope of practice and field of competence;
  - any drug(s) listed in the BNF provided that they are competent to do so and that they are working within the boundaries of a negotiated patient-specific clinical management plan.[4]

Information regarding prescribing by optometrists is not within the remit of this book but can be accessed at: ☒ http://www.collegeoptometrists. org/index.aspx/pcms/site.education.ex.cfa_2.IP2/ (accessed 28 April 2010).

1. *British National Formulary* (latest edn). British Medical Association and Royal Pharmaceutical Society of Great Britain, London.
2. Electronic Drug Tariff (2009). Compiled on behalf of the Department of Health by the NHS Business Services Authority, NHS Prescription Services. ☒ http://www.ppa.org.uk/ edt/October_2009/mindex.htm (accessed 19 October 2009).
3. Nurse Prescribers' Formulary for Community Practitioners (latest edn). Community Practitioners' and Health Visitors' Association, the Royal College of Nursing, British Medical Association, and the Royal Pharmaceutical Society of Great Britain.
4. Department of Health (2006). *Medicines Matters. A guide to the mechanisms for the prescribing, supply and administration of medicines.* ☒ http://www.dh.gov.uk/en/Publicationsandstatistics/ Publications/PublicationsPolicyAndGuidance/DH_064325 (accessed 19 October 2009).

Mixing drugs in syringe drivers

Mixing two licensed drugs together changes the properties of the drugs and creates a new product that has not undergone clinical trial. For a medicinal product to obtain a product licence it must undergo rigorous clinical trials. Therefore when two drugs are mixed together, as within a syringe or syringe driver, a new product is created that does not carry a product licence.

Changes to legislation in December 2009 enabled nurse, midwife, and pharmacist independent prescribers to prescribe unlicensed drugs as part of their clinical competence. This means that they can mix two drugs together in one syringe. For example, they can mix a local anaesthetic and an anti-inflammatory drug together for the purposes of an intra-articular injection. However, the legislation does not apply to controlled drugs.[1] This means that nurses working in palliative care as independent prescribers are not permitted to prescribe a controlled drug for mixing with any other drug within a syringe driver. For example, as nurse independent prescribers they are not permitted to prescribe diamorphine and an anti-emetic within a syringe driver.

Supplementary prescribers (nurses, midwives, pharmacists, podiatrists, physiotherapists, and radiographers) are permitted to prescribe controlled drugs and unlicensed drugs as part of an agreed clinical management plan. This means that nurses and health-care professionals who are qualified as supplementary prescribers may prescribe a combination of drugs for administration by injection or infusion via a syringe driver.

The National Prescribing Centre and the NMC have produced guidance that must be followed when practising as described above.[1,2]
When in practice always work to local policy and within the framework of professional standards.

Prescribing for cosmetic effect

The NMC have produced a fact sheet that provides guidance for prescribing injectable cosmetic treatments. This advice was last updated in November 2009 and must be followed by all non-medical prescribers who are working in this field of competence.[3]

Remote prescribing

The NMC have produced a position statement relating to the practice of remote online prescribing. This guidance must be followed by all non-medical prescribers who are likely to be prescribing remotely.[4]

1. ⌨ http://www.npc.co.uk/prescribers/faq.htm (accessed 1 February 2010).
2. ⌨ http://www.nmc-uk.org/Nurses-and-midwives/Advice-by-topic/A/Advice/Mixing-medicines/ (accessed 24 June 2010).
3. ⌨ http://www.nmcuk.org/aArticle.aspx?ArticleID=3525 (accessed 1 February 2010).
4. ⌨ http://www.nmc-uk.org/aArticle.aspx?ArticleID=3460 (accessed 1 February 2010).

Practical prescribing

History-taking

Taking a history to make a prescribing decision is a two-way process involving a complex interaction between the patient and the prescriber. A thorough systematic history and physical examination are fundamental before prescribing for any patient. The purpose of history-taking is to gather information from the patient to establish a trusting and supportive relationship with them, actively listening to their concerns, in order to provide holistic care. The prescriber is accountable for taking a history and making a prescribing decision.

When taking a history, start by asking open-ended questions. These questions can become more specific as the consultation progresses. Remember that the patient should be encouraged to tell his/her story.

To facilitate active listening
- Have an open and friendly posture.
- Use prompts, i.e yes, I see, tell me more….
- Ask the patient to clarify what they are saying/feeling.
- Show empathy and understanding.
- Check your understanding with the patient and summarize this back to him/her.
- Pick up on the patient's body language—what is this telling you about his/her complaint/expectations?
- Holistic assessment, p. 82.

You will need to record
- The date and time.
- Identifying data for the patient: age, gender, marital status, and occupation.
- Source of history or referral.
- Information from the patient, friend, family carer, etc.
- Reliability of information, if relevant.
- Chief complaints, where possible in the patient's own words.
- Present illness, including:
  - location of the complaint—where is it?
  - does it move?
  - quality—what is it like?
  - quantity or severity—how bad is it?
  - timing—when does it start?
  - how long does it last?
  - how often does it occur?
  - describe the pain?
  - is the pain always there or does it come and go?
  - how long have they had it?
  - have they had similar symptoms before?
  - what does the patient/carer think is wrong?
  - what are their health beliefs?
  - what do they want you to do for them?

Setting: environmental factors

- Which activities are associated with the complaint?
- Are there any emotional reactions which may have contributed to this illness?
- Are there factors that make it worse or better?
- Other associated manifestations.
- Current medications including:
  - home remedies;
  - over-the-counter medications (OTC);
  - herbs;
  - medicines/products borrowed from another person.
- Any known allergies?
- Any symptoms that could cause you to think that there is an underlying condition that could cause alarm? Identify as red flag symptoms.

📖 Over-the-counter (OTC) drugs, p. 422.

Past medical history

- Childhood illnesses
- Adult illnesses including mental health
- Current health status
- Smoking status
- Alcohol, drugs, and/or related substance abuse
- Other risk-taking leisure activities
- Exercise and diet
- Immunizations
- Screening tests.

Family history

- Note the age and health or age at death of each immediate family member.
- Information regarding the health of grandparents or grandchildren may also be of use.
- Note the occurrence within the family of any disease, e.g. diabetes, stroke, heart disease.

Personal, psychological, and social history are highly important. Remember that distress can manifest as physical ill health (disease). Remember to ask about:

- occupation;
- education;
- home situation and significant others;
- daily life;
- important experiences;
- religious/spiritual beliefs.

Remember that negative information from the patient is useful in helping to make the diagnosis by ruling out possibilities/potential diseases.

Red flags

These must always be considered when taking a history. A red flag is any associated symptom that is not directly a symptom of the presenting complaint but might be presenting alongside the main complaint. A red flag symptom may be a sign of a more serious or underlying condition.

Examples of red flag symptoms:
- chest pain;
- weight loss;
- bloody diarrhoea;
- vomiting blood;
- coughing up blood;
- fever;
- loss of appetite.

The patient might have had associated symptoms for some time or they might be presenting for the first time along with the complaint.

Making a diagnosis

A diagnosis has to be made before any prescribing can happen. Making a diagnosis can often be a complex and difficult exercise. You must only ever prescribe once a full history and assessment have been taken and a diagnosis has been made. Remember only work within your field of competence and scope of practice and if in doubt refer the patient onwards.

If you are working as an non-medical independent prescriber (V300 nurses, midwives, optomotrists, and pharmacists only), you are accountable for:
- taking a history;
- assessing your patient;
- making a diagnosis.

If you are working as a supplementary prescriber, the doctor acts as the independent prescriber in the prescribing partnership and is accountable for the intital history-taking and assessment and making the initial diagnosis. You are accountable for:
- agreeing or disagreeing with the diagnosis;
- assessing your patient before you prescribe.

You carry joint responsibility with the doctor who is the independent prescriber for negotiating and agreeing the clinical management plan. You cannot prescribe unless you agree with the diagnosis and with what has been agreed and documented as part of the clinical management plan.

You must take a history and assess your patient each time before prescribing under the clinical management plan as you are accountable for your prescribing decisions and actions.

📖 Using models of consultation for prescribing, p. 184.
📖 Using the medical model for clinical or physical examination, p. 178.

Using the medical model for clinical or physical examination

A structured and systematic approach needs to be taken to make a diagnosis, as outlined by the National Prescribing Centre (NPC):

> [the nurse prescriber] *takes a comprehensive medical history and undertakes the appropriate physical examination.[1]*

Competency frameworks for all non-medical prescribers can be accessed at 🖥 http://www.npc.co.uk/prescribers/competency_frameworks.htm.
Information needs to be gathered from three main sources:

- history-taking;
- physical/clinical examination;
- appropriate investigations.

📖 History-taking, p. 174

In addition to the comprehensive verbal history, which will be taken by the practitioner, prompting the patient to describe their experience of the presenting condition in a clear and factual way, close observation of the patient's physical and clinical condition is required. Note and record, as part of the assessment, the patient's:

- appearance;
- movement;
- demeanour.

Remember that a patient may be concerned about their tiredness and not think of swelling in their ankles and breathlessness as important. You will need to note these symptoms and address them after taking the patient's history.

Most provisional diagnoses will be made by the end of the history-taking process.

Clinical examination

Further evidence to support or reject the provisional diagnosis will be obtained by examining the patient.

The physical areas examined will depend on the provisional diagnosis. However, it is important to return to the history if the findings on examination do not support the provisional diagnosis.

Always be sensitive to the patient's:

- dignity;
- concerns;
- religious and cultural needs.

> **Remember**
>
> You are legally required to ask the patient's permission to carry out a physical examination. Do not do anything outside your area of competence. Always consider your training and experience.

---

1. National Prescribing Centre. 🖥 http://www.npc.co.uk/prescribers/competency_frameworks.htm (accessed 21 October 2009).

Further reading

Bickley, L. (2008). *Bates pocket guide to physical examination and history taking* (10th edn). Lippincott–Williams & Wilkins, Philadelphia, PA.

Crumbie, A. (2006). Taking a history. In M. Walsh (ed.), *Nurse practitioners: clinical skills and professional issues* (2nd edn). Butterworth Heinemann, Edinburgh.

Health beliefs

The Health Belief Model (HBM)[1] is a psychological model that was developed in 1950s in response to a failed screening programme for tuberculosis. The model is based on the premise that individuals tend to act to avoid the negative consequences of risk-taking. It examined motivation and what influenced individuals to take positive or negative actions that influenced their health. At the same time Rotter[2] was developing the theory of locus of control that was modified in the 1970s.

Individuals with an internal locus of control view events as resulting from their own actions. Persons with an external locus of control view events as being under the control of external factors such as luck.

The HBM was adapted in the 1970s and 1990s, and attempts to rationalize and predict health behaviours by focusing on the attitudes and beliefs of individuals (Table 10.1).[1,3] The model links in with others to the wider theories of change.

Criticism of the HBM

A criticism of the HBM is that its premise is that health behaviours are the consequence of individual responsibility, the cycle of change, and actions, and it does not take wider social and cultural influences into account.[4]

The Fishbein–Ajzen theory of reasoned action took this a step further and argued that a person's intentional behaviour (how they intend to act) is motivated by their own attitude towards that behaviour and that their motivation is modified by the attitudes and subjective norms of society and others.[5]

Attributional theory of emotional motivation

Weiner defined the attributional theory of emotional motivation[6] which-demonstrates how individuals attribute blame for their own lack of motivation to change to cause and effect based on external influences such as employment status or financial problems, and how they attribute successful change in behaviour to internal influences such as their own intelligence or skill.

Prochaska and DiClemente[7] developed a cycle of motivational change that is still used in a modified version to support motivational change, particularly in addiction.

📖 Cycle of change, p. 182.

Table 10.1 The key concepts of the health belief model

Concept (The idea)	Definition (What this means to the patient)	Application (What health professionals can do to help)
Perceived susceptibility	Individual belief in the odds of getting the condition	Define the at-risk population Personalize individual risk, and if the patient's perception of risk is too low, heighten it
Perceived severity	How bad is the risk to the patient? What are the consequences of chosing/continuing to take health-threatening risk or of ignoring disease symptoms?	Define and describe specific consequences
Perceived benefits	What are the benefits to the patient of chosing not to take the risk or to stop risk-taking behaviour?	Explain how to lessen/minimize the risk Clarify positive benefits Base explanation on evidence
Perceived barriers	To what extent does the patient believe that advice is effective?	Give encouragement, reassurance, and incentives
Cues to action	How ready is the patient to change and what have they done about it?	Use health-promotion strategies to give practical examples of how to change Prompt and support the patient through the stages of change
Self-efficacy	To what extent does the patient believe in their own ability to act and to change their behaviour?	Give practical training and support, and encourage steps to change

Adapted from Rosenstock et al.[3]

1. Becker, M.H. and Maiman, L.A. (1975). Sociobehavioural determinants of compliance with medical care recommendations. *Medical Care*, **13**, 10–24.

2. Rotter, J.B. (1954). *Social learning and clinical psychology*. Prentice-Hall, Englewood Cliffs, NJ.

3. Rosenstock, I.M., Stretcher, V.J., and Becker, M.H (1988) Social learning theory and the health belief model. *Health Education and Behavior*, **15**, 175–83.

4. Green, L.W. and Kreuter, M.W. (1991). *Health promotion planning: an educational and environmental approach* (2nd edn). Mayfield, Palo Alto, CA.

5. Fishbein, M. and Ajzen, I. (1975). *Belief, attitude, intention, and behavior: an introduction to theory and research*. Addison-Wesley, Reading, MA.

6. Weiner, B. (1986). *An attributional theory of motivation and emotion*. Springer-Verlag, New York.

7. Prochaska, J.O. and DiClemente, C.C. (1982).Trans-theoretical therapy: toward a more integrated model of change. *Psychotherapy: Theory, Research and Practice*, **19**, 276–88.

Cycle of change

Fig. 10.1 is a representation of the Prochaska–DiClemente[1] model illustrating how an individual or a group of individuals can bring about change either in themselves as individuals or as an institution. It reflects the experience that change in behaviour or attitude is not a linear process but can be beset by lapses and relapses. These slips should not be seen as failure but are to be expected as a person adapts to their new behaviour. It is also important to acknowledge that the cycle may only be completed over months or years rather than days or weeks.

1. The first stage of change is the 'pre-contemplative'. At this point an individual may not have considered the possibility of alternative behaviours or attitudes. It is important to stress that decisions are theirs and to encourage self-exploration and evaluation of current status.

2. The 'contemplative' stage is one of ambivalence. The person is in two minds. Should they change or try changing to a new pattern of behaviour? Consideration of the pros and cons of the change and the expectations of a positive outcome if the change is made.

3. 'Preparation' indicates the time where the decision to change has been made and the first steps to implementing the change are planned. Identify support systems and problem-solving activities.

4. 'Action' indicates that a change has been made and the person is engrossed in adaptation to their new behaviours or attitudes.

5. 'Maintenance' describes possibly the most challenging of the stages where the change is integrated in to a person's lifestyle.

6. This is often, but not inevitably, followed by a 'relapse'. Individuals often relapse several times before the new set of behaviours becomes (more or less) permanent. It may be helpful to identify triggers to relapse and to develop coping strategies to deal with these.

1. Prochaska, J.O., DiClemente, C.C., and Norcross, J.C. (1992). In search of how people change—applications to addictive behaviors. *American Psychologist*, **47**(9), 1102–1114.

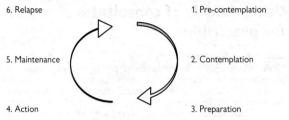

6. Relapse

5. Maintenance

4. Action

1. Pre-contemplation

2. Contemplation

3. Preparation

Fig. 10.1 The cycle of change. Adapted from Prochaska et al.[1]

Using models of consultation for prescribing

Consulting for prescribing

Models of consultation have been developed to support practice and until recently have been based on the biomedical tradition. A model can be viewed as a structural framework around which to build effective practice. To prescribe safely, you must develop and practise a safe, holistic, and effective consultation style that is patient focused and centred on their health beliefs. Patient/practitioner consultations have traditionally been medically led and, as such, paternalistic—the professional is in control of the consultation to which the patient is a passive recipient

Patients' choices within the consultation are affected by their 'health beliefs'. Health beliefs are influenced by many variables which must be viewed within the patient's cultural context. The health beliefs model[1,2] reviewed these as follows.

- The influence of the patient's social class, ethnicity, and personality.
- Patient's perception of the severity of the disease threat.
- Patient's perception of the risk–benefit of seeking treatment.
- Catalysts for action, e.g. severity of symptoms, pressure from family, information in the media.
- The patient's self-efficacy: how effective they are in influencing their own health.

Practitioner- and patient-centred models

In the disease–illness model,[3] the patient's condition is viewed as their primary concern, and it is the task of the practitioner to assist the patient in seeking a remedy. Information is gathered from the perspective of both the patient and the practitioner; integration of both agendas leads to shared decision-making and understanding.

Stott and Davis[4] suggested a systematic style of consultation which explored:

- management of presenting problems;
- modification of help-seeking behaviours, e.g. educating the patient in self-help methods;
- management of continuing problems, e.g. looking at long-term problems and solutions;
- opportunistic health promotion, e.g. screening, vaccination, brief intervention for smoking cessation.

Pendleton et al.[5] detailed seven tasks that would lead to a structured and effective consultation.

- Find out why the patient has come.
- Are there any other problems?
- In mutual doctor–patient consultation, act to address the problems.
- Work to achieve a mutual understanding of the problems.
- Involve the patient and encourage them to take responsibility.

- Efficient use of time and resources.
- Establish and maintain an ongoing relationship with the patient.

Byrne and Long[6] observed and described six phases that provided a logical framework for a consultation.

- Phase 1: establishing a relationship between the patient and the health professional.
- Phase 2: attempting to discover, or discovering, why the patient is consulting.
- Phase 3: conducting a verbal or physical examination—usually both are conducted within one consultation.
- Phase 4: mutual consideration of the condition.
- Phase 5: practitioner-led or joint detailing of the need for further treatment or investigation.
- Phase 6: practitioner-led termination of the consultation.

Heron[7] categorized the interventions of practitioners into six main styles.

- Prescriptive: using a directive advice-giving approach.
- Informative: sharing new knowledge—explaining this to the patient.
- Confronting: challenging existing attitudes and beliefs within a supportive environment.
- Cathartic: supporting the patient to release emotions.
- Catalytic: supporting patient exploration of thoughts and feelings.
- Supportive: comforting the patient and affirming their value.

Heron's model can be argued to be consumerist, in that the patient makes demands of the practitioner which are based on actual and perceived need. The patient is in control of the consultation.

Helman[8] placed the patient in charge and at the centre of their consultation and suggested that there were six common questions that patients asked.

- What is happening/has happened to me?
- Why is it happening to me?
- Why has it happened now?
- What would happen to me if nothing were done about it?
- What am I supposed to do about it and from whom should I seek advice?

Helman argues that the answers to these questions help to construct a 'folk model' of illness and that it is patient's folk beliefs about illness that affect their response to their underlying condition, for example whether they chose to adopt the sick role or not. This ties in with Lau,[9] who found that encounters with sickness in an individual's family have strong effects on the locus of control and controllability of health beliefs. Neighbour[10] categorized patient–practitioner consultation into five useful checkpoints.

- Connecting: establishing a practitioner–patient rapport.
- Summarizing: listening to the patient and eliciting information.
- Handover: mutual agreement/decision-making and action.

- Safety-netting: checking that all key points have been covered, and setting in place processes for record-keeping, review, and reflection.
- Housekeeping: caring for the needs of the practitioner.

In this model there is a mutuality/partnership—both parties have shared and equal control. This style is based on shared respect and works well for situations when negotiating a contract.

📖 Holistic assessment, p. 82.

📖 History-taking, p. 174.

1. Becker, M.H. (ed.) (1974). The health belief model and personal health behavior. *Health Education Monographs*, **2**, 324–473.

2. Rosenstock, I., Strecher, V., and Becker, M. (1994). The health belief model and HIV risk behaviour change. In R.J. DiClemente and J.L. Peterson (eds), *Preventing AIDS: theories and methods of behavioral interventions*, pp. 5–24. Plenum Press, New York.

3. Stewart, M. and Roter, D. (eds) (1989). *Communicating with medical patients*. Sage, Newbury Park, CA.

4. Stott, N. and Davis, R.H. (1979). The exceptional potential in each primary care consultation. *Journal of the Royal College of General Practitioners*, **29**, 201–5.

5. Pendleton, D., Schofield, T., Tate, P., and Havelock, P. (1984). *The consultation: an approach to learning and teaching*. Oxford University Press, Oxford.

6. Byrne, P. and Long, B. (1976). *Doctors talking to patients*. HMSO, London.

7. Heron, J. (1975). *Six category intervention analysis*. Human Potential Research Project, University of Surrey.

8. Helman, C.G. (1981). Disease versus illness in general practice. *Journal of the Royal College of General. Practitioners*, **31**, 548–52.

9. Lau R.R. (1982). Origins of health locus of control beliefs. *Journal of Personality and Social Psychology*, **42**, 332–4.

10. Neighbour, R. (1997). *The inner consultation*. Petroc Press, Reading.

Communication

The purpose of effective patient-centred communication in relation to prescribing is to promote concordance. Communication is a two-way process, involving giving and receiving, i.e: actively listening to the patient as well as imparting clear information to the patient. Patient-centred communication takes into account the patient's:
• hopes;
• beliefs;
• attitudes;
• expectations.
When communicating with patients, prescribers must always be sensitive and professional.
📖 Concordance, p. 84.
   The patient's agenda may differ from that of the prescriber. To prescribe effectively, listening must be balanced with the gathering of information:
• the patient's perception of the problem may be different from that of the prescriber;
• the patient may not be telling you the full story;
• the problem that they present with may not be the problem that they wish you to treat.

Effective communication: the role of the prescriber

• Respect the patient.
• Respect the patient's agenda.
• Be sensitive to the patient.
• Listening supportively.
• Show sensitive body language.
• Empathize.
• Establish the patient's hopes, fears, and expectations.
• Clarify.
• Listen actively.
• Ask open-ended questions.
• Give accurate feedback.
• Gather all the information.
• Ask the patient to fill in the gaps.
• Analyse the information.
• Seek the truth (perceived and actual).
• Give factual and easily interpreted evidence-based information.
• Explain all options.
• Explain the effects of drug.
• Explain any side effects.
• Negotiate efficiently.
• Communicate at a pace that is appropriate for your individual patient.
• Communicate with the wider team.
• Ensure that others who are caring for the patient are kept up to date with changes to the patient's prescriptions.

Information can be communicated via patient-held records and shared electronic records. 📖 Record-keeping, p. 192.

Equity and communication

Consider:
- effective communication for people for whom English is not their first language;
- effective communication for those with audio or visual impairment;
- effective communication for those with literacy deficits;
- effective communication for those with learning disabilities.

Websites to support communication with patients who are audio or visually impaired and for those with learning disabilities:

Royal National Institute for the Blind 🖥 www.rnib.org.uk
Royal National Institute for the Deaf 🖥 www.rnid.org.uk
Mencap 🖥 www.mencap.org.uk

Ensuring an effective consultation

Proceed in a sequence that is logical to yourself and to your patient.[1]

Before the consultation

- Ensure that adequate time is set aside to prepare for the consultation.
- Read the patient's records.
- Anticipate the patient's agenda, but do not set it for them.
- Give yourself space between patients.
- Tidy your desk space.
- Prepare the necessary documents and necessary equipment.
- Anticipate how long you will need to be able to complete the consultation.

Remember that first impressions count

To develop a relationship you need to employ verbal and non-verbal communication and to involve the patient at each stage of decision-making.

- Greet the patient:
  - ensure that you have got the patient you were expecting;
  - ask the patient to introduce themselves;
  - make eye contact;
  - make your patient comfortable;
  - establish a mutuality/rapport;
  - attend to their basic needs;
  - identify the purpose of the consultation.
- Explain and clarify your role:
  - introduce yourself by name and role;
  - clarify why the patient has come to see you;
  - explain what you do;
  - ask the patient what he/she expects from the consultation;
  - look for other underlying reasons for the patient to be attending the consultation.

Consider your patient

- Does your patient feel at ease?
- Is he/she comfortable?
- Why has he/she come?
- What does he/she want from the consultation?
- Can he/she talk to you?
- Is there mutual respect?
- Let the patient set the agenda.
- Is it the same as yours?
- Be aware of the patient's facial expressions and body language.
- Listen initially without interrupting.
- Use open questions to keep the consultation moving and closed ones to bring it to a controlled end.

📖 History-taking, p. 174.

---

1. Kurtz, S.M., Silverman, J.D., and Draper, J. (1998). *Teaching and learning communication skills.* Radcliffe Medical Press, Oxford.

Record-keeping

Follow your professional body's guidelines/standards for record keeping.[1–4] The Nursing and Midwifery Council state that:

> You must keep clear and accurate records of the discussions you have, the assessments you make, the treatment and medicines you give and how effective these have been.
>
> You must complete records as soon as possible after an event has occurred.
>
> You must not tamper with original records in any way.
>
> You must ensure any entries you make in someone's paper records are clearly and legibly signed, dated and timed.
>
> You must ensure any entries you make in someone's electronic records are clearly attributable to you.
>
> You must ensure all records are kept securely.[1]

When prescribing

Record prescribing decisions in patient-held records (if available) and in shared medical notes (paper or electronic) as in standard practice. Ensure contemporaneous record-keeping with a maximum time lapse of 24–48hr (72hr on bank holidays). Make sure that records are legible.

📖 Data Protection Act, p. 149.

What to record

- Time.
- Date.
- Purpose of the consultation.
- Outcome of negotiated decision-making.
- If you have prescribed or recommended medication to be bought from the pharmacist or as general sales list medication, and any instructions you have given the patient:
  - dose, frequency, how often, and how long to take medication for.
- What you have advised the patient to do in the event of unexpected side effects.
- Date of proposed review.

Negotiation within the team

- Inform fellow professionals of your role as a prescriber.
- It is important to maintain patient confidentiality but, in the interest of safe prescribing, other prescribers and clinicians who have access to the patient's medical records must be informed of prescribing decisions.
- In the case of supplementary prescribing, other prescribers can have access to a shared clinical management plan and, through access for professionals, to shared electronic records (where they are available).
- Patients and carers must be involved in negotiated decision-making and information should be recorded in patient-held records where available.

- Prescribing decisions must be documented in professional records, along with a copy of the clinical management plan.
- Avoid duplicating information that is already in the patient's notes.
- It is good practice to give a patient/carer a copy of the agreed clinical management plan.

Out of hours

It is vital that professionals who are involved in out-of-hours care have as near to contemporaneous as is possible access to medical records, which must clearly document prescribing decisions.

📖 NMC and HPC codes, p. 20.

1. Nursing and Midwifery Council (2009). *Record keeping guidance for nurses and midwives.* 🖳 http://www.nmc-uk.org/aDisplayDocument.aspx?documentID=6269 (accessed 21 October 2009).
2. 🖳 http://www.hpc-uk.org/publications/standards/
3. 🖳 http://www.rpsgb.org.uk/
4. 🖳 http://www.assoc-optometrists.org/search/site_search.html?query=record+keeping

Using the British National Formulary (BNF)

The BNF is revised, updated, and published on a six-monthly basis and informs the prescriber about 'the selection, prescribing, dispensing and administration of medicines'.[1] It is also available online. Information is linked to clinical conditions. The BNF, along with other commercially produced formularies and locally produced NHS formularies, contains information regarding dosages, formulations, and pack sizes, as well as the market cost of the drug/appliance.

Guidance provided by BNF:
• prescription writing;
• prescribing controlled drugs;
• prescribing for dependencies.

Each edition of the BNF indicates any significant changes that have been made since the previous edition, including:
• dose changes;
• classification changes;
• discontinued preparations;
• new preparations;
• name changes of drugs to conform to European law.

The inside front cover of the BNF contains useful contact numbers:
• regional and district Medicines Information Services;
• UK Medicines Information Pharmacists Group (UKMIPG);
• Driver and Vehicle Licensing Agency (DVLA);
• UK Sport;
• Poisons Information Services;
• travel information contact numbers.

The main text of the BNF is divided into 15 chapters covering comprehensive prescribing for each system of the body and related clinical conditions. Non-medical prescribers' formularies within the BNF include:
• nurse prescribers' formulary for community prescribers (CPF);
• dental practitioners' formulary.

Information regarding controlled drugs which can be prescribed by nurse independent prescribers can be found at in the latest edition of the Drug Tariff at 🖳 http://www.ppa.org.uk (accessed 21 October 2009).

As well as general information on prescribing, the BNF provides information on:
• prescription writing;
• emergency supply of medicines;
• controlled drugs and drug dependence;
• adverse reactions to drugs;
• prescribing for children;
• prescribing in palliative care;

- prescribing for the elderly;
- drugs and sport prescribing;
- emergency treatment of poisoning;
- index of manufacturers, contact addresses, and telephone numbers;
- Joint British Societies Coronary Risk Prediction Chart;
- Adult Advanced Life Support.

Appendices at the back of the BNF cover:
- drug interactions;
- liver disease;
- renal impairment;
- pregnancy;
- breast-feeding;
- intravenous additives;
- borderline substances;
- wound management products and elastic hosiery;
- cautionary and advisory labels for dispensed medicines;
- cautionary labels.

The pharmacist who supplies and dispenses the medication is required to supply it with the recommended informative wording and, if necessary, a cautionary label. Wording for cautionary labels can be found inside the back cover of the BNF together with abbreviations and symbols.

Wherever possible, the BNF uses internationally recognized abbreviations and symbols. A list of abbreviations can be found inside the back cover:
- symbols;
- Latin abbreviations;
- E numbers which are present in some medications.

Yellow card reporting (adverse drug reactions)

Detachable yellow cards for reporting adverse drug reactions (ADRs) to the Committee on Safety of Medicines (CSM) can be found at the back of the BNF. Yellow card reporting can also be filed on line via ⌨ www.mhra.gov.uk (accessed 21 October 2009)

Prescribing for special groups

Prescribing for older people

It is important to accept the diversity and individuality of the people who make up the group catagorized as older people. The term 'older people' is a descriptor which is economically and socially constructed and brings with it many disadvantages. However, for the purpose of this section we will take older people to be those with a chronological age over 60 years.

Homeostatic changes such as decreased renal function mean that older people are more sensitive to medicines and are more likely to have adverse reactions to prescribed medication. Table 11.1 shows other age-related pharmacokinetic changes.

Cotter and Martin[1] reported that studies have shown that adverse drug reactions may cause about 3–12% of hospital admissions in elderly patients. In addition, older people are prescribed more medicines (polypharmacy), facilitating greater chances for drug–drug reactions. For example, co-administration of NSAIDs and anti-hypertensives may lead to a reduction in the hypotensive effect caused by sodium retention induced by the NSAID. The BNF offers the following advice when prescribing for older people.

• Limit the range of medicines you prescribe from in order to be familiar with their effects in older people.
• Reduce the dose: generally, starting doses should be lower than for younger patients.
• Review regularly: the NSF for Older People[2] recommends reviewing every 6 months if on four or more medicines.
• Simple regimens: only give if there is a clear indication. Try to prescribe once- or twice-daily dosing.
• Explain clearly: give written instructions with every prescription so that containers are fully labelled.
• Repeat prescribing and disposal of unused medications: instruct patients on what to do when drugs run out and how to dispose of unneeded medicines. Try to prescribe matching quantities.

Polypharmacy

This is defined as being prescribed four or more medicines and brings an increased risk of drug interaction and/or adverse drug reaction (ADR).

Retrospective chart reviews were conducted on 283 randomly selected emergency department visits made by patients aged 65 and over during a 12-month period.[3] Of these patients, 257 (90.8%) were taking one or more medications (prescribed or over-the-counter). The number of medications used ranged from zero to 17, with an average of 4.2 per patient. Around 20% of people over 70 take five or more drugs.[4]

📖 Basic principles of pharmacology, pp. 53–64.

1. Cotter, L.E. and Martin, U. (2007). Prescribing for older people. *Student BMJ*, **15**, 337–82.
2. Department of Health (2001). *NSF for older people*. TSO, London.
3. 🔲 http://www.liv.ac.uk/~druginfo/csm/ADR_Bulletin21.pdf (accessed 29 October 2009).
4. Milton, J.C., Smith, L., and Jackson, S.H.D. (2008). Prescribing for older people. *BMJ*, **336**, 606–9.

Table 11.1 Some practical aspects of prescribing for older people

Problem	Result	Possibility
A frail older person may have difficulty in swallowing	Tablets remain in the mouth, causing: Localized ulceration Slowed availability of the drug	Consider prescribing as a liquid Encourage using sufficient fluid to facilitate swallowing Ensure the correct fluid, e.g. take with milk or take with water
Problems removing medications from packs	Prescribed items not taken	Blister packs may be problematic Consider: Foil-packed tablets Using a compartmentalized box with daily doses in each section
Difficulties reading the label	Missed doses or taken at inappropriate times Overdose ADR	Use large-print black-and-white labels
Forgetting to take medication	Missed doses	Consider using a compartmentalized box with daily doses in each section or a medicine reminder chart
Sensitivity to commonly used drugs	Nervous system may be sensitive to: Opioid analgesics Benzodiazepines Antipsychotics Antiparkinsonian drugs	Use with caution

Holistic assessment for older people

It is important to assess not only the presenting problem but also the altered pharmacodynamics and kinetics, which are part of the ageing process, as well as any underlying pathologies and/or polypharmacy.

Always check the use of herbal remedies, home remedies, and over-the-counter (OTC) medication for possible drug interactions and food–drug interactions (Table 11.2).

It is important that a comprehensive drug history is taken from the patient and/or their family and carers, and that any home remedies or herbal remedies are noted.

Note factors related to the patient, such as:
• cognition;
• capacity;
• swallowing;
• vision;
• manual dexterity;
• attitude to taking drugs.

These should inform your decisions in all aspects of treatment including selection of drugs, their formulation, times of taking them, and choice of container.

📖 Holistic assessment, p. 82.

Table 11.2 Common food–drug interactions

Food	Drug	Action
Orange juice (vitamin C)	Iron sulphate	Enhances the absorption of iron
Dairy produce	Tetracycline	Reduces the absorption of tetracycline
Foods rich in tyramine, e.g. cheese, meat extract, some alcohol	Monoamine oxidase inhibitors	Toxic effect such as sudden hypertensive crisis

Challenges when prescribing for older people

As we age, our bodies undergo changes that can affect the distribution, metabolism, and excretion of drugs. These changes included a reduction in renal clearance, liver size, and lean body mass.

Pharmacokinetic changes regarding the metabolism and excretion of drugs

- Delayed metabolism by the liver and excretion by the kidneys results in prolonged drug action:
  - older people may have a glomerular filtration rate (GFR) below 50mL/min because of reduced muscle mass, which may not be indicated by a raised serum creatinine. **This can result in prolonged drug action**;
  - follow local guidelines regarding monitoring renal function;
  - it is recommended to assume at least mild renal impairment when prescribing for older people. 📖 Prescribing for people with renal disease, p. 216.
- Complicated regimens may cause confusion and lead to excessive doses or overdose.
- Patients who are malnourished will have altered drug metabolism and distribution:
  - reduced plasma protein may result in an increase in the amount of drug available for activity;
  - insufficient dietary protein may lead to reduced enzyme activity and slow drug metabolism.
- Older people have altered body mass and body fat stores:
  - a leaner body mass, with reduced fat stores, limits the sequestration of a drug in the fatty layers, increasing the amount actively available.
- Further alterations are caused by declines in:
  - total body water—decreases by 10–15% between ages 20 and 80;
  - renal mass;
  - hepatic blood flow and mass decrease with age;
  - GFR—the number of nephrons decreases with age and they become less efficient.

This reduction in renal clearance, a natural process of ageing, is clinically significant and results in reduced excretion of water-soluble drugs. This is particularly important for drugs with a narrow therapeutic window (ratio of desired effect to toxic effect), such as digoxin, lithium, and gentamicin. 📖 Prescribing for people with renal disease, p. 216.

These alterations may be further exacerbated by routine illnesses, such as renal tract infection (RTI) or urinary tract infection (UTI), leading to the development of adverse effects or overdose in a patient previously stabilized on a drug with a narrow therapeutic margin (e.g. digoxin). First-pass metabolism may also be reduced, resulting in increased bioavailability. See Table 11.3 for other changes.

Table 11.3 Common age-related pharmacokinetic changes

Process	Age-related changes	Effect
Absorption	Gastric pH is higher because of a reduction in acid secretion, a decrease in gastric emptying, and a decrease in GI motility	These changes may lead to decreased absorption
Distribution	Total body water, proteins, and lean body mass decrease and total body fat increases	Lower body water may cause a reduced volume of distribution for polar drugs (e.g. aminoglycosides, digoxin)
		Increased fat stores may lead to a larger volume of distribution for lipid-soluble drugs (e.g. phenytoin, diazepam, flurazepam)
Metabolism	Hepatic oxidative pathways (phase 1) become less effective	May lead to reduced metabolism of drugs such as benzodiazepines
	Hepatic mass and blood flow are reduced—may be more important than enzyme activity	May lead to a reduced metabolism of many drugs in elderly people
Excretion	GFR is reduced and tubular function changes (Cockcroft–Gault calculation (Box 11.1)	This affects aminoglycosides, lithium, and digoxin; polar drug metabolites are excreted slowly, making patients more susceptible to nephrotoxic drugs

Box 11.1 The Cockcroft–Gault calculation

The Cockcroft–Gault calculation estimates renal function by estimating the creatinine clearance (CrCl) and therefore the residual renal function in patients with chronic renal failure:

estimated CrCl (men) =
{[140−age(years)] × weight(kg) × 1.23}/[serum creatinine (μmol/L)]

estimated CrCl (women) =
{[140−age(years)] × weight(kg) × 0.85}/[serum creatinine (μmol/L)]

Creatinine is influenced by intake of dietary protein, muscle mass, and activity. The inclusion of sex, age, and weight in the equation attempts to allow for this variation.

Improving prescribing for older people

The NSF sets out the following milestones to improve prescribing practice for this age group.

- Since 2002—all people over 75 years should normally have their medicines reviewed at least annually.
- Those taking more than four medicines should have a six-monthly review.
- All hospitals should have 'one-stop dispensing/dispensing for discharge' schemes where appropriate self-administration schemes for medicines for older people are available.
- Since 2004—every primary care trust should have schemes in place so that older people get more help from pharmacists in using their medicines.[1]

Beer's criteria, an American consensus guideline published in 1991 and updated in 2003,[2] provide a list of drugs that a panel of experts thought to be particularly problematic for older patients.

Further reading

Brack, G. and Franklin, P. (2007). Prescribing for older people. *Quarterly Journal of the Association for Nurse Prescribing*, **5**, 16–18.

1. Royal College of Physicians (2000). *Sentinel: Clinical audit of evidence based prescribing for older people*. RCP, London.
2. Fick D.M., Cooper, J.W., Wade, W.E., Waller, J.L., Maclean, J.R., and Beers, M.H. (2003). Updating the Beers criteria for potentially inappropriate medication use in older adults. *Archives of Internal Medicine*, **163**, 2716–24.

Prescribing for public health

Acheson defined public health as: 'the science and art of preventing disease, prolonging life and promoting health through the organised efforts of society'.[1] The umbrella term public health covers the following disciplines:

- health promotion;
- health education;
- health improvement;
- preventative medicine;
- social medicine;
- disease control;
- regulation of hygiene;
- environmental health;
- prevention of the transmission of communicable disease.

Prevention in public health involves the protection of communities from health risks that can be environmental, behavioural, social, or occupational. There is an implicit aim, as part of the public health agenda, to improve the health of the population through prevention of ill health and interventions to treat disease. Examples of public health interventions in relation to prescribing include:

- smoking cessation;
- sexual health screening;
- vaccinations;
- prescribing to prevent malaria;
- prescribing for the prevention of acute disease.

1. Department of Health (1998). *Report of the Independent Inquiry into Inequalities in Health (Acheson Report)*. TSO, London.

The determinants of health

These are the living conditions that influence a person's or society's life-style and choices.[1] Determinants of health are interrelated; for example, a person's ability to attain a standard of health and well-being is influenced by their genetic make-up, their socio-economic situation, and their lifestyle choices made as a consequence of their social setting. However, determinants can be categorized into social, biological, and wider determinants.

Social determinants of health
- Diet
- Exercise
- Sexual behaviour
- Use of recreational drugs
- Alcohol usage
- Smoking.

Biological determinants
- Communicable infectious diseases that have the potential to spread from one person or species to another (e.g. influenza).
- Biological/environmental hazards (e.g. pollution, weather conditions, and hazardous substances).

Some wider determinants of health
- Housing
- Employment status
- Transport
- Education
- Environment
- Income
- Social class
- Ethnic origin
- Living with the threat of terrorism or war.

The NHS Plan[2] set the template for modernization and improvement and for the standardization of high-quality public health intervention.

Prevention of chronic/long-term condition

Smoking cessation advice has proved to be one of the most economical and effective public health interventions for the prevention of many long-term conditions. The latest version of the BNF has a list of products that can be prescribed to support this intervention. 📖 Nicotine replacement therapy as an aid to smoking cessation, p. 365.

1. Wilkinson, R. and Marmot, M. (eds) (2003). *Social determinants of health: the solid facts* (2nd edn). World Health Organization, Copenhagen.
2. Department of Health (2000). *The National Health Service Plan*. TSO, London.

Policy drivers for public health

National Service Frameworks (NSFs)

As a result of a concerted strategic effort to improve the health of the population and reduce inequalities in health in the last 10 years, governments in England, Scotland, and Wales have produced a set of standards known as National Service Frameworks (NSFs). These are based on best available evidence.

The 10 year rolling programme of NSFs covers:

- children, young people, and maternity services;
- long-term conditions;
- diabetes;
- older people;
- mental health;
- paediatric intensive care;
- cancer;
- coronary heart disease;
- chronic obstructive pulmonary disease;
- renal services.

National Institute for Health and Clinical Excellence (NICE)[1]

The National Institute for Health and Clinical Excellence (NICE) formulates national guidelines for best evidenced-based health care practice. These guidelines inform the NSFs.

Opportunities for prescribing and public health

- Greater patient choice[2]
- Patient empowerment
- Reduced waiting times
- Improvements in local hospitals and surgeries[3]
- Introduction of national standards
- Demarcation professional roles.

Immunization as a means of disease prevention

The latest version of the BNF has an up-to-date list of vaccinations which can be prescribed to prevent disease. Information regarding vaccination can be obtained on line at ▣ http://www.dh.gov.uk/en/Publichealth/Healthprotection/Immunization/Greenbook/DH_4097254 (accessed 24 June 2010).
▣ Immune response, pp. 310–313.

1. National Institute for Health and Clinical Excellence (NICE). ▣ http://www.nice.org.uk/
2. Department of Health (2008). *Making connections: using healthcare professionals as prescribers to deliver organisational improvements.* ▣ http://www.dh.gov.uk/en/Publicationsandstatistics/Publications/PublicationsPolicyAndGuidance/DH_084514. (accessed 17 July 2009).
3. *Health Service Journal* in association with the Department of Health (2009). Ambition, action, achievement. How to deliver quality care closer to the patient. *Health Service Journal Supplement,* 9 July 2009, 1–9. ▣ http://hsj.co.uk (accessed 17 July 2009).

Over-prescribing of antibiotics

There is considerable concern about the over-prescribing of antibiotics for the treatment of self-limiting conditions. The Standing Medical Advisory Committee (SMAC) Subgroup on Antimicrobial Resistance[1] sought to reduce antibiotic usage and to promote international cooperation and consensus on the prescribing of antimicrobial drugs.

Antibiotic use has been demonstrated to:
• select for bacterial resistance which spreads from one bacterium to another;
• lengthen the patient's stay in hospital.

In the late 1990s hospital prescribing accounted for 20% of prescribing of antimicrobial agents. However, NICE notes that antibiotic prescribing has now reached its plateau.[2]

As a result of the increase in bacterial resistance to antimicrobial drugs, antibiotics are becoming less effective in the treatment of bacterial infections. There is mounting concern about the increasing resistance to antimicrobial agents of organisms such as *Mycobacterium tuberculosis*, *Streptococcus* and *Neisseria gonorrhoeae*. The over-prescribing of antibiotics for such conditions has led to antimicrobial resistance and an increased threat of adverse drug reactions. Hospital-acquired infections such as strains of *Staphylococcus aureus*, *Clostridium difficile*, and *Pseudomonas aeruginosa* are resistant to all antimicrobial agents.[3] Community-acquired resistance is a concern. Resistance to antifungal and antiviral agents is also developing. The Health Act 2006 introduced a code of practice for the prevention and control of health-care associated infections.[4]

Responsibilities of the non-medical prescriber when prescribing for infectious disease
• Resist pressure to prescribe antibiotics unnecessarily.
• Educate the public to change their expectations.
• The 1998 SMAC recommendations[1] are still relevant. They have been expanded by NICE[2] and CKS[5] and include:
  • no prescribing of antibiotics for simple coughs and colds;
  • no prescribing of antibiotics for viral sore throats;
  • limit prescribing for uncomplicated cystitis to 3 days in otherwise fit women;
  • limit prescribing of antibiotics over the telephone to exceptional cases.

Other factors which influence antimicrobial resistance
• Hygiene.
• Infection control and cross infection.
• Veterinary and agricultural use.
• Industrial use.

Further recommendations[6]
• Adherence to and harmonization between national and local prescribing evidence-based guidelines.
• International cooperation.

- Surveillance of resistance.
- Research.
- Education.
- Hygiene, infection controls, and limitation of cross-infection.

📖 Prescribing and sexual health, pp. 381–398.
📖 Prescribing for infections, pp. 309–316.
📖 Substance misuse and dependency, pp. 361–368.

Further reading

British National Formulary (latest edn). British Medical Association and Royal Pharmaceutical.
SIGN Clinical Guideline 88 (2006). *Management of suspected bacterial urinary tract infections in adults: a national clinical guideline.* Scottish Intercollegiate Guidelines Network.

1. Department of Health, Standing Medical Advisory Committee (1998). *Report of Subgroup on Antimicrobial Resistance.* TSO, London.
2. NICE (2008). *Respiratory tract infections: antibiotic prescribing. Prescribing of antibiotics for self-limiting respiratory tract infections in adults and children in primary care.* 🖳 http://www.nice.org.uk/ (accessed 20 September 2009).
3. Department of Health (2003). *Winning ways: working together to reduce healthcare associated infection in England.* TSO, London.
4. Department of Health (2006). *Health Act 2006. Code of practice for the prevention and control of health care associated infections.* Department of Health, London.
🖳 www.dh.gov.uk/PublicationsAndStatistics/Publications/PublicationsPolicyAndGuidance/ PublicationsPolicyAndGuidanceArticle/fs/en?CONTENT_ID=4139336&chk=6oAPfi (accessed 15 March 2007).
5. 🖳 www.cks.nhs.uk/
6. *British National Formulary* (latest edn). British Medical Association and Royal Pharmaceutical Society of Great Britain.

Prescribing for neonates (birth to 1 month)

The evidence for some treatments used for the neonatal population is conflicting and continuously developing. In addition, the wide use of unlicensed drugs heightens the hazards of prescribing for neonates.[1] Therefore non-medical prescribers prescribing for the neonatal population must be vigilant and use contemporaneous research findings as the basis for clinical prescribing decisions.

Historically, nursing staff in neonatal units guided and directed junior doctors in prescribing decisions for the neonates in their care. This 'proxy' prescribing accepted by doctors is not acceptable when non-medical prescribers undertake prescribing for the neonatal population.

Factors affecting drug disposition in neonates

Oral absorption
• GI contents
• Gastric emptying time is prolonged
• Increased gastric pH
• GI contents, posture, disease states, and therapeutic interventions, such as other drug therapy, can affect absorption.

Distribution
• Neonates require higher doses of water-soluble drugs on a mg/kg basis than adults because of their increased total body water (85% compared with 60% in young adults).
• The low serum albumin level decreases plasma protein binding.
• The high circulating bilirubin level potentially displaces drugs from albumin.

Metabolism
• Enzyme systems mature at different times and may be absent at birth, or present in considerably reduced amounts.
• Altered metabolic pathways may exist for some drugs.
• Metabolic rate increases dramatically in children and is often greater than that in adults.
• Compared with adults, children may require more frequent dosing or higher doses on a mg/kg basis.

Excretion
• Many sick neonates requiring intensive care will receive polypharmacy and may have poor renal function, thus increasing the half-life of many drugs and potentially causing toxicity. Remember that babies born prematurely will have less developed ability to excrete medicines and doses must be adjusted to reflect their stage of development (Table 11.4).

1. Conroy, S. and McIntyre, J. (2005) The use of unlicensed and off-label medicines in the neonate. *Seminars in Fetal and Neonatal Medicine*, **10**, 115–22.

Table 11.4 Drug clearance in premature babies

Post-conceptual age (compared with adults)	Clearance of drug
5%	24–28 weeks
10%	28–4 weeks
33%	34–40 weeks
50%	40–44 weeks

Immunizations
- Vaccinations should be administered as per the schedule in preterm neonates, which is at 2, 3, and 4 months of age.

Drug licensing:
- Many drugs are not specifically licensed for use in neonates and are used 'off-label'.

Information is available at ▣ www.medicines.org.

Concordance
- Non-medical prescribers must consider and respect the role of family members, carers, and advocates in prescribing decisions, resulting in shared decision-making for the baby as he/she is unable to participate actively in such decisions. Clearly document all conversations in patient's notes.

Prescription writing
- Calculate drug on baby's birthweight until this has been regained.
- Re-prescribe drugs on current weekly weight, especially for chronic conditions.
- Suitable formulations may not be available to allow precise dosing.
- Do not prescribe oral drugs to be added to milk feeds as it affects the osmolality.

Prescribing for children

Safety

Pharmacokinetics and pharmacodynamics are often different for children compared with adults and this can have surprising effects on the absorption, distribution, and metabolism of certain drugs. Refer to the *BNF for Children* (BNFC)[1] which provides advice on prescribing, dispensing, supply, administration, and monitoring for medicines for children of all ages. The NMC set the standards for non-medical prescribing and they state that it is crucial for prescribers to:

> *recognise the unique implications and developmental context of the anatomical and physiological differences between children, neonates and young people.*[2]

In addition they stipulate the following learning outcome that must be achieved in order to attain the recordable qualification of independent and supplementary prescriber.

> *Only nurses with relevant knowledge, competence and skills in nursing children should prescribe for children. This is particularly important in primary care (e.g out of hours, walk in clinics and general practice settings). Anyone prescribing for a child in these situations must be able to demonstrate competence to prescribe for children and refer to another prescriber when working outside of their area of expertise or level of competence.*[3]

And:

> *It is the responsibility of the employer to ensure that the registrant is able to apply prescribing principles to their own area of practice.*[3]

NB: never prescribe for children unless you are competent to do so.

📖 Basic principles of pharmacology, pp. 53–64.

📖 Seven principles of safe prescribing, p. 94.

📖 NMC and HPC codes, p. 20.

Key points

- Be extra vigilant when prescribing for neonates (babies under 30 days old).
- Allow for developmental differences in children of the same age.
- Calculate drug dosages with care.
- Absorption in the stomach in children under 2 years of age is different from that in older children and adults.
- Report all adverse drug reactions using the Yellow Card Scheme.
- Do not add the drug to the child's feed (there may be an interaction or the child might not complete their feed).
- In some cases children may require higher doses than adults because they have higher metabolic rates.
- Follow the BNF for Children (BNFC)[1] for frequency and duration of administration of medicines, especially in the case of potentially toxic drugs.

📖 Adverse drug reactions (ADRs), p. 68.

Calculating drug dosages in children

Doses are generally calculated using the child's body weight in kilograms.[2]

Age ranges for calculating drug doses[1]

- First month (neonates)
- Up to a year of age (infants)
- 1–5 years
- 6–12 years (BNFC).

NB: with obese children, calculate dosage on the basis of ideal height and weight for age. Greater accuracy in drug calculation can be achieved using body surface area (Box 11.2).

📖 Consent, p. 140

Box 11.2 Drug calculation

Formula to calculate surface area:
Surface area of patient (m^2) × adult dose/1.8

Formula to calculate drug dosage
(What you want/what you've got) x what it is in

Example

Drug A contains 500mg in 5mL. To give 600mg:
  (600/500) x 5 = 6mL.

📖 Prescribing and the law, p. 134

1. *British National Formulary for Children* (latest edn). British Medical Association and Royal Pharmaceutical Society of Great Britain, London.
2. Nursing and Midwifery Council (2007). *Prescribing for Children and Young People* 🖳 http://www. nmc-uk.org/aDisplayDocument.aspx?documentID=3431 (accessed 20 September 2009)
3. Nursing and Midwifery Council (2006) *Standards of proficiency for nurse and midwife prescribers.* NMC, London.

Achieving concordance when prescribing for children

Where appropriate (depending on the child's age, capacity and your assessment of their competence) involve the parent/carer.

Writing the prescription

Follow the guidelines in the BNFC (latest edition):[1]
- It is a legal requirement to write the child's age for children under 12 years.
- Always state the strengths and formulation of the medication (e.g. capsules, liquid or tablets).

NB: the prescriber is responsible for making sure that the parent/carer understands the instructions on the prescription and that, if they are an inpatient, the drugs are given as prescribed.

📖 Writing a prescription 1, p. 114

Advice for parents:

- Make sure that you follow the prescriber's instructions.
- Do not dilute the drug in the child's milk/water or add the drug to the child's food unless you are instructed to do so by the prescriber:
  - diluting the drug may lead to the child receiving a suboptimal dose if he/she does not complete the feed;
  - some drugs may interact with food or milk.
- Dispense the medicine using the device you have been provided with (e.g. a syringe or spoon).
- Keep all medicines out of reach of children.

NB: all drugs must be dispensed in a reclosable child-resistant container.

Prescribing for rare conditions

For prescribing for rare paediatric conditions see 'Prescribing for children' in the latest edition of the BNFC.[1]

Licensing

- Many medicines essential for treating childhood conditions are not licensed.
- Unlicensed medication can be prescribed by a supplementary prescriber as part of a clinical management plan (CMP) and by an independent prescriber provided there is a strong rationale for doing so.
- A nurse or pharmacist independent prescriber can prescribe outside of product license (off-label) if, for example, a medicine is licensed for use in adults but not in children.
- Useful information regarding the prescribing of unlicensed and off-label medication for children can be found in the latest edition of the BNFC.[1]

Crushing tablets

Crushing tablets alters the nature of the drug and makes it an unlicensed product. Therefore it is not recommended. The NMC states that:

> *The mechanics of crushing medicines may alter their therapeutic properties rendering them ineffective and not covered by their product license. Medicinal products should not routinely be crushed unless a pharmacist advises that the medication is not compromised by crushing, and crushing has been determined to be within the patient's best interest.*[2]

Disguising medication

The NMC do not consider disguising medication, and therefore deceiving the patient, to be good practice.

NB: regarding the administration of medicines, the prescriber is account-able for all directions they give to parents and others.[2]

1. *British National Formulary for Children* (latest edn). British Medical Association and Royal Pharmaceutical Society of Great Britain, London.
2. Nursing and Midwifery Council (2007). *Standards for medicines management.* NMC, London.

Prescribing for people with renal disease

Chronic kidney disease (CKD) is common, frequently undiagnosed, and often found with other pre-existing conditions, such as cardiovascular disease and diabetes.

NICE[1] has noted that on average 30% of people with advanced kidney disease remain undiagnosed or are diagnosed late. If untreated, CKD has a high risk of mortality. However, there is evidence that treatment can:
• prevent or delay the progression of CKD;
• reduce or prevent the development of complications;
• reduce the risk of cardiovascular disease.

The following conditions carry high risk factors for CKD.
• Diabetes
• Hypertension
• Cardiovascular disease:
  • ischaemic heart disease;
  • chronic heart failure;
  • peripheral vascular disease;
  • cerebral vascular disease.
• Structural renal tract disease
• Renal calculi or prostatic hypertrophy
• Multisystem diseases with potential kidney involvement (e.g. systemic lupus).
• A family history of stage 5 CKD (see below)
• Hereditary kidney disease
• Haematuria or proteinuria.

Pharmacokinetic considerations

Prescribing for people with renal impairment requires careful consideration as the metabolism of the drug may be altered.
• Drugs and their metabolites may not be excreted quickly enough to avoid toxicity (e.g. opioids and some antibiotics).
• Renal impairment may be made worse:
  • for example, patients who are prescribed NSAIDs may suffer increased sodium and water retention and further deterioration of renal function.
• Some drugs (e.g. potassium-sparing diuretics, ACE inhibitors, and NSAIDs) may cause hyperkalemia.
• Sensitivity to some drugs may be increased.
• Reduction of renal function, often present in older people, may affect the efficacy of some drugs.[1]

For further information, refer to the relevant appendix in the latest edition of the BNF.

Classification of chronic kidney disease (CKD)

NICE[1] has described the following stages of CKD which have superseded the three stages adopted in the NSF for renal services.

- Stage 1: estimated glomerular filtration rate (eGFR) 90mL/min—those with normal or increased GFR with other evidence of kidney damage.
- Stage 2: eGFR 60–89mL/min—those with slightly decreased GFR with other evidence of kidney damage.
- Stage 3A: eGFR 45–59mL/min—those with moderate decrease in GFR with or without other evidence of kidney damage.
- Stage 3B: eGFR 30–44mL/min—as for stage 3A.
- Stage 4: eGFR 15–29mL/min–those with a severe decrease in GFR with or without other evidence of kidney damage.
- Stage 5: eGFR <15mL/min—those with established renal failure.

Box 11.3 Normal values

GFR 100ml/min
Creatinine 70–150µmol/L

Additional information
The latest edition of the BNF will carry a table of drugs to be avoided or used with caution in renal impairment.

📖 Prescribing for older people, p. 198.

Further reading
Bardsley, A. (2003). Urinary tract infections: prevention and treatment of a common problem. *Nurse Prescribing*, **1**, 113–17.
Begg, E.J. (2003). *Instant clinical pharmacology*. Blackwell, Oxford.
Dunning, T. (2003) *Care of people with diabetes* (2nd edn). Blackwell, Oxford.
O'Callaghan, C. and Brenner, M. (2000). *The kidney at a glance*. Blackwell Science, Oxford.
Smith, T. and Thomas, N. (2002). *Renal nursing*. Ballière and Tindall, London.
Thomas, N. (ed.) (2004). *Advanced renal care*. Blackwell, Oxford.

1. NICE (2008). *Chronic kidney disease: Early identification and management of chronic kidney disease in adults in primary and secondary care*. NICE, London.
2. Department of Health (1998). *Health Survey for England*, Vol 1: *Findings*.TSO, London. Cited in Department of Health (2001). *Medicines and Older people*. TSO, London. 🖳 http://www.doh.gov.uk/nsf/medicinesop (accessed 5 May 2010).

Non-medical prescribing in mental health and learning disabilities

History and development

Non-medical prescribing in mental health arrived late. As recently as 2004 there were only around 300 qualified non-medical prescribers, mostly in three trusts.[1] Since then coverage has widened. Whilst non-medical prescribing in mental health and learning disabilities services is widely viewed as beneficial, it also presents a challenge to the existing balance of inter-disciplinary working and requires a team approach to implementation.[2,3]

The Department of Health expects that non-medical prescribing will ensure better use of existing skills and lead to efficiency gains.[4] It is linked to a wider initiative aimed at ensuring that mental health nurses use their skills to focus on those with the greatest need,[5] including introducing the new nursing role of advanced practitioner.[6]

Mental health professionals play a key role in multidisciplinary teams, having frequent and prolonged contact with users of the service.[3] It is also established practice that many mental health nurses already act as informal or 'proxy' prescribers,[1] making non-medical prescribing a safer and more robust alternative.[7]

Benefits

How non-medical prescribing is implemented depends on the service area. For example, supplementary prescribing is proving successful in Assertive Outreach[7] because it is suitable for the smaller caseloads; allows controlled drugs to be prescribed (through a CMP), and supports the management of complex cases. In other areas, such as specialist clinics, independent prescribing is considered the more appropriate option.[8]

Some of the key emerging benefits

- Quicker access to medication in the community.[7,9]
- More appropriate use of staff time.[7]
- CMPs can form an advance directive for medicines.
- Increased focus on physical health monitoring.[10]
- CMPs lead to improved documentation and audit trail.
- Improved management of as required medication.
- CMPs can form part of a more holistic approach to care.[9,10]
- Greater choice of medication.[10,11]
- Successful when linked to service development, and improved multi-disciplinary working.[7,9,11,12]
- Improved career prospects for prescribers.[11]
- Development of nurse-led clinics and services.
- Increased discontinuation of medicines no longer needed, through access to timely medicines reviews.[9,11]

Developing and supporting the role

Successful approaches include Peer Supervision Groups,[13] the use of workbooks,[14] and preceptorship pathways.[15] As roles for independent prescribers are being defined and built in to service plans, a need for further training on diagnostic assessment and neuropharmacology[16] has been identified. Many organizations are also developing interdisciplinary prescribing governance frameworks,[15] strategies, and policies.

1. Nolan P., Bradley, E., and Carr, N. (2004). Nurse prescribing and the enhancement of mental health services. *Nurse Prescriber*, **1**, 1–9.
2. Avery, A.J. and Pringle, M. (2005). Extended prescribing for nurses and pharmacists. *British Medical Journal*, **331**, 1154–5.
3. Gournay, K. and Gray, R. (2000). *Should mental health nurses prescribe?* Maudsley Discussion Paper No.11, Health Service Research Department, Institute of Psychiatry, London.
4. Department of Health (2005). *Improving mental health services by extending the role of nurses in prescribing and supplying medicines: good practice guide*. TSO, London.
5. Department of Health (2006). *From values to action: The Chief Nursing Officer's review of mental health nursing*. TSO, London.
6. Department of Health (2007) *Mental health: new ways of working for everyone*. TSO, London.
7. Turner, S. (2007). Non-medical prescribing in community mental health settings. *Mental Health Practice*, **11**, 29–32.
8. Jones, A. (2008). Exploring independent nurse prescribing for mental health settings. *Journal of Psychiatric and Mental Health Nursing*, **15**, 109–17.
9. Bradley, E., Wain, P., and Nolan, P. (2008). Putting mental health nurse prescribing into practice. *Nurse Prescribing*, **6**, 15–19.
10. Jones, M. and Gray, R. (2008). Time to wake up and smell the coffee: anti-psychotic medication and schizophrenia. *Journal of Psychiatric and Mental Health Nursing*, **15**, 344–8.
11. Green, B. and Coutney, H. (2008). Evaluating the investment: a survey of non-medical prescribing. *Mental Health Practice*, **12**, 28–32.
12. Latter, S., Maben, J., Myall, M., et al. (2005) *An evaluation of Extended Formulary independent nurse prescribing: executive summary*. University of Southampton School of Nursing and Midwifery on behalf of Department of Health.
13. Turner, S. (2008). Peer support in non-medical prescribing. *Association for Nurse Prescribing Journal*, **4**, 12–13.
14. Provan, V., Bennett, S, and Smith, E. (2007). Non medical prescribing workbook. Cumbria Partnership and North Cumbria Acute Hospitals NHS Trust ⬚ www.cumbriapct.nhs.uk/medicinesmanagement/NonMedicalPrescribingAndPGDs/nmp%20workbook.pdf (accessed 30 December 2008)
15. Jones, M. (2008). Nurse prescribing in mental health: a person-centred approach. *Nursing Standard* **22** (52), 35–38.
16. Skingsley, D., Bradley, E.J., and Nolan, P. (2006). Neuropharmacology and mental health nurse prescribers. *Journal of Clinical Nursing*, **15**, 989–97.

Prescribing in pregnancy

Physiological changes

Prescribing drugs in pregnancy can have an effect on both the mother and the fetus. Most drugs can cross the placental barrier which has a lipid barrier, meaning that lipophilic drugs cross the placenta more slowly and hydrophilic drugs cross it more easily. The many complex physiological changes that occur in the mother during pregnancy may have an effect on pharmacokinetics, and absorption, distribution, metabolism, and elimination can be affected. The dose prescribed might be affected by any or all of the above[1]. The general principle is only to prescribe if absolutely necessary after having fully assessed the patient and considered the need to prescribe. Only prescribe if competent.

Risk versus benefit

Drugs can harm the fetus throughout the gestational period. Because of the obvious risks, there is very little experimental research data on prescribing for pregnant women.

When considering whether to prescribe for a pregnant woman, the prescriber must always consider the risk–benefit ratio. Drugs are almost never tested on pregnant women.

Safe practice

- Only prescribe for pregnant women when it is essential.
- Counsel the mother on the risk versus benefit of prescribing.
- Where possible, avoid prescribing for pregnant women during the first trimester.
- Prescribe drugs that have been tried and tested as safe in pregnancy.

Teratogenic effects (harm to the fetus)

Because of the obvious risks to the fetus, and sometimes to the mother, there is very little experimental research data on prescribing for pregnant women[1]. Drugs that cross the placenta can harm the fetus throughout the gestational period, and their effects depend on the compounds in the drug and the gestational age of the fetus. Specific effects are complex and outside the scope of this book.

Appendix 4 in the latest edition of the BNF[2] provides an up-to-date table of the drugs that should be avoided, and at which trimester, during pregnancy.

First trimester

The greatest risk of the occurrence of congenital malformation is during the first trimester and between 3 and 11 weeks. When possible, avoid prescribing during this period.

Second and third trimesters

Drugs administered to the mother at these stages may have toxic effects on fetal tissue and may affect fetal growth.

Immediately before, during, and after labour

Drugs administered to the mother at this time may adversely affect the fetus and may have an effect on the duration and outcome of labour. They may also affect the new born baby. The National Teratology Service (UK Tel. 0191-232-1525) provides information for health professionals concerning poisoning and chemical exposures in pregnancy.

Drugs that are easily transported across the placenta include:

- narcotics;
- steroids;
- antibiotics;
- anaesthetics.

Risks versus benefits for epilepsy

- Anticonvulsants can cause congential abnormalities.
- Convulsions can cause fetal mortality or morbidity.

To manage epilepsy in pregnancy, give the lowest effective dose and monitor drug levels closely.

1. Warrell, D.A., Cox, T.M., Firth, J.D., and Benz, E.J., Jr (2005). *Oxford Textbook of Medicine* (4th edn). Oxford University Press, Oxford.
2. *British National Formulary* (latest edn). British Medical Association and Royal Pharmaceutical Society of Great Britain, London.

Prescribing for breastfeeding women

When considering prescribing for women who are breastfeeding remember that generally the advantages of breastfeeding outweigh the disadvantages. The risk–benefit ratio for the infant needs to be carefully considered when administering drugs to breastfeeding mothers. However, as drugs are only secreted in breast milk in small volumes, the benefits of breastfeeding generally outweigh the risks to the infant. Women should be advised to take drugs only if necessary; where possible, drug therapy should be delayed until the mother has completed breastfeeding. Always use the prescribing pyramid and apply the principles of good prescribing.[1] For breastfeeding patients, recommend or prescribe medication for necessity only.

- Consider the patient.
  - Is it appropriate to prescribe?
  - Can you give lifestyle/health promotion advice instead?
- If not, consider the product.
  - Is it safe?
  - Is it indicated for use for breastfeeding women?
  - Is it cautioned for use when breastfeeding?
  - Remember to ask the client about any OTC drugs she is taking.

For interactions and cautions and contraindications see Appendix 5 in the BNF (latest edition).[2]

- Many drugs are lipid soluble. Therefore the amount of drug which is secreted in breast milk depends to a greater or lesser extent on its lipid solubility.
- However, in many cases only small amounts of the drug are excreted in breast milk.
- Very few drugs are licensed for prescribing for breastfeeding.
- Remember that in some cases it is essential for the mother to continue with medication, e.g. prescribing for epilepsy, depression, and many chronic diseases.
- Some medication dosage may need to be adjusted to account for breastfeeding women.

Prescribing for mild to moderate pain while breastfeeding

Paracetamol is the drug of choice for mild to moderate pain. Some analgesic drugs pass less easily into breast milk than others. For instance, in the case of simple analgesia it is advisable for the breastfeeding mother to take paracetamol rather than aspirin which can pass into breast milk and the breastfeeding infant, causing a risk of Reye's syndrome in the baby.

Route of administration

- Drugs which do not undergo first-pass metabolism (intravenous drugs) pass to the infant in higher concentrations.
- Inhaled drugs have less tendency to pass into breast milk than oral drugs.

Volume of breast milk/drug concentration
- Production of breast milk is stimulated as a response to infant feeding.
- The concentration and amount of drug which is consumed by the infant is proportional to the volume of the baby's feed.

Time of administration
- It is advisable to take drugs immediately after feeding in order to maximize the length of time between taking the drug and the next feed.
- Drugs to be taken only once a day can be taken before the baby's longest sleep time.

Maturity of infant
- The baby has normal renal clearance by 3 days after birth.
- The maturation rate of liver enzymes can vary and some may take up to a year to mature.
- Caution needs to be exercised when administering liver enzyme inducers or liver enzyme inhibitors to the mother.

Molecular density/molecular weight
- Drugs with a high molecular weight and large plasma proteins can pass into breast milk for up to 1 week after birth.
- After 1 week only drugs with a low molecular weight can pass into breast milk.
- Drugs with a high molecular weight include heparin and insulin.

Plasma protein binding
- Plasma proteins which bind to drugs only pass into the breast milk in small amounts.
- Phenytoin is highly plasma protein bound.

Lipid solubility
- Drugs which are lipid soluble pass easily into breast milk.
- Diazepam is highly lipid soluble.

pH
- The pH of breast milk is 7.2 (neutral).
- Drugs with weak bases (slightly alkaline) have increased lipid solubility and pass more easily into breast milk.
- Drugs with weak bases include erythromycin and antihistamines.
- Weak bases can become ionized by an acid pH, leading to increased concentration of such drugs in the breast milk.

📖 Prescribing for children, p. 212.

Further reading

Banta-Wright, S.A. (1997). Minimising infant exposure to and risks from medications while breastfeeding. *Journal of Perinatal and Neonatal Nursing* **11**, 71–4.

Lawrence, R.A., and Lawrence, R.M. (2005). *Breastfeeding: a guide for the medical profession* (6th edn). Elsevier Mosby, Philadelphia, PA.

1. National Prescribing Centre (1999). The principles of prescribing. *Nurse Prescribing Bulletin*, N. 1. NPC, Liverpool.

2. *British National Formulary* (latest edn). British Medical Association and Royal Pharmaceutical Society of Great Britain.

Medical conditions

Prescribing for musculoskeletal conditions

Brief anatomy and physiology of the musculoskeletal structure

The musculoskeletal structure comprises:
• bones;
• muscles;
• joints.

Bones

Functions
• Provide framework for protection of the internal organs of the body.
• Enable movement.
• Store minerals and salts.

Structure
• 30% water.
• Soft and flexible:
• Three layers:
  • hard outer shell—compact bone, comprised of tiny cylindrical units called the Haversian system. The Haversian system provides strength as each cylinder lies orientated to the greatest stress for the bone, i.e. lies lengthways in the shaft of the femur;
  • inner—spongy, trabecular, or cancellous bone;
  • bone marrow—soft jellylike substance that lies centrally;
  • blood supply to bring nutrients.
• Nerve supply to enable sensory detection.

Skeletal muscles (striped/striated)

Functions
• Work in pairs one either side of a bone to facilitate movement.
• Work in groups, some relaxing and some contracting, to take the strain of complex movements—maintenance of position and body posture.

Structure
• Over 600 skeletal muscles in the body.
• Arranged in bundles with the cells forming a striped pattern.
• Under conscious control—voluntary muscles.

Joints

Functions
• Provide a framework.
• Provide an interface between two bones.

Structure
• Bones are linked to each other by ligaments to form a joint.
• Can be fibrous (skull), cartilaginous (vertebrae), or synovial (knee).

Movement

This is achieved through a series of levers. A lever is a way of moving a load by the application of pressure. The body has three main types of lever.

First-order lever (e.g. moving the head)

The fulcrum (pivoting point) of the lever is positioned between the load (skull and contents) and the effort (muscular contractions/relaxations of the neck muscles).

Second-order lever (e.g. standing on tiptoe)

The load (the body) is placed between the fulcrum and the effort (calf and foot muscle activity).

Third-order lever (e.g. bending the elbow)

The three-way effort (forearm muscular activity) is between the load (the hand and contents) and the fulcrum.

Soft tissue injuries

Sprains

Definition
Overstretching and tearing of ligaments, varying in severity from minor sparse fibrous tears to disruption of a complete ligament complex.

Signs and symptoms
- Pain
- Tenderness
- Soft tissue swelling.

Treatment of minor sprains
- Ice.
- Elevate.
- Compression with an elastic support or strapping.
- Progressive mobilization as symptoms allow.
- Pain relief such as paracetamol or NSAIDs.
- If inflammation is persistent a cortisone injection may be indicated.
- If a sprain has caused complete rupture of the ligaments associated with joint instability, surgery may be indicated.

Strains

Definition
Grade 1 and 2 strains involve torn muscle fibres but intact muscle sheaths. Grade 3 involves a partial rupture of the muscle sheath and Grade 4 is a complete muscle rupture.

Signs and symptoms
As sprains.

Treatment
- Grades 1 and 2 as sprains.
- Grades 3 and 4 may require surgery.

Minor contusions

Definition
Superficial soft tissue swelling and localized pain caused by a direct impact.

Signs and symptoms
As sprains.

Treatment
- Ice
- Analgesia
- Early mobilization.

Haematoma

Definition

An accumulation of blood resulting from a traumatic disruption of vascular structures within the bone, muscle, or soft tissues.

Signs and symptoms

As sprains.

Treatment

- Compression dressings
- Ice
- Massage
- Because of a risk of infection, if persistent may require surgical draining.

Skeletal muscular spasm in palliative care

Definition
A muscle spasm of long or short duration may arise in muscles close to bone metastasis, be drug induced, or caused by damage to nerve pathways.

Signs and symptoms
Painful and prolonged involuntary muscle contraction.

Treatment:
- Skeletal muscle relaxants
- Massage
- Relaxation techniques.

📖 Basic principles of pharmacology, pp. 53–64.
📖 History-taking, p. 174.
📖 Physical examination, p. 178.

Further reading:
Davies A. (ed.) (2007) *Cancer-related bone pain*. Oxford University Press: Oxford
Dean, M., Harris, J.D., Regnard, C., and Hockley, J. (2006). *A guide to symptom relief in palliative care* (5th edn). Radcliffe Medical Press, Abingdon.

Acute uncomplicated low back pain

Definition
Pain experienced in the back involving the lumbar, lumbar sacral, and sacroiliac areas.

Causes
Strain to the muscles or tendons caused by overuse or abnormal stress and exercise.

Assessment:
- History
- Age
- Sex
- Medical conditions
- Employment
- Exact nature of any injury
- Duration, position, and type of pain—is it radiating?
- Any unaccustomed activity?
- Has the patient had this before?
- If so when, and how often?
- What have they taken in the past which has worked?
- Have they tried anything to date?
- What is the impact of the symptoms?
- Stress
- Other symptoms.

Signs and symptoms
- Patient generally between 20 and 55 years old.
- Pain in the lumbar–sacral region, buttocks, and thighs.
- Pain of a mechanical type.

Treatment
- Pain relief: analgesia and/or NSAIDs.
- Advise to keep to normal activity.
- If symptoms are severe, prescribe muscle relaxants.
- Seek advice if limb numbness or weakness, or if any new bladder or bowel problems occur (Table 12.1).

📖 Basic principles of pharmacology, pp. 53–64
📖 History-taking, p. 174
📖 Physical examination, p. 178.

Table 12.1 Back pain which may be significant of more serious conditions

Additional symptoms	Possible diagnosis	Possible cause
Difficulty in passing urine	Cauda equine syndrome	Herniated lumbar discs
Loss of anal sphincter tone		Tumours: metastases, spinal tumours
Faecal incontinence		Trauma
Numbness around the anus, perineum, or genitalia		Spinal stenosis
		Infection including epidural abscess
Severe prolonged motor weakness		Congenital abnormalities
		Following spinal manipulation
		Later stages of ankylosing spondilitis
		Post-operative haematoma
		Inferior vena cava thrombosis
Unilateral leg pain which is more severe than the back pain	Nerve root pain	
Pain radiates to the foot and toes		
Pain is accompanied by numbness and paresthesia		
Pain is reduced by straight-leg raising, reflex, and sensory changes		

Acute uncomplicated neck pain

Definition

Pain caused by a sprain or persistent twisting of the neck.

Causes

Neck hyperextension as in whiplash.

History

- Any injury?
- When?
- Any visual disturbances?
- Any dizziness or tinnitus?
- Vertigo?
- Headache?
- Backache?
- Altered sensation?
- Lack of power?

Signs and symptoms

- Neck pain
- Stiffness.

Treatment

As for uncomplicated back pain.

📖 Basic principles of pharmacology, pp. 53–64
📖 History-taking, p. 174
📖 Physical examination, p. 178.

Prescribing for the circulatory system

A brief anatomy and physiology of the circulatory system

Blood flows around the body through a series of veins, venules, arteries, arterioles, and capillaries. The system comprises two circuits:
- systemic circulation—blood is transported from the heart around the body via the arteries and back to the heart via the veins;
- pulmonary circulation—blood is transported from the right ventricle of the heart into the lungs and back into the heart via the right atrium.

Veins
- Return deoxygenated blood to the right atrium of the heart.
- Contain approximately three-quarters of total blood volume.
- Take blood from the capillaries back to the heart.

Arteries
- Carry oxygenated blood away from the heart.
- Branch 15–20 times, reducing in size.
- Contain one-fifth of the blood volume.

Arterioles
- Small arteries.
- Arterioles lead into capillaries.

Capillaries
- Carry blood from the arterioles to the venules, facilitating the passage of oxygen and nutrients to surrounding tissues.
- Contain one-twentieth of the blood volume.
- Capillary walls consist of a single layer of endothelial cells.

The walls of arteries and veins are comprised of three layers of cells specific to their function (Table 12.2).

Table 12.2 Structure of the arteries

Name	Structure	Function
Tunica adventia	Outermost layer of vessel	Stability
	Generally thicker in veins than tunica media	Anchorage
	Forms a connective tissue sheath	
Tunica media	Involuntary muscle stimulated by involuntary nerve fibres	Alteration of lumen size
	Elastic fibres	
Tunica intima	Smooth endothelial cells	Lining and formation of valves and basement membrane

The venous system

Input mechanisms to enable the return of venous blood to the heart that comprise (Fig. 12.1):
* respiratory pump;
* venous pump;
* venous valves.

Respiratory pump

* On inhalation:
  * the thoracic cavity expands;
  * pressure is reduced (↓) in the pleural cavities;
  * air is pulled into the lungs;
  * simultaneously blood flows from the small veins in the abdominal cavity and lower body into the inferior vena cava and right atrium.
* On exhalation:
  * the thoracic cavity decreases in size;
  * pressure is increased (↑) in the pleural cavities;
  * air is forced out of the lungs;
  * venous blood is forced into the right atrium.

Venous pump

The venous system of the leg comprises:
* femoral, popliteal, and tibial deep veins, each encased in a tough muscle sheath;
* long and short saphenous veins and the superficial veins lie outside this sheath;
* short perforator veins connect through the sheath.

The pump works as follows:
* the weight of blood in the leg veins exerts ↑ pressure up to 90mmhg in the foot when standing still;
* this ↑ pressure is lower than that in the veins and capillaries;
* when standing and walking the calf muscles first contract becoming shorter and thicker;
* this compresses nearby blood vessels which move blood up towards the heart;
* calf muscles then relax, allowing vessels to refill;
* blood pools in the lower leg on standing still for a long time.

Venous valves

These are made from semilunar folds of endothelial tissue and form the valves present in the leg veins.
* The valves point in the direction of blood flow, allowing blood to flow in one direction only and preventing blood from flowing back to the capillaries.
* This compartmentalizes the vein, dividing the weight of blood evenly throughout it.
* Blood is then squeezed back towards the heart by the movement of skeletal muscle.
* Perforator connecting veins are important in this process.

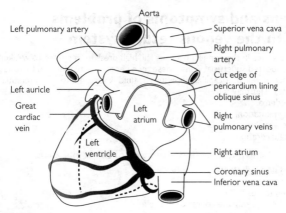

Fig. 12.1 The venous drainage of the heart—posterior view of heart.

Signs and symptoms of problems with the venous return system

If the valves in the connecting veins fail, high pressure is passed to weaker unsupported superficial veins. These then become distended and tortuous (varicose veins). If capillary pressure ↑, fluid is forced into the interstitial spaces. This may cause:

- oedema;
- pigmentation;
- eczema;
- leg ulceration.

Superficial phlebitis (inflammation of the vein walls)

Signs and symptoms

- Redness
- Tenderness
- Swelling along the course of the vein
- Fever
- Lymphangitis.

Treatment

- Heat
- NSAIDs
- Compression stockings (Table 12.3).

📖 Pain, p. 318.

Causes

Usually follows an injury to a vein followed by an inflammatory response.

Complications

Phlebitis can lead to venous thrombosis (a clot).

Table 12.3 Classes of compression hosiery prescribed in primary care

Class	Description of support	Pressure	Indications
Class I	Light	14–17mmHg at the ankle	Superficial varices
	Mild	≤80% of ankle pressure at calf	For use during pregnancy
		≤85% of calf pressure at mid thigh	
Class II	Medium	18–24mmHg at the ankle	Medium severe varices
	Moderate	≤70% of ankle pressure at calf	Ulcer treatment
		≤70% of calf pressure at mid thigh	Prevention of recurrence
			Mild oedema
			During pregnancy
Class III	Strong	25–35mmHg at the ankle	Gross varices
		≤70% of ankle pressure at calf	Post-thrombotic venous insufficiency
		≤70% of calf pressure at mid thigh	Gross oedema
			Ulcer treatment
			Prevention of recurrence

Problems with the venous return system: compression therapy

Compression therapy
- Graduated pressure from toe to base of knee
- Pressure highest at the ankle
- Pressure lowest at the knee.

Compression hosiery is one way of achieving this:
- below-knee or thigh-length socks, stockings, or tights which conform to the BSI made-to-measure standard sizes;
- stockings are classified according to pressure exerted at the ankle and the gradients at knee and thigh.

Types of hosiery
- Circular knit: nylon and cotton yarn—poor stretch.
- Flat bed knit: cotton, nylon, and nylon plated—greater stretch.
- Net stockings: seamed net fabric, one-way stretch—class I only.

Selection of compression hosiery
- Patient's age
- Dexterity or disability
- Skin condition
- Appearance of hosiery
- Type usually worn by patient (tights or stockings).

Measurement points for compression hosiery
Circumference
1. Top of thigh
2. Midpoint between 1 and 3
3. Knee at widest point
4. Base of knee
5. Widest calf circumference
6. Midpoint between 5 and 7
7. Ankle at narrowest point (2–4cm above ankle bone)
8. Widest point on foot for stocking to pass over
9. Toe base.

Length
1. Draw around patient's foot whilst they are standing on a piece of paper
2. Measurement from toe to back of heel
3. Measurement between each of the nine points above.

Fitting
- Turn stocking inside out at heel.
- Pull up two-handed with thumbs inserted in either side.
- Check heel is in correct position.
- Ease up over the leg.
- Check that there are no ridges or tight bands.
- Take off at night and apply first thing in the morning.

- Patients may need to start by wearing the stocking for a short time only.
- If the hosiery is effective in reducing oedema re-measure and re-prescribe.
- If unable to tolerate class III hosiery, try two pairs of class I hosiery worn at the same time.[1] Pressure is cumulative.

Advice on washing hosiery

- Handwash at 40°C
- Frequent washing improves shape
- Should provide pressure for 3–4 months.

Points to consider when prescribing:

- The quantity—single or pair?
- Article/style/type and any accessories.
- Compression class I, II, or III.
- Patient's measurements, if made to measure hosiery is required.
- Issues of concordance—no point in prescribing if hosiery is not going to be worn.

Contraindications

- Severe arteriosclerosis or other ischaemic vascular disease
- Skin lesions, allergies, or gangrene
- Recent vein ligation.

Further reading

RCN (1998) Clinical practice guidelines. *The management of patients with venous leg ulcers*. RCN, London.

▣ www.cks.nhs.uk/prescribing/compression_stockings/choice_of_compression_stockings_for_prevention (accessed 3 February 2010).

1. Fentern, P.H. (1986). Elastic hosiery. *Pharmacy Update*, **5**, 200–5.

Haemorrhoids (piles)

A common condition affecting about 50% of the population aged over 50 years.

Definition
Varices in the veins of the anorectal canal.

Causes
- Elevated venous pressure causes these vessels to stretch and dilate.
- Commonly, straining to pass a stool when constipated.
- Pregnancy.[1]
- Ageing.[2]
- Hereditary factors, possibly due to a congenital weakness of the venous walls.[3]

Signs and symptoms
- Painless bright red rectal bleeding
- Blood on stool around the toilet pan
- Prolapsing perianal lump, blue coloured
- Localized swellings in the perianal region
- Acute perianal pain due to thrombosis
- Faecal soiling or pruritus ani (itching).

Classification
External and or internal[4,5]
- External haemorrhoids occur below the dentate line 2cm from the anal verge marking the transition between the upper anal canal, which has no pain fibres, and the lower anal canal which is richly innervated with pain fibres.
- Internal haemorrhoids occur above the dentate line and are usually painless unless they become strangulated. They are further classified as follows:[3]
  - first degree—projecting into the lumen of the anal canal;
  - second degree—prolapse on straining but spontaneously reduce;
  - third degree—prolapse on straining but require manual reduction;
  - fourth degree—prolapse and cannot be reduced (incaserated).

Advice
Avoid constipation and straining:
- information on high fibre and fluid intake;
- episodes tend to worsen with time.

Only 10% of people eventually require surgery.

Non-surgical treatment

Suppositories and ointments

- Many symptomatic episodes settle with conservative measures such as corticosteroids combined with local anaesthetic. This treatment should not be used for more than 7 days.

1. Quijano, C.E. and Abalos, E. (2005). *Conservative management of symptomatic and/or complicated haemorrhoids in pregnancy and the puerperium (Cochrane Review)*. Cochrane Library Issue 3.
⬚ www.thecochranelibrary.com
2. Studd, P. (2005). Haemorrhoids: prevention and treatment. *Nursing in Practice*, **25**, 50–3.
3. Davies, R.J. (2006). *Haemorrhoids: clinical evidence*. BMJ Publishing, London.
4. Nisar, P.J. and Scholefield, J.H. (2003). Managing haemorrhoids. *British Medical Journal*, **327**, 847–51.
5. Alonso-Coello, P. and Castillejo, M.M. (2003). Office evaluation and treatment of hemorrhoids. *Journal of Family Practice*, **52**, 366–74.

Prescribing for the ear

Brief anatomy and physiology of the ear

Structure of the ear

There are three main parts: external ear, middle ear, and inner ear (Fig. 12.2).

External ear

- The pinna is a skin-covered flap which protects and channels sound waves into the external auditory meatus.
- The external auditory meatus is about 2.5cm long in the adult and is protected by fine hairs and wax-secreting ceruminous glands.
  - the function of these secretions and hairs is to prevent airborne particles from reaching the inner ear canal;
  - with a pH of 6.0, the cerumen (earwax) provides a defence against micro-organisms (see below);
  - this area ends at the tympanic membrane.

Middle ear

- The thin transparent tympanic membrane stretches across the entrance to the middle ear and vibrates when sound waves impinge on it.
- The air-filled middle ear, facilitated by the auditory ossicles (the malleus, incus, and stapes) transports these vibrations to the fluid-filled inner ear.
- The barrier between the middle and inner ear is the oval window to which the stapes is attached.
- Movements of the stapes cause the oval window to bow and flex, facilitating transference of vibrations into the inner ear.

Inner ear

Vibrations transported through the inner ear are interpreted and perceived as sound by the central nervous system (CNS).

Earwax

Earwax is a combination of:
- desquamated keratin squames (dead flattened skin cells);
- cerumen (wax produced by ceruminous glands which are modified sweat glands);
- sebum (from sebaceous glands);
- various foreign substances (e.g. cosmetics and dirt).

Earwax can be classified as wet or dry, and wet earwax may be soft or hard.

Wet earwax

Soft wet earwax is:
- moist and sticky;
- comprised of small sheets of keratin squames;
- more common in children.

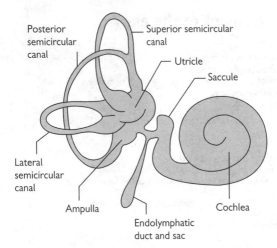

Fig. 12.2. Diagram of the inner ear.

Hard wet earwax is:
- dry and desiccated constituency;
- sheets of keratin are large and dense;
- more common in adults and more likely to become impacted.

Dry earwax
- Flaky
- Golden-yellow
- More common in people from Asia.

Functions of earwax
- It aids removal of keratin from the ear canal (earwax naturally moves out of the ear, aided by the movement of the jaw).
- It cleans, lubricates, and protects the ear canal, trapping dirt and repelling water.
- It is mildly acidic with antibacterial properties.

Further reading

Action on ENT Steering Board (2007). *Guidance document in ear care*. Primary Ear Care Centre. ☐ http://www.cks.nhs.uk/earwax/evidence (accessed 7 Octber 2009).

Baer, S. (2005). Knowing when to treat ear wax. *Practitioner*, May 11, 328.

Burton, M.J. and Doree, C.J. (2003) *Ear drops for the removal of ear wax (Cochrane Review)*. Cochrane Library, Issue 3. ☐ www.thecochranelibrary.com

Assessment of the ear

History

Difficulty with hearing:
- duration of the problem;
- onset of the problem—was it gradual or sudden?
- previous history;
- any trauma?

Routine physical examination

Look for:
- foreign bodies;
- reported irritation or itching;
- infection;
- build-up of wax which can obstruct the lumen of the ear canal;
- scaliness;
- narrowing of the ear canal because of swelling;
- redness;
- pain;
- discharge;
- hearing loss.

Common conditions of the ear

Conductive hearing loss

Definition
Difficulties in hearing as sound waves are not transferred to the inner ear.

Prevention
Earwax is a normal secretion. Warn patients to avoid impacting the wax by using implements such as hairpins and matchsticks as probes.

People are most at risk of impacted earwax if they:
- have narrow or deformed ear canals;
- have numerous hairs in their ear canals;
- have benign bony growths in the external auditory canal (osteomata);
- have a dermatological disease of the peri-auricular area or scalp;
- produce hard wax, as this more likely to become impacted;
- are older, because as a person ages the cerumen glands atrophy, causing the earwax to become drier;
- have a history of recurrent impacted wax;
- have learning disabilities—the reason for this is not known;
- have recurrent otitis externa;
- use cotton buds—these push the earwax deeper into the canal;
- wear a hearing aid or ear plugs—this prevents the wax from being excreted.

Causes
- Most common cause is a build-up of earwax
- Blockage of the outer ear by foreign body
- Infection of the inner ear
- Perforation of the tympanic membrane
- Immobilization of one or all of the auditory ossicles.

Signs and symptoms
Hearing loss.

Treatment
- Instill drops, i.e. almond or olive oil ear drops (ceruminolytics), to soften the wax (see below).
- If ear syringing is required following softening of the wax, it should be undertaken by a practitioner who is proficient in the technique.

Otitis externa

Definition
Inflammation of the outer ear. affecting the pinna and/or external auditory meatus. It may vary in severity from mild to severe. It may be acute or chronic.

Causes
- Infection:
  - usually bacterial but sometimes secondary fungal infections.
- Reaction to materials found in earrings or earphones (contact dermatitis).

Signs and symptoms
- Scaliness
- Narrowing of the ear canal because of swelling
- Redness
- Pain
- Discharge
- Hearing loss.

Treatment
- Clean, remove. or treat any precipitating or aggravating factors (often enough).
- Prescribe or recommend an analgesic for symptomatic relief.
- Prescribe a topical ear preparation for 7 days. Options include preparations containing:
  - both a non-aminoglycoside antibiotic and a corticosteroid;
  - both an aminoglycoside antibiotic and a corticosteroid (contraindicated if the tympanic membrane is perforated);
  - only an antibiotic (gentamicin ear drops are contraindicated if the tympanic membrane is perforated).

If there is sufficient earwax or debris to obstruct topical medication, consider cleaning the external auditory canal (patient may require referral). If there is extensive swelling of the auditory canal, consider inserting an ear wick (patient may require referral).

Drugs for the ear

Drugs for the ear belong to the following categories:
• astringent preparations;
• anti-inflammatory preparations;
• anti-infective preparations;
• earwax softeners.

They may be in the form of ear drops instilled into the ear or as a soak on a piece of ribbon gauze with which the ear is packed.

Instillation of ear drops
• Warm the drops to body heat prior to instillation.
• Encourage the patient to lie with the affected ear uppermost for 5–10 minutes after the drops have been instilled.

NB: do not prescribe to patients with a history of ear disease, those complaining of dizziness, or those with a discharge from the ear.

Prescribing for the eye

NB: the advice given in this chapter is for non-medical prescribers who are not optometrists

Brief anatomy and physiology of the eye

Assessment of the condition of the eye rests on an understanding of the normal protective functions and a history of the duration of the presenting condition.

Structure of the eye

Eyelids (palpebrae)

- Epithelial tissue.
- Their function is to protect the eye by keeping the surface clear and lubricated.
- Lubrication is provided by a lipid-rich secretion of the meibomian glands (modified sebaceous glands) and the lachrymal caruncle.
- The eyelashes prevent contamination of the eye.
- The conjunctiva covers the inner surface of the eye (palpebral conjunctiva), the outer surface of the eyeball (bulbar conjunctiva), and the cornea.

Eyeball (see Fig. 12.3)

Kept moist and clean by secretions of the accessory glands and goblet cells.

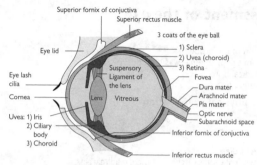

Fig. 12.3 Diagram of the eye.

Assessment of the eye

History

- Duration of the problem
- Onset of the problem—was it gradual or sudden?
- Full medical history
- Any trauma?

Routine physical examination

Look for:
- redness;
- discharge;
- foreign bodies;
- reported irritation or itching of the eyelid margins;
- gritty sensation;
- stye (chalazion);
- scales attached to the eyelids;
- appearance of the sclera (cobblestone appearance of the lining of the upper lid may indicate allergic conjunctivitis);
- patient complains of feeling a foreign body in the eye;
- visual acuity (VA);
- pupil size and reaction.

Visual acuity

Visual acuity is assessed in order to assess the limits of visual perception. A Snellen chart (Figure 12.4) is used to estimate VA.

Procedure

Carried out in a well-lit area place with the patient, initially wearing their distance correction glasses, 6m from the chart.
- Test each eye separately.
- Occlude the eye not being tested (do not apply pressure to eyeball when occluding).
- Test with and without distance glasses.
- Begin at the top of the chart and read progressively down.
- If the acuity is below 6/6, correct for any refractive error using a pinhole.
- Vision expressed as a fraction:
  - distance from chart in metres/lowest line read;
  - upper number: the distance from chart (conventionally 6m);
  - lower number: the distance at which an individual with no refractive error should see the chart.

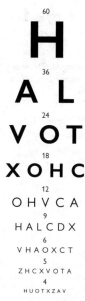

Fig. 12.4 Snellen chart. Reproduced from Denniston, A. and Murray, P. (2006), *Oxford Handbook of Ophthalmology*, with permission from Oxford University Press.

If the top line cannot be read at 6m, it is moved towards the patient 1m at a time until it can be read. If the patient is unable to read the top at 1m, the tester will check:
• counting fingers (CF);
• hand movement (HM);
• perception of light (PL).

NB: If VA is worse with pinhole consider maculopathy as cause.

📖 Clinical and physical examination, p. 178.
📖 History-taking, p. 174.

Conditions of the eye 1

Blepharitis

Definition

Inflammation of the eyelid margins. There are two main types:
- staphylococcal, caused by either *Staphylococcus aureus* or *Staphylococcus epidermidis*;
- seborrhoeic, associated with *Pityrosporum ovale*.

These are often found in combination.

Signs and symptoms
- Soreness of the eyelids
- Irritation
- Itching of the eyelid margins
- Gritty sensation
- Stye
- Scales on the lower lid margins and lashes.

Treatment:
- Keep lids clean: patients may need instructions on how to clean the eye and apply ointment.
- Treat any infection with antibiotic ointment usually 3–4 times daily.
- Topical eye treatments may cause transient blurring of vision or stinging pain. Warn patients of these possibilities.
- If eyes are dry, keep moist with artificial tears.
- Severe cases may need oral antibiotics.
- Prevent inflammation returning by continuing to treat for 1 month after the cessation of symptoms.

Acute glaucoma

NB: if left untreated, this condition will lead to blindness.

Causes
- The drainage system of the eye becomes blocked.
- Fluid builds up, resulting in an increase in intraocular pressure.

Signs and symptoms
Early symptoms such as sub-acute-angle glaucoma may occur, where the patient is aware of:
- halos around lights at night accompanied by aching in the eye;
- blurring of vision;
- acute pain;
- redness of the eye;
- headache;
- tenderness around the eye.

Treatment
• Treatment is urgently required and the patient should be referred to a specialist.

Additional information regarding acute glaucoma can be obtained from ⊞ www.glaucoma-association.com

Further reading

National Prescribing Centre (2010). ⊞ http://www.npc.co.uk/prescribers/faq.htm (accessed 3 February 2010).
Royal College of General Practitioners and Royal College of Ophthalmologists (2001). *Ophthalmology for general practice trainees.* Medical Protection Society, London.
Yanoff, M. and Duker, J.S. (eds) (2004). *Ophthalmology* (2nd edn). Mosby, St. Louis, MO.

Conditions of the eye 2

Conjunctivitis
This is the most common eye condition in the world.
Definition
- Inflammation of the conjunctiva, sometimes called 'red eye'.
- The causative agent can be either allergic or infective.

Allergic conjunctivitis

Causes
- Often associated with allergic reactions such as asthma and hay fever (allergic rhinitis).
- Sometimes resulting from contact with chemicals (e.g. eye make-up).
- Use of contact lenses.

Signs and symptoms
- Itching
- Redness
- Oedematous clear discharge
- 'Cobblestone' appearance inside the upper lid due to oedema
- Feeling of a foreign body in the eye
- VA is normal
- Pupils react normally.

Treatment
- Apply topical antihistamines or mast cell stabilizers.
- Instruct patients on how to:
  - clean the eye;
  - apply ointment or drops.
- Warn patients that eye treatments may cause transient blurring of vision or stinging pain.
- Oral antihistamines may be necessary.
- Topical corticosteroids may be used, but there is a risk of steroid-induced cataracts and glaucoma with these.
- Soft contact lenses should not be worn during treatment with eye drops as they may absorb either the active medication or preservatives within the drops.

Infective conjunctivitis
Infection may be viral or bacterial.

Bacterial conjunctivitis
Causes:
- Commonly due to *Staphylococcus*.
- Often infection by *Streptococcus pneumoniae* and/or *Haemophilus influenzae*.

Signs and symptoms
- Purulent exudates (indicative of bacterial infections).
- Sticky eyelids on waking.

CONDITIONS OF THE EYE 2 **265**

- Usually starts in one eye and is spread by the patient's hands or fomites to the other.
- It also spreads from person to person in this way.
- Feeling of a foreign body in the eye.
- Visual acuity is normal.
- Pupils react normally.

Treatment
- Apply topical antibiotics, usually one drop every 2hr initially, with the timing between drops extended as the infection abates.
- Continue eye drops for up to 48hr after the infection is controlled.
- Eye ointment is usually applied at night and eye drops during the day. If ointment is used alone, it should be applied 3–4 times daily.
- Instruct the patient on how to clean the eye and apply ointment or drops.
- Warn patients that eye treatments may cause transient blurring of vision or stinging pain.

Prevention
Strict hygiene measures are required to prevent the spread from one eye to the other and from person to person. Advise patients:
- to use their own pillowcase, flannel, and towel;
- to administer their own drops and ointment where possible;
- to wash their hands before and after touching the eyes;
- always clean an uninfected eye first and then move to the infected eye;
- to avoid eye make-up;
- not to wear contact lenses.

Viral conjunctivitis
Causes
- More common than bacterial conjunctivitis.
- Commonly caused by adenoviruses.
- Some viral serotypes may cause severe kerato-conjunctivitis.

Signs and symptoms
- Eyes feel gritty.
- Watery discharge (indicative of viral infections).
- Feeling of a foreign body in the eye.
- VA is normal.
- Pupils react normally.
- Sometimes associated with sore throat, upper respiratory tract infection, and fever.
- May persist for weeks—longer duration than bacterial conjunctivitis.
- Severe kerato-conjunctivitis may result in lasting visual disturbances, photophobia, and discomfort.

Treatment:
- Apply topical antibiotics to prevent secondary bacterial infection.
- As for bacterial conjunctivitis.

Prevention
As for bacterial conjunctivitis.

Administration of drugs for the eye

Eye drops
- Penetrate the globe, probably through the cornea.
- Some systemic absorption follows instillation into the eye, but this is variable and often undesirable.
- Usually instilled into the pocket formed by pulling the lower lid forward.
- The eye should be kept closed for as long as possible to allow absorption.
- Eye-drop dispensers are for repeated use by individual patients only.

Eye ointments
- A small amount of ointment is smeared along the inside of the lower lid.
- Blinking helps to spread the melted ointment.

Eye lotions
- Flush out foreign bodies from the conjunctival sack.
- Used for first-aid treatment.

When more than one product is being used to treat the eye, it is advisable to leave ~5min between instillations.

Prescribing for problems within the endocrine system

Introduction

The functioning and development of the human body depend on a complex and sequential interaction of chemicals. The three main players which ensure these processes are the immune system, the hormonal system, and the nervous system. In this chapter we concentrate on pre-scribing for problems within the hormonal or endocrine system.

Definition

The endocrine system maintains a stable environment within the body. It consists of glands which produce chemical substances called hormones. The glands comprising this system are as follows:

- pituitary gland;
- thyroid gland;
- parathyroid glands;
- pancreas;
- adrenal glands;
- ovaries;
- testis;
- thymus;
- pineal gland.

The kidneys also secrete hormones.

Hormones

These are chemical messengers that are secreted directly from the glands into the bloodstream and are carried to their specific targets where they exert a metabolic influence. Some hormones (e.g. thyroxin from the thyroid gland) affect nearly all cells, whereas progesterone, from the ovaries, specifically causes a reaction in the thickness of the uterine walls.

By maintaining, accelerating or slowing enzyme activity in receptor cells, hormones control growth and development, metabolic rate, sex hormone sequences, and reproduction.

The amounts of hormone secreted depend on complex feedback mechanisms which rely on the action of other hormones. For example, insulin secretion is controlled by the regulatory hormone glycogen.

The management of diabetes mellitus

Diabetes mellitus is a chronic and progressive disease which alters the body's management of carbohydrate, protein, and fat metabolism. It is described as being either type 1 diabetes, previously known as insulin-dependent diabetes mellitus (IDDM), or type 2 diabetes, previously known as non-insulin-dependent diabetes (NIDDM). Gestational diabetes (diabetes during pregnancy) and impaired fasting glucose or the pre-diabetic state also occur.

Type 1 diabetes is characterized by an absence of insulin production. Type 2 diabetes is caused by the body's inefficient use of endogenous insulin (insulin resistance) and/or insufficient production of insulin.

The two main hormones produced in the pancreas, a leaf-shaped gland that lies across the back of the stomach, are insulin and glucagon. Insulin lowers and glucagon raises the circulating blood glucose levels.

Somostatin is secreted by the pancreas, tissue in the intestinal tract and the CNS (outside the hypothalamus). It inhibits the secretion of both insulin and glucagon and suppresses pancreatic exocrine secretions which are vital for completing digestion of food.

Diabetes can affect people of all ages and races. Poor people in affluent societies and people of South Asian, African, and African Caribbean descent are particularly at risk.

Diabetes impacts on both physical and psychological health. Physical long-term complications can lead to both micro- and macrovascular disease including:

* stroke;
* heart disease;
* amputation;
* renal failure;
* neuropathy;
* blindness.

Diabetes, through restricted job choices, driving restrictions, and the decisions of financial institutions, can affect the material well-being of both the individuals with the disease and their families.

Further reading

Avery, L. and Beckwith, S. (2009) *Oxford Handbook of Diabetes Nursing*. Oxford University Press, Oxford.

Type 1 diabetes

Type 1 diabetes is due to the destruction of the β cells (insulin-producing cells) in the pancreas by the body's autoimmune system. It is usually diagnosed in children, teenagers, and young adults who present with:

- unexplained weight loss;
- thirst (polydipsia);
- frequent urination (polyurea);
- fatigue;
- poor healing;
- itchy skin;
- fungal infections;
- frequent urinary tract infections;
- hyperglycaemia (raised circulating blood glucose levels);
- abdominal pain and vomiting;
- ketoacidosis;
- ketotic coma.

However, some individuals present later in life with late-onset type 1 diabetes, also referred to as latent auto-immune diabetes of adults (LADA). LADA has the following clinical features:

- onset >40 years of age;
- may be moderately overweight (e.g. body mass index (BMI) ~27);
- poor response to sulphonylurea therapy;
- coexistent autoimmune diseases—typically thyroid disorders;
- definitive diagnosis is made by the presence of anti-GAD antibodies.

Further reading

Department of Health (2001). *National Service Framework for Diabetes: standards*. Department of Health, London.

Department of Health (2003). *National Service Framework for Diabetes: delivery strategy*. Department of Health, London.

Expert Committee on the Diagnosis and Classification of Diabetes Mellitus (2003). Report of the expert committee on the diagnosis and classification of diabetes mellitus. *Diabetes Care*, **26**, S5–20.

National Clinical Director for Diabetes and National Diabetes Support Team (2007). *Improving diabetes services: the NSF four years on. The way ahead: the local challenge*. Department of Health, London.

NICE Guidelines (latest edn). 🖳 www.nice.org.uk (accessed 3 February 2010).

Table 12.4 Insulin types and actions
N.B. all timings are approximate and vary from preparation to preparation

Type of insulin	Examples	Onset	Peak	Duration
Rapid-acting insulin analogues Soluble	Insulin lispro Insulin aspart Insulin glulisine	Inject immediately before meals or with meals Onset of action immediate	Peak action 2hr	Up to 4–6hr
Short-acting Soluble	Humulin S® Actrapid® Insuman Rapid®	Inject 15–30min before a meal	2–4hr	8hr
Intermediate and long-acting	Insulin glargine	–	–	24hr
	Insulin zinc suspension	1–3 hr	7–16hr	23–30hr
	Insulin zinc suspension (crystalline)	4–8hr	8–24hr	24–28hr
	Isophane	30min–2hr	1–12hr	11–24hr
	Protamine zinc suspension	4–6hr	10–20hr	25–35hr
Biphasic	Biphasic insulin aspart	–	8hr	13hr
	Biphasic insulin lispro	–	8hr	13hr
	Biphasic Isophane insulin	5–15min	Depends on mix	20–24hr

See current edition of BNF for all insulin preparations

Treatment of type 1 diabetes

- Physiological insulin replacement (Table 12.4).
- Self blood glucose monitoring.
- Where necessary diet and lifestyle modifications.
- Structured education to promote and support self-care.

Physiological insulin replacement

The aim of insulin replacement therapy for people with type 1 diabetes is to mimic as closely as possible the normal endogenous insulin production and release which comprises:

- a constant delivery of insulin to manage hepatic glucose output;
- peak of insulin delivery post meals to limit post-prandial hyperglycaemia;
- avoidance of hypoglycaemia (low circulating blood glucose levels).

Insulin replacement can best be achieved by regimens which mimic the bodies normal insulin production, e.g. continuous insulin infusion via an insulin pump or the basal bolus regimen which comprises four injections a day:

- a background insulin injection, often referred to as basal insulin, given at night;
- three injections of fast-acting insulin with meals, referred to as bolus insulin.

Some patients may not wish to commence on four injections per day. Other types of insulin are available, including premixed insulin (Table 12.4).

Self blood glucose monitoring in type 1 diabetes

People with type 1 diabetes are subject to a wide variability of blood glucose levels, and have an increased risk of hypoglycaemia. Frequent monitoring of blood glucose levels enables the person with type 1 diabetes to:

- adjust insulin doses according to carbohydrate intake allowing more flexibility with meal sizes and timing;
- prepare for and manage blood glucose levels when enjoying sporting activity;
- adjust insulin doses according to trends and patterns of blood glucose monitoring;
- optimize blood glucose levels to achieve target pre- and post-prandial blood glucose levels and target HbA1c results;
- reduce risk of hypoglycaemia;
- cope with minor illnesses such as sickness, colds, and flu.

Dietary advice for people with type 1 diabetes

In addition to sustaining our activity, choosing the food we eat reflects cultural and social influences. It is usually a source of pleasure and self-expression. People with type 1 diabetes also need to balance the carbohydrate, fat, and protein composition and the timing of their meals with the action of their injected insulin.

Increasingly patients are again being taught to count carbohydrate intake and adjust their insulin accordingly. This is known as the insulin-to-carbohydrate ratio and is calculated using the following simple relationship:

1 unit of insulin is given for each 10g of carbohydrate eaten.

Drugs used to treat type 1 diabetes

- Insulin (see Table 12.4 and current BNF for different types)
- GlucaGen® HypoKit
- GlucoGel®.

Other prescribable items

- Hypodermic injection equipment
- Pen injectors (check that these are compatible with insulin cartridge prescribed)
- Needles
- Syringes
- Lancets
- Needle clippers
- Blood glucose monitoring equipment
- Ketone monitoring blood and urine testing sticks.

Type 2 diabetes

Type 2 diabetes is usually diagnosed in adults over the age of 40 years, although there has been an increase in the number of young people being diagnosed with the disease. People of South Asian descent are six times more likely and those of African or African Caribbean decent are three times more likely to have type 2 diabetes than members of the white population. The initial treatment for type 2 diabetes is a combination of increased exercise, dietary control, and, if the patient is overweight, weight reduction. Most people with type 2 diabetes will progress to require oral hypoglycaemics and other anti-diabetic drugs either as monotherapy or combination therapy. Some may require a combination of oral hypogly-caemic drugs and insulin.

Drugs used to treat type 2 diabetes

Oral hypoglycaemics and anti-diabetic preparations (Table 12.5)

- Metformin reduces the amount of glucose produced and stimulates the amount used by the body.
- Sulphonyureas stimulate insulin production.
- Thiazolidinediones increase the effect of insulin to reduce circulating glucose.
- DPP-4 inhibitors or incretin enhancers increase glucose-dependent secretion of insulin and suppress glucagon secretion.
- GLP-1 (mimetic) or incretin (mimetic) increases insulin secretion, reduces glucagon secretion, and slows gastric emptying.
- Alpha-glucosidase slows the digestion of complex carbohydrates, limiting absorption.
- Insulin—NICE[1] recommends commencing with:
  - human NPH insulin at bedtime or twice a day;
  - if the person needs help with injecting consider a long-acting insulin analogue such as insulin determir or insulin glargaine initially and review.

Medications to treat associated conditions

- Hypotensive medication
- Statins
- Nicotine replacement therapy
- GlucoGel®
- Anti-obesity medication/meal replacements.[2,3]

Other products

- Blood and urine testing sticks for glucose and ketones.
- Finger prickers, lancets and needle clippers.
- Hypodermic devices (see above).

1. 🖳 http://www.nice.org.uk/nicemedia/live/12165/44318/44318.pdf (accessed 11 June 2010).
2. *National Obesity Forum guidelines on management of adult obesity in primary care.*
🖳 www.nationalobesityforum.org.uk
3. NICE guidelines. 🖳 www.nice.org.uk

Table 12.5 Examples of oral hypoglycaemics or oral glucose-lowering drugs and anti-diabetic drugs

Type and generic name	Action time	When taken
Biguanide		
Metformin	12hr	2–3 times a day with or after food
Sulphonyureas		
Chlorpropamide	36–72hr	Once a day with food
Glibenclamide	16–24hr	Once a day with or immediately after the first meal of the day
Gliclazide	12–18hr	Once or twice a day with or shortly before food
Glimepiride	18–24hr	Once a day shortly before the first meal
Glipizide	12–18hr	Once or twice a day before food
Tolbutamide	6–8hr	1–3 times a day with or immediately after food
Prandial glucose regulators		
Nateglinide	1–4hr	Before each meal*
Repaglinide	1–6hr	1–3 times a day with or immediately after food
Thiazolidinediones (glitizones) PPAR-agonists		
Pioglitizone		Once at the same time each day with or without food
Rosiglitazone		Once or twice at the same times each day with or without food
Rosiglitazone and metformin		Twice daily
Alpha-glucosidase inhibitor		
Acarbose		Chewed with the first mouthful of each meal
DPP-4 inhibitors (gliptins)		
Sitagliptin (licensed as both a monotherapy and 2nd-line therapy and as a 3rd-line alternative to insulin)		Once daily
Vildagliptin (licensed as a 2nd-line therapy)		Once or twice daily
GLP-1 (mimetic)		
Exenatide (3rd-line therapy)		Injection twice daily

* Nateglinide is intended to be taken with a meal – if the meal is missed the dose is missed.

Help available: 🖥 www.rcn.org.uk/development/practice/diabetes

Pregnancy and diabetes

Diabetes during pregnancy may be pre-existing type 1 or type 2 diabetes or gestational diabetes. Pregnant women with gestational diabetes experience high circulating blood glucose levels during pregnancy which resolve following their delivery. These high glucose levels will cross the placental membrane and detrimentally compromise the safety and development of the fetus. Gestational diabetes occurs in 3–12% of the pregnant population and can be an indicator of type 2 diabetes later in life.

Pre-conceptual care is vital for women with diabetes. The NICE guidelines recommend that information, care, and advice are offered from the adolescent years to all women with diabetes who are planning to become pregnant before they discontinue contraception. The advice should cover:

- the reasons for baby and mother of avoiding an unplanned pregnancy;
- the risks of diabetes in pregnancy:
  - fetal macrosomia (very large baby);
  - birth trauma (to mother and baby);
  - the need for induction of labour or Caesarean section;
  - miscarriage;
  - congenital malformation;
  - stillbirth;
  - transient neonatal morbidity;
  - neonatal death;
  - obesity and/or diabetes developing later in the baby's life.

These risks may be reduced but not eliminated by:
- good glycaemic control before and during pregnancy;
- care with diet;
- body weight and exercise, including weight loss for women with BMI $>27\text{kg/m}^2$;
- hypoglycaemia and hypoglycaemia awareness.

Advice should also include:
- how to cope with pregnancy-related nausea/vomiting and glycaemic control;
- the reasons for and implications of retinal and renal assessment;
- when to stop contraception;
- taking folic acid supplements (5mg/day) from preconception until 12 weeks of gestation;
- review of, and possible changes to, medication, glycaemic targets, and self-monitoring routine;
- frequency of appointments;
- local support, including emergency telephone numbers.

The current NICE guidelines[1] are that all women with diabetes who are trying to become pregnant or who have a confirmed pregnancy should:
• stop oral hypoglycaemic agents, apart from metformin;
• commence insulin if required;
• stop ACE inhibitors, angiotensin-II receptor antagonists, and statins;
• consider alternatives to anti-hypertensive medication.

1. NICE (2008). *Diabetes in pregnancy: management of diabetes and its complications from pre-conception to the postnatal period.* ⌨ http://www.nice.org.uk/nicemedia/pdf/CG063QuickRefGuide1 (accessed 10 September 2009).

The thyroid

The thyroid-stimulating hormone (TSH) is produced by the pituitary gland and regulates the production of hormones from the thyroid gland. Among other functions the thyroid gland produces T_4 (thyroxine) and T_3 (tri-iodothyronine) which are carried in the bloodstream. On reaching the cells, T_4 is converted to T_3, the active form of the hormone.

Problems with the thyroid

These happen when the body's metabolism is affected by the under- or overproduction of thyroid hormones.

Thyrotoxicosis

This occurs when the T_4 and T_3 levels are raised.

Symptoms
- Sweating
- Heat intolerance
- Diarrhoea
- Tremor
- Weight loss despite increased appetite
- Rapid heart beat
- Tremor
- Irritability
- Frenetic activity
- Emotionally labile
- Psychosis
- Itching.

Signs
- Raised pulse
- Warm peripheries
- Fine tremor
- Palmar erythema
- Thinning hair, eyelashes, and eyebrows
- Eyelids lag behind the eye's descent when watching the finger slowly descend
- Eyelid retraction, causing stare
- On physical examination: goitre, thyroid nodules, or bruit depending on the cause.

Hypothyroidism (myxoedema)

TSH is raised and T_4 is lowered.

Symptoms
- Tiredness
- Lethargy
- Depression
- Dislike of the cold
- Weight gain
- Constipation
- Menorrhagia
- Hoarse voice
- Poor cognition/dementia
- Myalgia.

Signs
- Bradycardia
- Dryness of the skin and hair
- Non-pitting oedema of the eyelids, hands, or feet
- Slow relaxing reflexes
- Peripheral neuropathy
- Cerebella ataxia:
  - unsteadiness;
  - lack of balance;
  - clumsiness.

Prescription of thyroid hormones (Table 12.6)

These are used to treat:
- hypothyroidism (myxoedema);
- diffuse non-toxic goitre;
- Hashimoto's thyroiditis (lymphadenoid goitre);
- cancer of the thyroid.

Table 12.6 Thyroid hormones and antithyroid drugs

Condition	Medication
Hypothyroidism	**Thyroid hormones**
	Levothyroxine sodium/thyroxine sodium
Hyperthyroidism	**Antithyroid drugs**
	Carbimazole
	Iodine and radio-iodine
	Propylthiouracil

Corticosteroids

In a healthy person the adrenal cortex produces steroids.

- Glucocorticoids which affect carbohydrate, lipid, and protein metabolism. Excessive production causes Cushing's syndrome.
- Mineralocorticoids which control sodium and potassium balance (e.g. aldosterone). Excessive production causes hyperaldersteronism.
- Androgens: sex hormones which become potent on peripheral conversion to testosterone and dihydrotestosterone.

Adrenal insufficiency causes Addison's disease.

Replacement therapy

- In corticosteroid deficiency a combination of hydrocortisone and the mineralocorticoid fludrocortisone are prescribed.
- Following an adrenalectomy or in Addison's disease, hydrocortisone is prescribed.
- In acute adrenocortical insufficiency, hydrocortisone is given intravenously.

Glucocorticoid therapy

See current BNF for dose recommendations, indications, advantages, cautions, and contraindications.

Sex hormones

Female sex hormones

Oestrogens

These are required for:
- the secondary female sexual characteristics;
- the stimulation of myometrial hypertrophy;
- endometrial hyperplasia.

Hormone replacement therapy (HRT)

Natural oestrogens are more appropriate for HRT. If long-term therapy is needed, progesterone should be added to the oestrogen to reduce the risk of:
- cystic hyperplasia of the endometrium as this may be a pre-cancerous state;
- diabetes (and increased risk of coronary heart disease);
- breast nodules;
- breast cancer (if there is a family history with a first-degree relative);
- increased risk of deep vein thrombosis (DVT) in women who have predisposing risk factors;
- increase in size of uterine fibroids;
- exacerbation of the symptoms of endometriosis.

Progestogens

There are two groups of progestogens:
- progesterone and its analogues;
- testosterone analogues.

Progestogens are used to treat:
- endometriosis;
- menorrahagia;
- severe dysmenorrhoea.

They are also used:
- for alleviation of premenstrual symptoms;
- for prevention of spontaneous abortion in women with a history of recurrent miscarriage;
- as an oral contraceptive.

Male sex hormones and antagonists

Androgens

- In the healthy body, androgens inhibit pituitary gonadotrophin secretion, leading to the production of anabolic steroids and depression of spermatogenesis.
- They are required for masculinity and may be used as a replacement therapy for castrated adult males and those who are hypogonadal due to either pituitary or testicular disease.

Replacement therapy
- Depot intramuscular injections of testosterone esters are the preferred preparations for replacement therapy.
- Implants of testosterone can be given to menopausal women as an adjunct to HRT in order to alleviate symptoms.
- Preparations are also available as patches, as gel, and for oral administration.

Anti-androgens
These inhibit spermatogenesis and result in reversible infertility. As they can reduce male characteristics, they can be used to treat male pattern baldness and acne. They are also used to treat specific cancers.

Anabolic steroids
These can be used in the treatment of some aplastic anaemias.

Other hormonal preparations and their uses

Anti-oestrogens

These can be used as a treatment for infertility in women who have oligomenorrhoea or secondary amenorrhea (associated with polycystic ovary disease). By occupying the oestrogen receptors in the hypothalamus they interfere with the feedback mechanism causing gonadotrophin release.

Anterior pituitary hormones

Corticotrophins

These are used to test adrenocortical function. If the plasma cortisol concentration fails to rise after their administration, this is an indication of adrenocortical insufficiency.

Gonadotrophins

These are used in the treatment of infertility in women with proven hypopituitarism or those who have failed to conceive after receiving other infertility treatments. They have also been used to treat delayed puberty in young males.

Antidiuretic hormone antagonist

These can be used to treat hyponatraemia by blocking the renal tubule response to antidiuretic hormone.

Drugs affecting bone metabolism

Calcitonin and teriparatide

Calcitonin is involved with the parathyroid in the regulation of calcium balance and homeostasis in the body. It is used in severe Paget's disease for the relief of pain and some of the neurological symptoms. It is also used to lower plasma/calcium concentrations in patients with hypercalcaemia associated with cancer.

Teriparatide is a recombinant fragment of the parathyroid hormone and may be prescribed for post-menopausal women who have osteoporosis.

Bisphosphonates

These slow the rate of bone growth and dissolution, thus reducing the rate of bone turnover. They are used prophylactically for osteoporosis, and are also used in the treatment of Paget's disease and hypercalcaemia associated with cancer.

Further information

For further information and help, see the current edition of the BNF.

Links to journals, guidelines, patient handouts and research for endocrine disease are available from 🖥 http://omni.ac.uk

Prescribing for gastrointestinal problems

Many of the medications for treatment of the conditions included in this section are available as over-the-counter (OTC) medications at less cost than a prescription and prescribers should consider this before writing a prescription. 📖 Over-the-counter (OTC) drugs, p. 422.

Anatomy and physiology of the gastrointestinal (GI) tract

The GI tract is shown in Fig. 12.5.

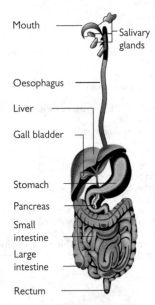

Mouth

Salivary glands

Oesophagus

Liver

Gall bladder

Stomach

Pancreas

Small intestine

Large intestine

Rectum

Fig. 12.5 Brief anatomy and physiology of the GI tract. Reproduced from Glasper, E.A., McEwing, G., and Richardson, J. (2006). *Oxford Handbook of Children's and Young People's Nursing*, by kind permission of Oxford University Press.

Oral cavity

The oral cavity comprises:
• cheeks;
• lips;
• teeth where present;
• gums;
• tongue.

Function of the oral cavity

• Speech
• Ingestion
• Chewing (mastication)
• Taste
• Lubrication
• Digestion of starch
• Swallowing (deglutition)
• Respiration.

Xerostomia (dry mouth)

Can result from the following.
• Medication:
  • antiparkinsonian drugs;
  • antihistamines;
  • lithium;
  • monoamine oxidase inhibitors;
  • tricyclic antidepressants;
  • clonidine;
  • antimuscarinic drugs.
• Dehydration
• Emotional stress
• Radiotherapy
• Renal failure
• Shock.

Oral candidiasis

Those most at risk have altered or compromised autoimmune responses:
- debilitated infants and children;
- older people;
- people with diabetes;
- those with an indwelling venous or urinary catheter;
- those receiving corticosteroid therapy;
- those receiving/recently completed antibiotic therapy;
- those with immunodeficiency (e.g. HIV, AIDS, chemotherapy for cancer treatment).

Oral assessment

See Table 12.7.

Preparations for the treatment of oral candidiasis

Fluconazole capsules and oral solution
- Contraindications:
  - hepatic impairment;
  - previous hypersensitivity;
  - increases the effect of warfarin, sulphonylureas, and antiepileptics;
  - use with caution in pregnancy.
- Adverse effects:
  - nausea;
  - abdominal discomfort;
  - flatulence;
  - diarrhoea;
  - impaired liver function;
  - anaphylaxis.

Miconazole oral gel and dental lacquer
- Contraindications:
  - hepatic impairment;
  - previous hypersensitivity;
  - use with caution in pregnancy.
- Interactions:
  - increases prothrombin time when given with warfarin;
  - increases blood levels of phenytoin;
  - prolongs the serum half-life of sulphonylureas;
  - potentiates anti-epileptics;
  - antagonizes the effect of amphotericin.
- Adverse effects:
  - oral preparation may cause GI upset if used for a long time;
  - nausea;
  - vomiting;
  - diarrhoea;
  - headache;
  - rash.

Table 12.7 Oral assessment

Area	Normal appearance	Problems
Lips	Smooth	Bleeding
	Pink	Ulceration
	Moist	Cracks at the edges of the mouth
Buccal mucosa	Pink	Reddening
	Moist	Coated (oral candidiasis)
		Ulcerated
Saliva	Clear	Dryness (xerostomia)
Tongue	Pink	Reddening
	Moist	Coated (candidiasis)
	Papillae present	Papillary loss
		Blisters
		Ulceration
		Cracking
Gums	Pink	Bleeding
	Firm	Bleeding with pressure
		Reddened (gingivitis)
		Puffy and pale (oedema)
Teeth	White	Broken teeth
	No evidence of dental caries	Teeth with rough edges
		Plaque
		Dental abscess
Dentures	Well-fitting	Rubbing
	Clean	Uneven
		Broken

Nystatin pastilles and oral suspension
- Contraindications:
  - previous hypersensitivity.
- Adverse effects:
  - oral irritation;
  - large doses may cause, nausea, diarrhoea, and/or vomiting.

The pharynx and oesophagus

This hollow muscular tube links the mouth and stomach.

Heartburn

This region may be affected by heartburn—a retrosternal or epigastric burning sensation which spreads upwards into the pharynx and may spread across the chest. It may be related to hunger, eating specific foods, or the time of day, and there may be demonstrable acid reflux.

The carbon-13 (^{13}C) breath test is an accurate non-invasive test for *Helicobacter pylori (H.pylori)*, and may be indicated if the symptoms persist in an individual:
- without a previous history of peptic ulceration;
- who has tried treatment for a month with anti-reflux measures such as magnesium trisilicate mixture or alginates (e.g. Gaviscon®).

Provided that there are no alarm symptoms or signs such as:
- anaemia (iron deficiency);
- weight loss;
- melaena;
- haematemasis;
- swallowing symptoms;
- and the patient does not exhibit the signs of:
  - non-specific tenderness in the epigastrium;
  - any mass felt on examination.

Mild to moderate heartburn may be helped by the following lifestyle changes:
- weight loss;
- smoking cessation;
- reduction in alcohol consumption;
- avoiding large meals, especially late at night;
- raising the head of the bed;
- avoiding foods known to precipitate the condition.

Mild to moderate heartburn can be treated with antacids and alginate–antacids which can be purchased as OTC medication. If there is minimal or no response to these an H_2-receptor antagonist may be considered (Table 12.8). H_2-receptor antagonists reduce the volume of gastric acid secretion by blocking the action of histamine on the parietal cells in the stomach.

However, these have been superseded by proton pump inhibitors (PPIs) which are more effective. PPIs act by irreversibly blocking the hydrogen/potassium adenosine triphosphatase enzyme system, commonly called the gastric proton pump. The proton pump is the terminal stage in gastric acid secretion, being directly responsible for secreting H^+ ions into the gastric lumen, which makes it an ideal target for inhibiting acid secretion.

Table 12.8 Contraindications and adverse effects of H_2-receptor antagonists

Contraindication	Adverse effects
Hepatic impairment	Diarrhoea
Renal impairment	Altered liver function test results
Pregnancy	Headache
Breastfeeding	Rash
Cimetidine inhibits the action of:	Dizziness
• warfarin	Tiredness
• phenytoin	Rare effects include:
• aminophylline	• bradycardia
• theophylline	• acute pancreatitis
	• confusion
	• depression
	• atrioventricular block
	• impotence
	• older people may be affected by hallucinations

Small intestine

The small intestine is referred to as 'small' as the lumen has a diameter of only 2.5cm, although it measures over 6.0m in length. It comprises three regions:

- duodenum (~25cm long) which receives secretions via the pancreatic and bile ducts;
- jejunum (~2.5m long);
- ileum (~3.5m).

Most of the digestion and absorption of food and many drugs takes place in the small intestine. When nutrients are present in the small intestine the hormone cholecystokinin is produced, and this triggers the release of the pancreatic enzymes. Secretin is also produced and this stimulates the pancreas to release bicarbonate in order to neutralize the potentially harmful acid coming from the stomach.

Digestion

The three major classes of nutrients that undergo digestion in the small intestine are:

- proteins;
- lipids;
- carbohydrates.

Proteins

The chemical breakdown of proteins and peptides begins in the stomach and continues in the small intestine as they are degraded into amino acids. The pancreas produces the proteolytic enzymes which gradually break down the proteins into their amino acid components:

- trypsin and chymotrypsin start the process;
- carboxypeptidase splits one amino acid at a time;
- aminopeptidase and dipeptidase- finish the breakdown.

Lipids

Lipids (fats) are degraded into fatty acids and glycerol, and pancreatic lipase breaks down triglycerides into free fatty acids and monoglycerides. Pancreatic lipase works with the salts from the bile secreted by the liver and the gall bladder. Bile salts emulsify triglycerides, enabling access by pancreatic lipase.

Carbohydrates

Carbohydrates are broken down into simple sugars—monosaccharides (e.g. glucose). Pancreatic amylase breaks down carbohydrates into oligosaccharides which are further degraded by dextrinase and glucoamylase.

Absorption

The digested food can now be absorbed into the blood vessels in the wall of the intestine. Any food that remains undigested and unabsorbed passes into the large intestine. Absorption of the majority of nutrients takes place in the jejunum with the following exceptions:

• iron is absorbed in the duodenum;
• vitamin B12 is absorbed in the terminal phase of the ileum;
• water and lipids are absorbed by passive diffusion throughout the small intestine.

Absorption of orally administered medication

Most drugs are absorbed by passive diffusion which allows chemicals from a concentrated source in the gut to pass across the gut mucosa to a weaker source in the splanchnic circulation (vessels which supply the abdominal vicera). Examples of exceptions are:
- methyldopa;
- levodopa.

Weakly acidic drugs are absorbed from the GI tract at a lower pH because more of the drug is in a non-ionized or un-ionized form and therefore is more lipophilic (lipid soluble). Lipophilic drugs diffuse readily across cell membranes.

The converse is true for weakly alkaline (base) drugs. Ionized drugs are highly water soluble (hydrophilic) but have low lipid solubility and high electrical resistance and cannot penetrate cell membranes easily.

The proportion of the non-ionized form is determined by the drug's pH (acid or alkaline) and pK_a (acid dissociation constant):
- the pK_a is the pH at which the non-ionized and ionized forms are equal;
- if the pH is lower than pK_a, the non-ionized form of a weak acid predominates and the ionized form of a weak base predominates.[1]

In practice this means that when a weak acid medication (e.g. aspirin) is given orally, most of the drug in the stomach is non-ionized which facilitates absorption through the gastric mucosa. Conversely, if the medication is a weak base (pK_a 4.4), most of the drug in the stomach is in the ionized form.

Theoretically, weakly acidic drugs are more readily absorbed from the stomach (an acidic medium) than weakly base drugs.

However, whether a drug is an acid or a base, most absorption occurs in the small intestine because the surface area is larger and the membranes are more permeable.

Having food in the gut

Food in the gut may:
- increase;
- decrease;
- delay;
- the absorption of drugs by altering the pH of the GI tract. Hot food and fatty meals delay gastric emptying to a greater extent than high-protein or carbohydrate meals and alter drug metabolism by:
  - increasing the time the drug spends in the stomach and prolonging the time for its disintegration and dissolution;
  - delaying the time to peak concentrations for drugs absorbed from the small bowel.

Therefore to optimize the efficacy of a medication it is important to check that a drug is administered in accordance with the manufacturer's instructions regarding the timing of medications:
• Is it to be taken on an empty stomach, with food, or after food?

Sublingual or buccal administration

Drugs absorbed from under the tongue (sublingually) or placed between the gum and the cheek (buccal), e.g. glyceryl trinitrate for angina, are absorbed straight into the small blood vessels of the oral mucosa. The drugs are neither metabolized by the gut wall nor by the liver before entering the blood stream. This route is unsuitable for many drugs as absorption may be erratic or incomplete.

Rectal administration

Many drugs that are administered orally can also be administered rectally as a suppository. In this preparation the drug is mixed with a waxy substance that dissolves or liquefies after insertion into the rectum. The drug is readily absorbed as the rectum has a good blood supply.

1. Medicines complete.
☒ http://www.medicinescomplete.com/mc/index.htm (accessed 16 October 2009)

Gastroenteritis

Gastroenteritis is caused by infection of the GI tract through the ingestion of bacteria, viruses, and toxins from food and/or water.

Symptoms

- Abdominal pain
- Diarrhoea
- Vomiting
- Abdominal cramps
- Bloating
- Flatulence
- Nausea
- Fever
- Faecal urgency
- Tenesmus (painful spasm of the anal sphincter with the feelings of a desire do defecate without results).

Both the young and frail older people are at risk of becoming dehydrated and salt depleted. Dehydration in infants is a medical emergency, and referral will be indicated if symptoms do not abate within 24hr. Presenting symptoms of dehydration and salt depletion may be:

- lassitude;
- anorexia;
- light-headedness;
- postural hypotension;
- nausea.

Assessment

- Obtain a full history, including the following.
- Has the patient been canoeing or swimming?
- What types of food and water were ingested?
- What cooking methods were used?
- How long between ingestion and onset of symptoms?
- Were others who shared the food or water affected?
- Assess state of hydration.
- Assess frequency and consistency of bowel motions.
- If more than one person is affected, or if symptoms have persisted for more than 4 days, a referral may be indicated.
- Referral is indicated if patients have:
  - fever;
  - abdominal pain;
  - blood in the diarrhoea;
  - tenesmus;
  - severe dehydration;
  - shock;
  - vomiting to the extent they are unable to retain oral rehydration solution (ORS).
- Consider the possibility that a recent course of antibiotics may have destroyed the normal gut flora, leading to diarrhoea.

Treatment of gastroenteritis

Rehydration

Give advice and a proprietary ORS, such as Dioralyte®, Electrolade®, or Rehidrat®. Once rehydrated, further prevention of dehydration should be avoided by encouraging normal fluid intake and use of ORS to replace additional losses due to vomiting and diarrhoea. Infants should be offered breast or formula feeds in addition to ORS drinks.

Antimotility agents

These are useful in non-infectious diarrhoea. Bowel motility is decreased as these narcotic analgesics act upon the opioid μ-receptors on the mesenteric neurons in the intestinal wall, reducing the release of acetylcholine (📖 Pain, p. 318), resulting in suppression of peristaltic action.

Contraindications
- Diarrhoea caused by infection because diarrhoea enables pathogens to be eliminated.
- Not shown to be useful in children or infants.

Adverse effects
- Associated with CNS toxity and paralytic ileus in the young.

Codeine phosphate

Contraindications
- Acute diarrhoea conditions (e.g. ulcerative colitis)
- Hypersensitivity to opioids
- Respiratory depression
- Severe respiratory disease
- Acute alcoholism
- Risk of paralytic ileus.

Adverse effects:
- Lethargy, drowsiness, and sedation
- Dizziness
- Mood changes (e.g. agitation)
- Dependency
- Hallucinations,
- Bradycardia, palpitations, tachycardia
- Hypotension
- Nausea
- Constipation
- Urinary retention
- Flushing
- Rash
- Hypothermia
- Respiratory depression.

Loperamide

Loperamide is a synthetic opioid which does not readily cross the brain–blood barrier.

Contraindications

- Those with ulcerative colitis or abdominal distension, where peristaltic inhibition should be avoided.

Adverse effects

- Abdominal cramps
- Drowsiness
- Dizziness
- Skin reactions
- Abdominal bloating
- Paralytic ileus.

Antibiotics

Antibiotics are indicated if infection is shown to be caused by:

- *Salmonella*
- *Shigella*
- *Campylobacter*
- *Clostridia*.

Advice on likely pathogens should be sought from the Public Health Department.

NB: food poisoning is a notifiable disease and should be reported to the UK Health Protection Agency at: 🖳 www.hpa.org.uk.

Bowel colic

This abdominal pain is caused by spasmodic contractions of the intestine. It can be treated by administration of antimuscarinic (formerly known as anticholinergic) drugs which both decrease gastrointestinal secretions and act as a smooth muscle relaxant (see Table 12.9).

Table 12.9 Cautions, contraindications, and adverse effects of antimuscarinic preparations

Cautions	Contraindication	Adverse effects
Antimuscarinic drugs are not to be used for people with Down syndrome, children, or older people		These are increased in this group
Caution with their use for people with:	Angle-closure glaucoma	Constipation
• gastro-oesophageal reflux disease	Myasthenia gravis	Transient bradycardia (followed by tachycardia, palpitations, and cardiac arythmias)
• diarrhoea	Paralytic ileus	
• ulcerative colitis	Pyloric stenosis	Reduced bronchial secretions
• acute myocardial infarction	Prostatic enlargement	
• tachycardia		Urinary retention and urgency
• hyperthyroidism		
• cardiac insufficiency following cardiac surgery		Pupil dilation with loss of accommodation
• pyrexia		Photophobia
• pregnancy		Dry mouth and skin
• breastfeeding		Flushing
• receiving anti-parkinsonian treatments.		Confusion sometimes occurs in older people

For interactions see BNF

Helminths

Helminths (multicellular parasitic worms), both *Enterobius vermicularis* (threadworms or pinworms) and, more rarely, *Ascaris lumbricoides* (roundworms), are found within the digestive tract. They may be classified as nematodes (roundworms), cestodes (tapeworms), or trematodes (flatworms and flukes).

It is estimated that about 40% of UK schoolchildren under 10 years of age have an infestation of threadworms.[1,2] Transmission rates are particularly high for children living in dense populations with poor sanitary conditions.

Roundworm infestations have a much lower incidence and more serious consequences as they may cause intestinal obstruction or pulmonary eosinophilia. It is most likely that they will have been contracted abroad.

Threadworms

Clinical features:
- Nocturnal pruritus
- Worms (8–12mm long) visible on the perianal skin or in the stools
- Vulvovaginitis
- Vaginal discharge.

Treatment
Anthelmintic preparations are available which either prevent the uptake of glucose by the worm (mebendazole), which becomes depleted in energy and dies, or paralyze the worm by blocking the neurotransmitter acetylcholine (piperazine). The paralyzed worm is then removed from the intestine by the normal peristaltic activity of the host. A third type of anthelmintic (Pripsen®—piperazine and sennoside) kills the paralyzed worm which is expelled along with the faeces.

Re-infestation is common, and so two doses of mebendazole may be required, the second dose 2–3 weeks after the first. The second course of piperazine is usually given for 7 days, 14 days after the first course.

Advice to avoid re-infestation includes the following:
- Treat the whole family if possible.
- Cut fingernails short.
- Handwashing and scrubbing after using the toilet and before preparing food and eating.
- Bath or shower on rising to wash away any eggs that have been laid during the night.
- Pants or pyjamas to be worn at night and washed daily.
- Mittens or gloves may be worn to avoid scratching and carrying the eggs to the mouth. These also need daily laundering.

Preparations for the treatment of helminth infection

Mebendazole

- Contraindications:
  - pregnancy—teratogenesis has been shown in rats;
  - not licensed for those under 2 years old because there is insufficient information regarding safety in these patients.
- Adverse effects:
  - can cross the placenta and may be found in small amounts in breast milk (the manufacturer advises avoiding use when pregnant or breastfeeding);
  - rare occurrence of abdominal pain or diarrhoea.

Piperazine

- Contraindications:
  - avoid in the first trimester of pregnancy;
  - lactating women should not breastfeed within 8hr of taking piperazine;
  - avoid in those with liver disease, renal disease, epilepsy (piperazine lowers the seizure threshold).
- Adverse effects:
  - nausea;
  - blurred vision;
  - vomiting;
  - bronchospasm;
  - diarrhoea;
  - rash;
  - abdominal cramps;
  - anorexia.
- Rarely, causes:
  - drowsiness;
  - lack of muscle coordination (worm wobble);
  - convulsions;
  - nystagmus;
  - vertigo;
  - blurred vision;
  - confusion.

1. The Royal College of General Practioners (1996). *Fact sheet 32*. RCGP, London
2. ▨ http://www.fredworm.co.uk/resources/downloads/Factfile.pdf (accessed 7 October 2009).

Large intestine

The large intestine is the last part of the digestive system and is about 1.5m long. Its function is to absorb water from the remaining indigestible food matter, and then to pass useless waste matter from the body. The large intestine starts in the right iliac fossa of the pelvis, from which it continues up the abdomen, then across the width of the abdominal cavity, before turning down and continuing to its endpoint at the anus. It consists of the following.

- Caecum:
  - a blind-ended pouch from which the appendix projects;
  - receives chyme from the ileum via the ileo-caecal valve.
- Ascending and transverse colon; sodium is reabsorbed along with chloride and water.
- Descending colon.
- Rectum.
- Anus.

Haustral contractions move back and forth along the large intestine, aiding absorption and storing material until the colonic contents are moved into the rectum. Stimulation of the stretch receptors in the rectal wall initiates the defecation reflex (the call to stool).

Constipation (difficulty in passing stools)

Constipation may be caused by:
- stools of poor bulk, sometimes caused by a diet which is low in fibre;
- hard stools due to increased time in the intestine or poor hydration.

Assessment (Table 12.10)

Assessment of constipation requires the following.
- A full history
  - what is the normal pattern for the individual?
  - are the changes in bowel habit recent?
  - family history of bowel cancer?
- Medical history
  - is there anything which might predispose to constipation, e.g. drug action (opiates, aluminium antacids, oral iron, and antimuscarinics can all cause constipation)?
  - what other symptoms does the patient have?
  - is fluid intake sufficient?
  - what are the frequency and nature of the stools?
  - is there any blood in or on the stools?
  - is there a pattern of diarrhoea alternating with constipation?

Abdominal examination

- A tender abdomen with guarding and rigidity.
- Rebound tenderness may indicate an acute condition. When present consider:
  - is the pain is radiating, shifting?
  - where is it, what relieves it?
  - are bowel sounds absent?

Rectal examination
- A full rectum suggests nerve damage or failure to heed the 'call to stool'.
- An empty rectum suggests a chronic obstruction or laxative abuse.

NB: only undertake abdominal and rectal examinations if competent to do so and with the patient's permission. 📖 Consent, p. 140.

Treatment
Constipation can be treated with lifestyle changes, such as an increase in exercise, foods with dietary fibre (18–30g/day), and fluid intake (1.5–2L) where these have been low. It is important to encourage a response to the 'call to stool', usually shortly after mealtimes, as ignoring this will allow more fluid to be absorbed from the stools, making them difficult to pass. If there is a poor response to these interventions, laxatives and rectal preparations may be needed.

Laxatives and rectal preparations
Laxatives are medicines that promote bowel evacuation, and may be mild (aperients) or strong (purgative or cathartic). Rectal preparations are either suppositories or enemas.

Bulk-forming laxatives
These laxatives are used for those with a low-fluid low-fibre diet. They increase the volume of faecal matter, stimulating peristalsis, but may take to several days to act and must be taken with plenty of fluids. Some trap water by forming a viscous gel, softening faeces and decreasing transit time. They are useful for those with a colostomy or ileostomy.
- Generic names: bran, ispaghula (husk granules and powder), sterculia (granules), methylcellulose.

Contraindications
- Difficulty in swallowing
- Intestinal obstruction
- Atonic colon
- Faecal impaction.

Adverse effects
- Flatulence
- Abdominal distention.

Table 12.10 Possible explanations for constipation symptoms

Symptom	Possible reason
Increased bowel sounds, abdominal distension, and/or pain	Structural lesion
Thin pencil-shaped stools	Lesion in the descending colon
Abdominal mass, jaundice, weight loss, and fatigue	Advanced colon cancer
Black or malaena stool	High intestinal lesion
Blood mixed with stool	Colonic bleeding
Stool covered with blood	Lower colonic or rectal disease
Blood on toilet paper	Anal fissure, haemorrhoids

Laxatives and rectal preparations

Osmotics

Lactulose
- Mode of action:
  - osmotic laxative—a semi-synthetic disaccharide, which is not absorbed from the bowel.
- Contraindications:
  - intestinal obstruction;
  - galactosaemia.
- Adverse effects:
  - abdominal cramps;
  - flatulence.

Macrogols
- Mode of action:
  - retain water in the large intestine;
  - undergo fermentation in the colon, producing gas and short-chain fatty acids stimulating peristalsis;
  - discourage the formation of ammonia-producing organisms.
- Contraindications:
  - intestinal obstruction;
  - paralytic ileus;
  - Crohn's disease;
  - ulcerative colitis;
  - toxic megacolon.
- Adverse effects:
  - abdominal distension;
  - nausea;
  - abdominal pain.

Magnesium hydroxide, phosphate enema, sodium citrate enema
- Contraindications:
  - colic, bowel irritation.

Stimulants

Oral and rectal preparations for those on prolonged bed rest with neurological dysfunction, or to counteract other constipating drug therapies. Induce peristaltic action by stimulation of the nerve plexuses to produce propulsive waves.

Senna, dantron, sodium picosulfate
- Contraindications:
  - avoid in intestinal obstruction;
  - avoid with children;
  - use with caution in pregnancy.
- Adverse effects:
  - gripe;
  - abdominal cramps.

Bisacodyl
- Contraindications:
  - avoid in intestinal obstruction;
  - avoid with children;
  - use with caution in pregnancy.
- Adverse effects:
  - gripe;
  - abdominal cramps;
  - may cause rectal irritation.

Docusate (tablets, oral solution, or enema)
Docusate sodium reduces the surface tension of stools, allowing fluid to enter and soften them, in addition to stimulation of peristalsis.
- Contraindications:
  - do not use oral formula in intestinal obstruction or for those with nausea, vomiting, or abdominal pain;
  - avoid rectal preparations if rectal fissures or haemorrhoids are present.
- Adverse effects of oral formulation:
  - cramps;
  - nausea;
  - anorexia.

Faecal lubricants/softeners
Soften faeces and lubricate bowel to promote motility. Softeners are used for patients who need to avoid straining, e.g. after surgery or myocardial infarction.

Arachis oil
Use warmed as an enema to soften impacted faeces.

Glycerin suppositories
Lubricate and inset into the rectum.

Liquid paraffin
Liquid paraffin is no longer used because of:
- impaired fat-soluble vitamin absorption;
- potential inhalation of droplets causing lipid pneumonia;
- anal seepage of oil;
- prolonged use has a risk of cancer.

Further reading
National Prescribing Centre (2003/04) *The management of constipation.* MEREC Bulletin 14.6
🖥 http://www.cks.nhs.uk/constipation (accessed 2 January 2010).
🖥 http://www.nhs.uk/Conditions/Constipation/Pages/Introduction.aspx (accessed 2 January 2010).

When and how to take laxative preparations (Table 12.11)

Table 12.11 When and how to take laxative preparations

Type of product	When to take	Specifics
Bulk formers	Do not take before bed	Should be taken with water and consumed as soon as the fibres swell
Osmotics	Lactulose: take with water or fruit juice	Lactulose: may take 48hr to work
	Magnesium hydroxide: shake well before taking and take with water	Magnesium hydroxide: 2–4hr before effect
		Avoid macrogols in pregnancy and breastfeeding. Discontinue if fluid or electrolyte imbalance
Stimulants	Senna: take with fluid	Senna: may take 8–12hr to work
	Bisacodyl: take after food and 1 hr after or before other medications	Bisacodyl: orally, effect in 10–12hr; suppository, 20–60min
	Dantron: take at bedtime	Dantron: effect in 6–12hr Incontinent patients: avoid prolonged contact with skin (risk of irritation/excoriation). Avoid in pregnancy and breastfeeding
		Glycerin suppositories: moisten with water and insert into faeces
Stimulants/ softeners/lubricants	Oral docusate sodium: take alone or 1hr after or before other medications	Oral docusate: take with water, effect in 1–2 days
		Arachis enema: warm to body heat. Needs to be retained for as long as possible for maximum effect

Prescribing for the prevention and treatment of infections

Immune response: 1

Specific immunity

T and B cells, which are provided by the lymphocytes, act as a co-ordinated response to specific antigens. T cells are responsible for the mediation of cell immunity, providing defence against abnormal cells and pathogens inside cells. B cells respond to antigens and pathogens in body fluids, providing humeral or antibody-mediated immunity (Table 12.12).

Vaccines

Vaccines provoke a response to a particular pathogen, which is intentionally administered in order to sensitize the immune cells for a subsequent exposure and protect the individual. Immunoglobulin refers to antibodies of a human origin. Antiserum refers to materials prepared in animals. (Table 12.13).

Adverse effects

These vary from a few symptoms to a mild form of the disease, including fever, malaise, and discomfort at the site of the injection.

Pregnancy and breastfeeding

The current BNF recommends that live vaccines should not be administered routinely during pregnancy because of the theoretical risk of fetal infection. However, where there is a significant risk of exposure to disease (e.g. to yellow fever or influenza), the need to administer an inactivated virus vaccination usually outweighs any possible risk to the fetus. Termination of pregnancy following inadvertent immunization is not recommended by the BNF.

If a breastfeeding woman has a significant risk of exposure to a disease, vaccination is not contraindicated despite a theoretical risk of live vaccine being present in breast milk.

Evidence of risk for pregnant or breastfeeding women has not been found when using inactivated viral or bacterial vaccines or toxoids. For specific vaccines use during pregnancy or breast-feeding, see under individual vaccines in the current BNF.

📖 Prescribing for breastfeeding women, p. 222.

Table 12.12 Forms of immunity

Type of immunity	How acquired
Innate immunity	Present at birth. Genetically determined. No relationship to exposure to antigens
Acquired immunity	Not present at birth. Either active or passive
Active acquired immunity	Naturally acquired immunity following exposure to an antigen within the environment, or induced active immunity following deliberate exposure to an antigen (i.e. vaccination or immunization)
Passive acquired immunity	Natural passive immunity following the transfer of antibodies from another person (i.e a mother to her baby either in utero via the placenta or in breast milk), or induced passive immunity when antibodies are administered in the form of antisera to prevent or fight infection

Table 12.13 Types of vaccine

Type of vaccine	Characteristic	Number of doses
Inactivated preparation	The organism is treated with heat or chemically in order to render it safe. Stimulates antibody response but not cell-mediated immunity	May require an initial series of administrations followed by boosters
Attenuated organisms (e.g. poliomyelitis)	Viable organisms which cause infection but not disease. Stimulates both cell-mediated and humoral immunity	Immunization generally achieved by a single dose
Extracts of detoxified exotoxins	In some organisms the disease is caused by a reaction to toxins. The vaccination is by a chemically treated toxin so that toxicity is lost but antigenicity remains	Requires an initial series of administrations followed by boosters

Immune response: 2

Post-immunization pyrexia—Joint Committee on Vaccination and Immunization recommendation

Parents should be informed if pyrexia develops following childhood immunization, and the child should be given a dose of paracetamol suitable to their age and weight. This may be followed by a second dose 6–8hr later if symptoms persist (Table 12.14). Medical advice should be sought if pyrexia persists after the second dose. See literature accompanying the product for full details of side effects and contra-indications.

Table 12.14 Doses of paracetamol for post-immunization pyrexia in children

Age	Dose by mouth	Comments
2 months	60mg (10mg/kg if jaundiced)	For post-immunization pyrexia only. Otherwise, do not give to a baby under 3 months of age. Repeat once after 6 hours if necessary
3 months–1 year	60–120mg	
1–5 years	120–250mg	
6–12 years	250–500mg	

NB: doses may be repeated every 4–6hr when necessary. Do not exceed more than 4 doses in any 24hr period.

Anaphylactic reactions

These are rare but serious as they may prove fatal.

Route of administration

Most vaccines are given by the intramuscular route. However, some are given other routes:
• intradermal route for BCG vaccine;
• deep subcutaneous route for Japanese encephalitis and varicella vaccines;
• oral route for cholera, live poliomyelitis, rotavirus, and live typhoid vaccines.

Vaccines should **not** be given intravenously.

NB: children with bleeding disorders such as haemophilia or thrombocytopenia should not be given their vaccinations by the intramuscular route but by a deep subcutaneous injection.
📖 Prescribing for public health, p. 205.

Note

The Department of Health has advised ***against*** the use of jet guns for vaccination because of the risk of transmitting blood-borne infections such as HIV.

Prescribing tips

- Vaccines which are available for prescribers who are trained and competent in their administration and the contraindications and recognition and management of anaphylaxis are listed in the current BNF.
- In general, if the patient is suffering from an acute illness postpone vaccination.
- A severe reaction to a preceding dose is a contraindication for further doses and boosters.
- Hypersensitivity to hen's eggs contraindicates influenza vaccine.
- Live vaccines should not be routinely administered to individuals with impaired immune response or with leukaemia.
- Oral syringes can be obtained from the pharmacy to ensure that the correct dose/volume is given.

Additional information can be found on ⊞ http://www.medicinescomplete.com/mc/bnfc/current/6451.htm (accessed 2 February 2010).

Further reading:

Salisbury D., Ramsey M., and Nokes K. (2006). *Immunisation against infectious disease*. TSO, London.
⊞ http://www.dh.gov.uk/en/Publichealth/Healthprotection/Immunisation/Greenbook/DH_4097254

Treatment of bacterial infections

Know your bacteria

The cell walls of bacteria contain a substance called peptidoglycan. Penicillin, penicillinase-resistant penicillins, and cephalosporins disrupt the formation of the peptidoglycan layer of the cell wall, thus inhibiting the maintenance of the cell's osmotic gradient so that the cell ruptures and dies. Polymixins bind to phospholipids within the cell membrane, altering its permeability and allowing holes to form within the membrane resulting in the cell rupturing.

Bacterial cells differ in other ways from those of the human body:
- the permeable cell membrane contains no sterols;
- the cell lacks a nucleus;
- the genetic material (DNA) is found within a single chromosome lying in the cell cytoplasm;
- quinolones disrupt the replication of cell DNA, in particular blocking the activity of DNA gyrase essential for DNA replication and repair;
- similarly, metronidazole breaks down and inhibits synthesis of bacterial DNA;
- both preparations which stimulate the immune system providing protection from an assault and those which treat an established infection are listed in the BNF.

Table 12.15 explains how antibiotics work.

Choice of a suitable drug

There are two main considerations: the patient and the probable causative agent.

The patient
- History of allergy
- Hepatic and renal function
- Are they immunocompromised?
- Ability to tolerate oral medication
- If female, are they pregnant, breastfeeding, or taking an oral contraceptive
- Ethnic origins
- Age.

Probable causative organism
- Sensitivity
- Safety for a particular patient group
- Local antibacterial policies
- Is it a notifiable disease?

Other considerations
- Duration of treatment
- Dosage according to age, weight, renal function, and severity of the infection
- Route of administration
- Contraindications.

Remember
- Viral infections should not be treated with antibacterials.
- Antibacterials should not be prescribed prophylactically.
- There are specific timings for administation of some antibacterials (Table 12.16).

Prescribing antibiotics

Having reviewed the available evidence, NICE have published guidelines on prescribing of antibiotics for self-limiting respiratory tract infections.[1] They note that although antibiotic prescribing fell during the 1990s it is still at a higher level in the UK than other European countries.

📖 Prescribing for public health, p. 205.

Further reading

Salisbury, D., Ramsay, M., Noakes, K. (2006). *Immunisation against infectious disease*. TSO, London.

1. NICE (2008). Respiratory tract infections—antibiotic prescribing.
🖥 http://www.nice.org.uk/nicemedia/pdf/CG69FullGuideline.pdf (accessed 2 February 2010).

Table 12.15 How antibacterial drugs work

Classification	Mode of action	Mechanism	Examples
Bacteriostatic	Inhibit bacterial growth without killing the cell The human immune system will eventually destroy the bacteria	Modification of bacterial energy metabolism	Trimethoprim
		Protein synthesis inhibitors (e.g. macrolides)	Tetracyclines
		Macrolides accumulate within leucocytes and are transported to the root of the infection	Erythromycin Clarithromycin Roxithromycin
Bactericidal	Kill the bacteria	Inhibition of synthesis and damage to the cell wall or membrane	Penicillin
By chemical structure	Quinolones (synthetic antimicrobial agents) inhibit replication of bacterial DNA and prevent the bacteria from replication and repair. Others bind to the subunits of the bacterial ribosomes where proteins are synthesized (RNA)	Modification of bacterial nucleic acid or protein synthesis	Ciprofloxacin

Table 12.16 Optimal administration times and methods

Preparation	Timing	Reason
Tetracycline Demeclocycline Oxytetracycline	1hr before or 2hr after meals Should be swallowed whole, whilst sitting or standing	Absorption is adversely affected by: dairy products antacids zinc, calcium, iron, magnesium, and aluminium salts
Nitrofurantoin	After meals	To avoid gastric irritation

Prescribing for pain

Pain

People culturally and psychologically experience pain in different ways. When prescribing for pain it is important to remember how it is intensified by fear.

The physiology of pain

Physiologically sensations of pain are transmitted from nociceptors to the central nervous system (CNS). Nociceptors are found in the epidermal layer of the skin, the joint capsules, the periosteum of bone, and the walls of blood vessels. Nociceptors have a large receptive field and this makes it difficult to pinpoint the exact source of a painful sensation. Pain may be perceived as sharp and localized, diffuse, or referred.

Nociceptors may be sensitive to:
- extremes of temperature;
- mechanical damage;
- chemicals such as those which signal damaged cells.

Strong stimuli may excite all of these receptors.

During injury, tissue damage occurs to the cell membrane which releases arachidonic acid into the interstitial fluid in the injured area. This is converted by the enzyme cyclo-oxygenase into different types of prostaglandins.

Prostaglandins coordinate cellular activity and stimulate nociceptors in the area surrounding the injury. Thus the initial reaction to an injury is sharp localized pain followed by a more diffuse discomfort.

Assessing for pain
- Identify and treat or refer for treatment any underlying pathology.
- Prescribe and advise administration of regular doses of analgesia rather than a prn (as-required) regime.
- Choose the optimal route for the administration of the analgesia.
- Accompany prescribed analgesia with explanation and reassurance.
- Develop a concordant and trusting rapport with your patient and where possible allow them to control their pain relief.
- Liaise with the acute pain service if necessary.

Examples of some online pain assessment tools are given in Box 12.1.

Box 12.1 Online pain asessment tools

Children

⊟ http://www.gosh.nhs.uk/gosh/clinicalservices/Pain_control_service/
Custom%20Menu_02/

⊟ http://www.rcn.org.uk/development/practice/pain

Palliative care

⊟ http://www.hospicecare.com/resources/pain-research.htm

⊟ http://whocancerpain.wisc.edu/?q=node/112

Adults (including those with dementia)

⊟ http://pain-topics.org/clinical_concepts/assess.php

Older people

⊟ http://www.biomedcentral.com/1471-2318/6/3

Emergency and urgent care

⊟ http://www.library.nhs.uk/Emergency/ViewResource.
aspx?resID=266669

(All accessed 3 February 2010)

Aspirin

Aspirin (acetylsalicylic acid) acts reversibly. It inactivates cyclo-oxygenase which is responsible for the production of prostaglandins and the inflammatory response to injury. Therefore action is local rather than central, involving the brain.

The body's response to pyrexia is the release of prostaglandins in the brain, which causes the hypothalamus to reset the body's thermostat at the new higher level in an attempt to preserve stasis. Aspirin enables the normal body temperature to be restored.

Therefore aspirin is suitable for use with:
• mild to moderate pain such as:
  • headache;
  • muscular pain;
  • dysmenorrhea.
• pyrexia.

Minimize gastric irritation by taking after food and/or prescribing enteric-coated aspirin. The adult dose is 300–900mg every 4–6hr, with a maximum of 4g daily. Use aspirin with caution for older people.

📖 Basic principles of pharmacology, pp. 53–64.
📖 Prescribing for special groups, pp. 197–223.

The interactions and side effects of aspirin are shown in Tables 12.17 and 12.18.

Table 12.17 Drugs that interact with aspirin

Drug	Effect of aspirin
Anticoagulants	Increased risk of bleeding due to antiplatelet effect
Antacids and adsorbents	Increased urine alkalinity
	Increased excretion of aspirin
Anti-epileptics, e.g. phenytoin and valproate	Enhances the effect of phenotoin and valporate
Corticosteriods	Increased risk of:
	gastrointestinal bleeding
	gastrointestinal ulceration
Cytotoxics	Reduced excretion rate
	Increased toxicity
Diuretics	Antagonism of diuretic effect of spironalactone
	Reduced excretion of acetazolamide (risk of toxicity)
Metoclopramide	Increased rate of aspirin absorption
Mifepristone	Avoid aspirin until 8–12 days after taking mifepristone
Uricosurics	Reduction in effects of probenecid and sulfinpyrazone.

Table 12.18 Side effects and contraindications of aspirin

Area	Side effects	Comments
Gastric	Irritates gastric mucosa Can cause nausea and vomiting Gastric ulceration Gastric bleeding Exacerbation of peptic ulceration Erosive gastritis	Inhibits prostaglandin production, decreasing production of gastric mucus Can lead to mucosal damage and bleeding (blood loss of 10–30ml per day) To reduce these effects take after food
Anticoagulation	Blood vessels damaged in tissue injury By inhibiting the enzyme cyclo-oxygenase, aspirin inhibits platelet aggregation	Has an anticoagulatory effect In large doses may prolong the bleeding time Should not be prescribed for people with haemophilia
Hypersensitivity	Attacks of asthma, angio-oedema, urticaria, and rhinitis have been precipitated by aspirin	Caution: 1 in 10 patients with asthma or allergic conditions may be hypersensitive to aspirin
Renal and hepatic disease	Can cause liver and kidney impairment	Those with these conditions should avoid aspirin
Pregnancy	Can cause fetal abnormalities if taken in the 3rd trimester Can prolongs pregnancy and labour Can cause excessive bleeding before, during, and after delivery	Avoid if possible in the last few weeks of pregnancy
Reye's syndrome	Can cause Reye's syndrome in children under 16 years Symptoms involve a combination of: • swelling of the brain • liver inflammation Avoid using aspirin during or following a viral infection as this may trigger Reye's syndrome in children under 16 years of age	Do not give aspirin to children under 12 years Do not give aspirin to breastfeeding mothers
Toxicity	Tinnitus Hearing loss Hyperventilation Respiratory acidosis Fever	Toxicity occurs when daily dosage exceeds 4g

Other NSAIDs

Most other NSAIDs act reversibly. They reduce prostaglandin production by inhibiting the enzyme cyclo-oxygenase. Pain relief starts soon after taking the first dose and the full analgesic effect should normally be obtained within a week. However, their anti-inflammatory effect may not be achieved for up to 3 weeks.

Administration routes

NSAIDs may be administered by several routes.
- Orally.
- Some topically.
- Diclofenac: rectally or orally. Diclofenac **must not be administered intravenously (IV)** as this may cause venous thrombosis.
- Some by injection for musculoskeletal pain (e.g. acute low back pain). The side effects are the same as for oral administration with the additional problem of painful injections.
- Ketorolac may be given IM or slowly IV (see latest BNF).

Adverse effects

As with aspirin, NSAIDs can cause gastrointestinal irritation, bleeding, and perforation, with increased risk at higher doses and in those over 60 years of age or with a history of peptic ulcer. NSAIDs may:
- exacerbate asthma;
- precipitate renal failure in those with heart failure, cirrhosis, or renal insufficiency.

Contraindications

- Use with caution for older people.
- Contraindicated for those with allergic disorders:
  - asthma;
  - urticaria;
  - rhinitis.
- Contraindicated for those with a hypersensitivity to aspirin or angio-oedema.
- Contraindicated during pregnancy and breastfeeding.
- Contraindicated for those with impaired coagulation.
- Long-term use may cause reduced fertility in women, which is reversed on cessation of treatment.

Interactions

See NSAID interactions in the latest BNF:
🖥 http://www.medicinescomplete.com/mc/bnf/current/5183.htm

Many NSAIDs can cause serious side effects, but ibuprofen, diclofenac, and naproxen are relatively safe. Ibuprofen has the lowest incidence of side effects, is the cheapest, and can be purchased as an OTC medication. Ibuprofen is useful as both an analgesic and an antipyretic in children when paracetamol is insufficient.

📖 Over-the-counter (OTC) drugs, p. 422.

NICE quick reference guides

NICE quick reference guides contain clinical guidelines that provide recommendations about the treatment and care of people with specific
diseases and conditions in the NHS in England and Wales, e.g. pain in
rheumatoid arthritis (Table 12.19).

• The guidance represents the view of NICE arrived at after careful
  consideration of the evidence available
• Health-care professionals are expected to take it fully into account
  when exercising their clinical judgment
• The guidance does not override the individual responsibility of
  healthcare professionals to make decisions:
  • appropriate to the circumstances of the individual patient;
  • in consultation with the patient and/or guardian or carer;
  • informed by the summary of product characteristics of any drugs
    they are considering.

A table listing the available quick guides can be obtained from
📖 http://www.nice.org.uk/Guidance/CG/Published (accessed 10 October
2009).

Table 12.19 NSAID dosage for rheumatoid arthritis

NSAID	Timing	Adult doses	Child doses
Ibuprofen	3–4 divided doses	Oral dose 1.6–2.4g daily (max. 2.4g daily)	According to body weight e.g. over 5kg–5mg per kg 3–4 divided doses
Diclofenac (oral or rectal)	2–3 divided doses	Oral dose 75–150mg daily Rectal dose 75–150mg daily	–
Naproxen	1–2 divided doses	Oral dose 0.5–1g daily (max. 1.25g daily)	–

Paracetamol

Paracetamol has similar analgesic and antipyretic properties to aspirin but is not an anti-inflammatory agent. It is thought to work by inhibiting the production of cyclo-oxygenase in the CNS and to have an effect on peripheral pain receptors. It is suitable for mild to moderate pain. Recommended dosages are given in Table 12.20.

Adverse effects

Paracetamol has relatively few adverse effects compared with aspirin. However, the toxic level is only slightly greater than the therapeutic level, and overdosage is particularly dangerous as it may cause liver damage which is sometimes not apparent for 4–6 days. In overdose, the liver is unable to provide sufficient amounts of the protein glutathione which counteracts the highly toxic metabolite acetyl-benzo-quinoneimine formed during the breakdown of paracetamol in the liver.

There is a possibility of accidental overdose as many OTC medications for pain, sinus problems, or cold and flu symptom relief contain paracetamol alone or in combination with other drugs. It is vital to ask patients to check the active ingredients in any other remedy they may be taking and not to take more than one paracetamol-containing preparation at a time.

Paracetamol can be used safely for children and for pregnant and breastfeeding women, and is also suitable for use with older people.

Contraindications

There are no contraindications. However, use is cautioned for those with hepatic or renal impairment or those who suffer from alcohol dependence.

Interactions

See current BNF appendix regarding paracetamol.

Table 12.20 Paracetamol dosage

Age group	Dose (PO)	Timing	Maximum dose
Adult	0.5–1g	4–6 hourly	4g daily
Children: 2 months (post-immunization pyrexia)	60mg (10mg/kg if jaundiced*)		
3 months–1 year	60–120mg	4–6 hourly	4 doses in 24hr
1–5 years	120–250mg	4–6 hourly	4 doses in 24hr
6–12 years	250–500mg	4–6 hourly	4 doses in 24hr

*📖 Post-immunization pyrexia, p. 312

Opioid analgesics

Opioids act on receptors in the CNS which are designed for the body's endogenous opiods and therefore have no anti-inflammatory effects. The opioid receptors suppress pain messages from the periphery to the CNS. Each receptor has been designated a letter of the Greek alphabet, mu (μ), kappa (κ), epsilon (ε), and delta (δ) (Table 12.21).

Adverse effects of opiates

Morphine, codeine, and pethidine all mimic the action of endogenous opiates, providing both pain relief and unwanted effects such as:
- respiratory depression;
- constipation;
- drowsiness;
- visual disturbances and/or hallucinations;
- bradycardia or tachycardia;
- sedation;
- miosis (constriction of the pupil of the eye);
- anorexia;
- flushing;
- urticaria;
- nausea;
- urinary retention;
- postural hypotension.

Opioids are used for the relief of moderate to severe pain. With repeated administration, there is a risk of the patient becoming tolerant or dependent on these drugs. This should not be a deterrent for their use in the management of pain in terminal illness.

Contraindications of opioid analgesics

Opioids should be used with caution in patients with:
- impaired respiratory function;
- hypotension;
- shock;
- myasthenia gravis;
- prostatic hypertrophy;
- obstructive or inflammatory bowel disorders;
- diseases of the biliary tract;
- convulsive disorders.

Opioids should be avoided in those with chronic obstructive pulmonary disease (COPD) and those suffering an asthma attack.

Codeine phosphate (a morphine salt) is contraindicated in respiratory disease and for those with respiratory depression or a hypersensitivity to opioids.

Opiod doses should be reduced for:
- older people or debilitated patients;
- those with hepatic impairment (avoid opiods if severe);
- those with renal impairment (avoid opiods if severe).

Table 12.21 Opioid receptors and the corresponding endogenous opioid

Receptor	Position	Endogenous opioid	Action
Mu (μ)	Dorsal horn of the spinal chord and thalamus	Endogenous endorphin	Analgesia Respiratory depression Euphoria
Kappa (κ)	Hypothalamus	Dynorphin	Analgesia Sedation Miosis Hypothermia
Epsilon (ε)	Hippocampus and amygdala	Enkephalin	Some psychotic effects Dysphoria
Delta (δ)	Limbic system	Unknown	Behavioural change Hallucinations

Palliative care

The cautions listed above should not necessarily be a deterrent to the use of opioid analgesics for palliative care in the control of pain in terminal illness.

Interactions

- See appendix in the latest BNF.
- There is a special hazard with pethidine and possibly other opioids and monoamine oxidase inhibitors (MAOIs).

Repeated use of opioid analgesics is associated with the development of psychological and physical dependence. This is rarely a problem with therapeutic use, but caution is advised if prescribing for patients with a history of drug dependence. Avoid abrupt withdrawal after long-term treatment.

Prescribing for neuropathic pain

Neuropathic pain results from damage to neural tissue. It includes conditions such as:
- post-herpetic neuralgia;
- phantom limb pain;
- compression neuropathies;
- peripheral neuropathies;
- pain following stroke;
- spinal chord injury;
- syringomyelia;
- idiopathic neuropathy.

Treatment
- Tricyclic antidepressants are usually used for treatment of neuropathic pain.
- Some anti-epileptic drugs may also be suitable.
- Opioids are only partially effective for this type of pain but may be considered if other treatments fail (e.g. methadone, tramadol, and oxycodone).
- The use of transcutaneous electrical nerve stimulation (TENS) may help.
- Topical application of capsaicin cream.
- Compression neuropathy may be eased by the use of corticosteroid preparations.

Analgesic ladder
The WHO's conceptual framework of an analgesic ladder (Fig. 12.6) suggests that, when pain occurs, initially there should be prompt oral administration of drugs in the following order until the patient is free from pain:
- non-opioids (aspirin and paracetamol);
- mild opioids (codeine);
- strong opioids such as morphine.

To calm fears and anxiety, additional drugs or 'adjuvants', which speed up or delay the action of others, should be used. To maintain freedom from pain, drugs should be given 'by the clock' (i.e. every 3–6hr) rather than 'on demand'.

This three-step approach of administering the right drug in the right dose at the right time is inexpensive and 80–90% effective.[1]

1. WHO (2008). Pain relief ladder. ☐ http://www.who.int/cancer/palliative/painladder/en/ (accessed 10 October 2009).

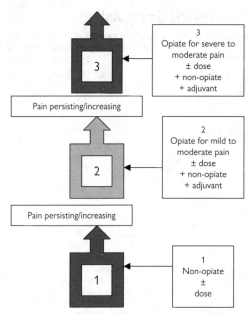

Fig. 12.6 WHO analgesic ladder (reproduced with permission).

Local anaesthetics (LAs)

LAs may be applied to the mucous membrane or injected causing a reversible block to the transmission of pain signals along a nerve pathway. The variation of preparation determines its applicability to the route of administration:
• topical;
• epidural;
• local infiltration;
• nerve blocks.

Administration

Consider:
• the rate at which the LA preparations are absorbed and excreted;
• the potency of the product;
• the duration of the procedure;
• the patient's:
  • weight;
  • age;
  • clinical condition;
• vascularity in the area to be anaesthetized.

Contraindications

• Poor cooperation or refusal by the patient.
• Allergy to LA—anaphylaxis is rare but can occur:
  • check specific details of any reported allergy;
  • check if allergic symptoms were a response to overdose, or fainting caused by pain or fear rather than a reaction.
• Infection at the proposed site of injection:
  • injecting into this area could spread the infection;
  • inflammation may cause high tissue acidity which reduces the effectiveness of LA drugs which are bases.
• Bleeding disorders, anticoagulant therapy and thrombocytopenia are contraindications for nerve block procedures.

Side effects

Risk of toxicity in:
• small children;
• older people;
• people in poor clinical condition;
• people with:
  • heart block;
  • low cardiac output;
  • epilepsy;
  • myasthenia gravis;
  • hepatic impairment;
  • porphyria;
• anti-arrhythmic or B-blocker therapy (risk of myocardial depression)
• cimetidine therapy (inhibits the metabolism of lidocaine).

Prescribing for the respiratory tract

Brief anatomy and physiology of the respiratory tract

The respiratory tract comprises:
- upper respiratory tract—nose, nasal cavity, and pharynx;
- lower respiratory tract—larynx (voice box), trachea (windpipe), bronchi, and lungs containing bronchioles and alveoli.

Structure of the upper respiratory tract (Fig. 12.7)

The nose and nasal cavity
- Two nasal passages.
- Rich blood supply and secretory cells to provide warm and moist air to the lungs.
- Produce up to 1L of mucus in 24hr.
- Lined with nasal hairs and cilia to remove dust particles.

The pharynx
This muscular tube leads from the oral cavity and nose to the larynx and oesophagus. It contains lymphoid tissue:
- the nasopharyngeal tonsils (adenoids);
- the palatine and lingual tonsils.

These lymph glands filter out invading micro-organisms.

Structure of the lower respiratory tract

The larynx
This is cartilaginous box containing:
- the epiglottis, which stops ingested materials from entering the bronchi;
- the vocal chords.

The trachea
- Kept open by C-shaped cartilage ribs.
- Lined with secretory cells.

The lungs
- Cone-shaped and divided into lobes.
- Right lung has three lobes; left lung has two lobes.

The bronchi
- Divided into the right and left branches to the corresponding lungs;
- Kept open by C-shaped cartilage ribs.
- Tree-like configuration.
- Each bronchus divides to form narrower passages called bronchioles.

The bronchioles
- The most distant branches are called terminal bronchioles.
- These divide into finer tubes called respiratory bronchioles which terminate in the alveoli.

The alveoli
- Rich capillary blood supply to facilitate gas exchange.
- Approximately 150 million alveoli in each lung.

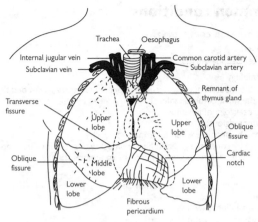

Fig. 12.7 The respiratory system.

Drugs and treatments for the respiratory system

- Respiratory stimulants
- Pulmonary surfactants
- Oxygen
- Mucolytics
- Aromatic inhalers
- Cough suppressants
- Expectorants and demulcent preparations
- Mouthwashes.

Common conditions

The common cold (coryza)

Definition
- Acute nasopharyngitis

Epidemiology
This is the most frequently occurring upper respiratory tract condition and is the most common infection experienced by healthy children[1] who act as reservoirs of infection:[2]
- very contagious;
- spread by droplets when sneezing and coughing;
- spread by contact, e.g. direct hand contact with secretions from an infected person or indirectly from environmental surfaces.

Causes
- Viral—often rhinoviruses but may be:
  - adenoviruses;
  - para-influenza viruses;
  - respiratory syncytial virus (RSV);
  - coronaviruses;
  - human meta-pneumovirus;
  - enteroviruses.[1]
- Local inflammation caused by immunological response.
- Micro-organisms are contained in the mucus produced in response to the inflammation.

Signs and symptoms
- Red and swollen nose
- Extra secretion of clear fluid
- Coughing, sneezing, hoarse voice
- Low-grade fever and general malaise
- Muscular aches.

Treatment:
- Pain relief
- Relief of fever
- Topical nasal decongestants
- OTC cold remedies containing decongestant and pain relief combinations
- Steam inhalation.

Further advice obtainable from 🖳 http://www.npsa.nhs.uk/search (accessed 7 May 2010).

Acute sore throat (pharyngitis, laryngitis, or tonsillitis)

Definitions
- Tonsillitis: acute inflammation of the tonsils.
- Laryngitis: acute inflammation of the larynx.
- Pharyngitis: acute inflammation of the pharynx.

Causes
- Tonsillitis:
  - usually viral;
  - if bacterial, commonly group A B-haemolytic streptococcus.
- Laryngitis:
  - often occurs in individuals with respiratory infections such as pneumonia or bronchitis.
- Pharyngitis:
  - oedema of the vocal chords.

Signs and symptoms
- Sore throat
- Inflammation of the larynx leading to hoarse voice
- Extra secretion of clear fluid
- Coughing
- Sneezing
- Low-grade fever
- Muscular aches.

Treatment
- Pain relief
- Gargling
- Mouthwash
- Treat symptoms
- Increase fluid intake
- If confident bacterial case, treat with antibiotics.[3]

Allergic rhinitis
May be self-limiting and not require any treatment.

Definition
Nasal passage has hypersensitive responses to allergens such as pollen.

Causes
- Pollen activates mast cells in the nasal passages.
- Mast cells release histamine and other mediators.
- Histamine acts on receptors in the lining of the nasal passage.
- This causes vasodilation and increased capillary permeability.

Signs and symptoms
- Sneezing
- Watery discharge
- Swollen mucous membranes which lead to narrowing of the airways
- Itchy eyes
- Watering eyes.

Treatment
- Topical nasal corticosteroids.
- Oral and topical antihistamines.
- Systemic nasal decongestants.
- If seasonal condition, begin treatment 2–3 weeks before the triggering pollen is in the environment.

Further reading

Department of Health (2003). *Immunisation against infectious diseases—pneumococcal*. Department of Health, London.

File, T.M., Jr (2002). New millennium: new antimicrobial agents for respiratory infections: but an old plea. *Current Opinion in Infectious Diseases*, **13**, 141–3.

Low, D.E. (2000). Trends and significance of antimicrobial resistance in respiratory pathogens. *Current Opinion in Infectious Diseases*, **13**, 145–53.

Public Health Laboratory Service (1997). *Clostridium difficile infection. Prevention and management*. Department of Public Health, London.

Redding, S.W. (2001). The role of yeasts other than Candida albicans in oropharangeal candidiasis. *Current Opinion in Infectious Diseases*, **14**, 673–7.

Wood S.F. (2003). Sneezing, runny, blocked or itchy nose: is it hay fever a cold or something else? *Nurse Prescribing*, **1**, 86–91.

1. Kesson, A. (2007). The common cold. *Paediatrics Respiratory Review*, **8**, 240–8.
2. Tolan, R.W. (2009). *Rhinovirus infection*. ⬚ http://emedicine.medscape.com/article/971592-overview/ (accessed 21 September 2009).
3. Practical antibiotic prescribing guidelines. ⬚ http://www.cks.nhs.uk (accessed 13 October 2009).

Prescribing for skin problems

Brief anatomy and physiology of skin

Structure and purpose of the skin (Fig. 12.8)

- Skin is the largest organ in the human body.
- In adults the surface area is approximately 2m^2.
- Skin limits water loss through this surface area to ~500mL each day.
- Skin comprises 16% of an individual's body weight.
- Skin is composed of the outer epidermis and the inner dermis.
- The structure varies depending on the position in the body, e.g. hairy areas such as the scalp have a thin epidermis, and the non-hairy palms of the hands and soles of the feet have a thicker epidermis.
- Skin structure varies depending on age, environment, and ethnicity.
- Accessory structures, such as hair, nails, sweat, and sebaceous glands, are located within the dermis but protrude through the epidermis.

Epidermis

- Provides protection from mechanical and micro-organism assault.
- Outermost layer—stratum corneum.
- Innermost layer—stratum germinativum—is attached to the basement membrane which forms the barrier between epidermis and dermis.
- The stratum germinativum generates new cells to replace those shed at the epithelial surface.
- As cells move towards the surface of the skin their structure and functions change:
  - initially at the basement membrane they begin forming a protein, keratin;
  - during their journey to the surface they continue this protein synthesis;
  - on reaching the surface some 15–30 days later, their internal organelles have gone and they are flattened capsules of protein.
- They remain in the stratum corneum for 14 days, providing a protective barrier:
  - first, this lipid-rich barrier limits the loss of water through the skin surface;
  - secondly, the keratin within each flattened cell enables water molecules to be retained.

Dermis

- Consists of a network of proteins, collagen, and elastin:
  - elastin provides flexibility to the skin;
  - collagen provides strength.
- Accessory structures, e.g. sweat glands, are found throughout the dermal area, whereas sebaceous glands are found only in hairy areas.

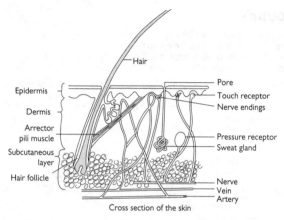

Fig. 12.8 Brief anatomy and physiology of the skin. Reproduced from Glasper, E.A., McEwing, G., and Richardson, J. (2006). *Oxford Handbook of Children's and Young People's Nursing*, by kind permission of Oxford University Press.

Function of the skin

- Protection of underlying structures
- Maintenance of body temperature
- Storage of nutrients
- Excretion of waste (i.e. salt, water)
- Sensory detection of temperature, pain, etc.
- Protection from mechanical and micro-organism assault.

Wounds

Wounds are classified depending on their depth.
- Superficial wounds affect the epidermis.
- Partial-thickness wounds extend as far as the dermis.
- Full-thickness wounds involve fat or deeper layers.

A break in the external integrity of the dermis leads to a loss of function of the skin, depending on the nature of the wound.
- Burns lead to loss of fluid, with extensive burns this may be a life-threatening loss.
- Lacerations and punctures allow micro-organisms to enter the deeper tissues and cause infection.

Causes of wounds
- Trauma, which may be chemical, physical, or mechanical
- Surgery
- Ischaemia (e.g. arterial leg ulcers)
- Pressure (e.g. pressure sores, corns, foot ulcers)
- The above in combination.

Healing
- Primary intention: formation of limited amounts of new tissue (e.g. wounds closed by sutures).
- Secondary intention: wounds caused by trauma may involve new tissue to fill the gap and a covering of epithelium.
- The healing processes of both primary and secondary intention have three overlapping phases:
  - inflammation—red, hot, swollen, and painful;
  - proliferation;
  - maturation.

Inflammation
- Initial bleeding at the wound site delivers fibrinogen, which brings the edges into close approximation, and fibrin, which forms the blood clot.
- The blood clot dries to a scab, preventing bacterial invasion and further fluid loss.
- Serum proteins and white cells leak from adjacent blood vessels, which gives rise to the appearance of inflammation.
- Neutrophils and macrophages move into the area to clear any debris and bacteria.

Proliferation
- New blood vessels are formed in a collagen matrix (granulation).
- The wound contracts.
- Epithelialization: epithelial cells on the wound surface grow down under the dried scab.

Maturation
- The number of blood vessels decreases.
- Collagen and scar tissue gradually reshape to normal tissue.

Assessment of wounds

Patient history
- General health
- Social circumstances
- Environment.

Routine physical examination
- Position, size, and depth of the wound.
- Is the tissue sloughy covered or filled with soft yellow slough?
- Is the tissue necrotic—covered with a hard black layer?
- How much exudate?
- Any there signs of infection?
- Presence or absence of pain?
- Is the wound clean with significant tissue loss (granulating)?
- Is the wound clean and superficial (epithelializing)?

Wound dressings

Functions
- Maintenance of high humidity (speeds up epithelial growth, reduces pain, and breaks down necrotic tissue).
- Dries excess exudates, preventing tissue maceration.
- Allows gaseous exchange which is thought to be beneficial.
- Thermal insulation—a temperature of 37°C promotes macrophage and mitotic activity during granulation and formation of epithelial tissue.
- Impermeability to bacteria by reduction of contact with the air.
- Freedom from contaminates and particles.

  Dressings need to be replaced without causing trauma to the healing wound.

Assessment
- Essential to fit the type of dressing to the needs of the wound.
- Physical examination.
- Must concord with patient's wishes.

📖 History-taking, p. 174.
📖 Clinical and physical examination, p. 178.

Further reading

Dealey, C. (2005). *The care of wounds* (3rd edn). Blackwell Science, Oxford.
Moffatt, C., Martin, R., and Smithdale, R. (2007). *Leg ulcer management: essential skills for nurses.* Blackwell, Oxford.

Eczema

Atopic eczema (atopic dermatitis) is a chronic, relapsing, inflammatory, and itchy skin condition. Atopic means sensitivity to allergens. Atopic eczema may vary in severity from reddened and occasionally itchy skin to painful cracked and bleeding skin.

Aetiology
Eczema is characterized by:
- an itchy red rash, often in skin folds such as the elbows and back of the knee;
- associated with other atopic diseases such as:
  - asthma;
  - hay fever.
- the majority of cases develop in childhood or infancy;
- often familial.

Causes
May be triggered by allergens or irritants such as:
- soaps, detergents, shower gels;
- skin infections;
- contact allergens (e.g. pet fur, pollen);
- food allergens (e.g. cow's milk, hen's eggs, nuts, soya, wheat);
- inhalant allergens (e.g. house dust mites);
- emotional stress;
- fluctuations of hormone levels.

Diagnosis
Holistic assessment:
- Onset
- Pattern
- Severity
- Response to previous/current treatments
- Identify possible trigger factors (e.g. changes in washing powder, soap)
- Impact of condition on patient and family/carers
- Dietary history—may require a food diary
- General health
- Children—growth and development
- Personal and family history of atopic disease.

Clinical criteria

Persistent itchy skin in addition to three or more of the following:
- Itchiness and irritation in skin creases:
  - front of elbows;
  - behind the knees;
  - front of ankles;
  - around the neck;
  - around the eyes.
- Have asthma or hay fever, or have had them in the past. If a child, have a parent or sibling with asthma or hayfever.
- Dry skin over the preceding year.
- Condition started when 2 years old or younger.
- Reddened inflamed areas on the skin covering joints such as elbows, knees and wrists.

Further reading

http://www.cks.nhs.uk/eczema (accessed 13 January 2010).

Treatment of eczema

Childhood eczema often improves with age.

Self-care
- Avoid scratching as this may cause infection.
- Keep nails short.
- Use anti-scratch mittens for babies.
- Avoid known trigger factors where possible.
- Try using a soap substitute.
- Keep the home cool if heat is a trigger factor.

Emollients
Emollients reduce the symptoms caused by skin dryness by improving the depleted lipid barrier of the skin which reduces water loss. This lessens dryness and itch and increases the skin's resistance to irritants. Therefore emollients are indicated for use where there is a diagnosis of eczema. They are made in three preparations:
- lotions (lipid content lowest);
- creams;
- ointments (lipid content highest).

The type of emollient may be varied depending on the response (Table 12.22). Emollients should always be generously smoothed into the skin (in the same direction as the hairs grow) after showering or bathing, and initially three times daily. Some emollients may be added directly to bath water. However, these leave the bath slippery and care must be taken to avoid slips and falls.

The current BNF contains a full list of emollients available. A Prodigy quick reference guide for emollient use in eczema is also available.

Treating an eczema 'flare-up' in an infant or child
Flare-up inflammation should be treated with topical corticosteroids[2] in addition to emollients. It may be necessary to change the emollient to one with a higher lipid content. Wait for 30min after applying corticosteroid before applying emollient.[3]

Initially a mildly potent corticosteroid such as hydrocortisone 1% should be applied once daily using finger-tip units (FTUs):
- One FTU is the amount of cream or ointment which can be squeezed from a standard nozzle onto an adult finger tip to the first crease of the finger.
- One FTU is sufficient to treat an area of skin equivalent to twice that of the palm of an adult's hand.[4]

Table 12.22 Types of emollient to use

Considerations	Type	Notes
Hairy skin	Lotion	
Mildly dry skin	Cream/lotion	
Moderate to severely dry skin	Ointment/cream	
Weeping eczema	Cream	
Individual preference	May want an additional emollient for use during the day	Ointment may be used at night and cream during the day
Intolerance	Some emollients may cause skin reactions	Sensitivity to: preservatives fragrances lanolin

Further reading

NICE. Guidelines for eczema treatment
<svg> http://www.nhs.uk/Conditions/Eczema(atopic)/Pages/Treatment.aspx (accessed 10 October 2009).
NICE. Guidelines for treatment of eczema in children.
<svg> http://www.nice.org.uk/guidance/index.jsp?action=byID&o=1190 (accessed 10 October 2009).

1. PRODIGY quick reference guide. *Emollient use in eczema.* <svg> www.nelm.nhs.uk/en/NeLM- (accessed 10 October 2009).
2. Hoare, C., Li Wan Po, A., and Williams, H. (2000). Systematic review of treatments for atopic eczema. *Health Technology Assessment* **4**(37) 1–191.
3. PRODIGY quick reference guide. *Atopic eczema: managing flare-ups in children.* Version 1.1. <svg> www.nelm.nhs.uk (accessed 10 October 2009).
4. MeReC (1999). Using topical corticosteroids in general practice. *McRec Bulletin* **10**(6) 21–4.

Infected eczema

The Clinical Knowledge Summaries (CKS) suggest that *Staphylococcus aureus* or *Streptococcus pyogenes* are the most likely invading organisms.[1]

Diagnosis

The patient:

• may be unwell;
• may be feverish;
• pustules may develop and become moist and weepy.

A swab should be taken for culture and sensitivity.

Treatment

Treat clinically.

• Treat apparent bacterial infection with oral antibiotics. Flucloxacillin (or erythromycin if the patient is allergic to penicillin) is the preferred recommendation.[1]
• Continue emollients.

NB: topical corticosteroids and emollients used during the infection should be disposed of as they may be contaminated.

Differential diagnosis

It is important to distinguish infected eczema from eczema herpeticum where the eczema is infected with type 1 or type 2 herpes simplex virus (HSV). Eczema herpeticum may cause significant morbidity and death. Eczema herpeticum may be suspected if:

• the patient is unwell and feverish;
• the eczema is worsening and painful;
• the appearance may be of clusters or blisters;
• erosion appears to be punched out;
• erosions form large areas with a haemorrhagic crust.

Eczema herpeticum may require systemic or IV antiviral therapy in addition to antibiotics for any secondary infections.[2]

1. Clinical Knowledge Summaries (CKS) (2007). ▣ http://cks.library.nhs.uk/eczema_atopic (accessed 10 October 2009).
2. McKenna, J. and Krusinski, P. (2007) *Karposi varicelliform eruption.* ▣ http://tinyurl.com/oxcezk (accessed 15 May 2009).

Rashes

Terms used to describe different rashes are listed in Table 12.23.

Table 12.23 Terms used to describe different rashes

Common name	Medical term	Description
Nettle rash or hives	Urticaria	Red itchy weals or swellings
Spots	Papule	Small circumscribed elevated area of skin
	Age spots	Small areas of pigmented skin often associated with ageing
	Koplik spots	Small red spots with blue-white centres which appear on the buccal mucosa prior to the disseminated rash in measles
	Macula	Small reddened area
	Pustule	Collection of pus visible in the epidermis
Redness	Erythema	Redness of the skin produced by congestion of the capillaries
Boil	Furuncle	Infection (often staphylococcal) which involves a hair follicle
Group of boils	Carbuncle	
Cold sore	Herpes	Clusters of small vesicles on or above the lip caused by infection by the herpes virus
Rash	Impetigo	Discrete vesicles surrounded by an erythematous border which may exude an amber liquid which dries to form a yellow crust
	Dermatitis	Inflammation of the connective tissue underlying the skin
	Annular	A rash that is ring shaped
Itch mite	Scabies	Contagious dermatitis cause by *Sarcoptes scabiei*

Table 12.23 (Contd.)

Common name	Medical term	Description
Birthmarks Strawberry mark Port wine stain	Naevus	Localized capillary-rich area of the skin.
Whitlow	Onychia	Ulceration at the base of a fingernail or toenail
Bruise	Contusion	An injury which has caused discoloration without breaking the skin
Blood blister		A collection of blood within a skin blister caused by pinching

Further reading

Barankin, B., Metelitsa, A.I., and Lin, A.N. (2004). *Stedman's illustrated dictionary of dermatology eponyms*. Lippincott Williams & Wilkins, Philadelphia, PA.

Skin conditions

Terms used to describe different skin conditions are listed in Table 12.24.

Table 12.24 Terms used to describe skin conditions

Term	Definition	Treatment
Abrasion	A scraping injury which produces a break in the epithelium	Clean Cover or leave open depending on severity
Animal or human bites	Abrasion, laceration, or puncture wound caused by an animal or human bite	As for abrasion Consider tetanus cover Consider antibiotic cover
Atopic dermatitis or eczema	Inflammatory skin disorder	Emollients Creams Ointments
Boils Carbuncles Folliculitis Furuncles	Bacterial infection of the hair follicles which may spread to deeper tissues	Generally resolve without treatment Consider pain relief If spreading consider antibiotics
Burns:	Tissue damage or loss caused by exposure to:	As for abrasion Consider pain relief Consider tetanus cover
thermal	flame, steam, or hot liquid	
chemical	acid or base	
electrical	electrical current	
radiation	sunburn or radiation treatment	
Candidiasis	Infection of the skin usually caused by *Candida albicans*	Imidazoles Corticosteriods Topical antifungals Clean the skin
Chronic skin ulcer	Blistered, broken, or necrotic skin lesions which may extend to underlying structures	Metronidazole Silver sulfadiazine
Pressure sores (decubitus ulcer)	Impaired mobility causing long-term pressure on bony prominences	Move the patient frequently

Table 12.24 (Contd.)

Term	Definition	Treatment
Leg ulcers	Loss of skin of the leg which takes more than 6 weeks to heal	Use appropriate mattress aids etc.
Foot ulcers	Loss of skin of the foot which takes more than 6 weeks to heal	If ankle brachial pressure index at least 0.8 multilayer compression bandaging is indicated
Dermatitis		Identify and avoid cause where possible
Contact	Localized inflammatory reaction caused by chemical irritant, hypersensitivity, or an allergen	Emollients Topical corticosteroids
Seborrhoeic (cradle cap in infants)	Inflammatory disorder involving the scalp, eyebrows, eyelids, ear canals, nasolabial folds, axillae, and trunk	From age 1 year: topical antifungals, corticosteroid gels and lotions, ketoconazole 2% shampoo For cradle cap in infants: soft brushes and baby shampoo/baby oil
Dermatophytosis (ringworm)	Fungal infection of the stratum corneum of the skin, the nails, and the hair	Topical application of: Imidazoles Clotrimazole
Tinea corporis	Annular lesion with a raised scaly edge with the centre clear	Topical application of: Clotrimazole 1% / Hydrocortisone 1% cream
Tinea cruris (rare in women, common in young males)	Scaly erythematous rash of the inner aspects of both thighs and sometimes the buttocks	Terbinafine cream
Tinea pedis (athlete's foot)	Itchy flaky area of skin, often between the fourth and fifth toes	Miconazole Sulconazole
Herpes labialis	Lesion found on the face and mouth caused by the herpes simplex virus	Usually self-limiting Aciclovir 5% cream Penciclovir 1% cream Consider analgesia

(Continued)

Table 12.24 (*Contd.*)

Term	Definition	Treatment
Impetigo	*Staph. aureus* vesicular infection with a honey-coloured discharge which dries to a crust	Tetracycline hydrochloride 3% ointment is discontinued. Fusidic acid 2% cream is commonly used Flucloxacillin capsules
Nappy rash	Rash caused by degradation of urine to release ammonia Often accompanied by bacterial or fungal infections	Frequent nappy changing Barrier creams Topical mild corticosteroids with antifungals if necessary
Pediculosis (lice infestation)	Infestation of *Anoplura* or sucking parasites of humans	Malathion Carbaryl
Pediculus humanus capitis (head lice)	Itchy scalp with lesions caused by scratching which may become infected	Pyrethroids May also be treated by mechanical clearance using a fine-toothed comb
Pediculus corporis (body lice)	A red itchy rash with excoriated skin and pigmented eczema	Wash clothes and bedding
Pthirus pubis (pubic lice)	Itching	Malathion lotion Permethrin cream
Sarcoptes scabiei (scabies)	Infestation by the female mite, which burrows into the stratum corneum and lays its eggs at the boundary of the dermis and epidermis, causes itching	Malathion Alcoholic lotion or aqueous lotion Permethrin dermal cream
	Itching is an allergic reaction to the mite's coat, saliva, and faeces	Treat the entire household Launder clothing and bedding
	Areas which have been scratched may become infected	
Urticaria (hives or nettle rash)	Allergic skin reaction causing oedema with surrounding erythema and itching	Oral histamines

For more information: 🖥 www.nurse_prescriber.co.uk, current BNF or BNF for Children, 🖥 www.npc.co.uk/nurse_prescribing, or 🖥 www.cks.nhs.uk/seborrhoeic_dermatitis/evidence

Further reading

HPA (2006). Fungal diseases in the UK. The current provision of support for diagnosis and treatment: assessment and proposed network solution. Health Protection Agency, UK Clinical Mycology Network. ⌨ www.hpa.org.uk

O'Connor, N.R., McLaughlin, M.R., and Ham, P. (2008). Newborn skin. I: Common rashes. *American Family Physician*, **77**, 47–52.

Sheffield, R.C., Crawford, P., and Wright, S.T. (2007). What's the best treatment for cradle cap? *Journal of Family Practice*, **56**, 232–3.

Types of dressing 1

Suitable dressings for different wound types are listed in Table 12.25.

Alginates

• Contain calcium alginate, a derivative of seaweed.
• Exudate from the wound causes the dressing to change from a fibrous structure to a gel.
• Different forms:
  • flat dressings;
  • rope or ribbon;
  • some are extra-absorbent with an adhesive backing.
• Depending on the product used, the resultant gel can either be lifted off as a sheet or rinsed off.
• A secondary dressing is required to preserve moisture.
• Used for wounds with a heavy exudates and odour.
• May be left in place for up to 7 days.
• If heavy exudates or infection, the dressing may require changing daily.

Contraindications
• Not to be used for infected wounds.
• Unsuitable for dry necrotic wounds.
• Not to be used with topical antimicrobial or antibiotic agents as these may prevent the gelling process.

Problems
Certain alginates cause excoriation and maceration of the surrounding skin (Kaltostat® dressings should be cut and folded to fit the wound).

Foam dressings

• Promote healing by absorbing exudates and maintaining a moist environment.
• Different preparations are available for wounds with light and heavy exudates.
• A secondary dressing is required.

Products
Lyofoam®
• Suitable for smelly, moderately exudating wounds.
• Has an adhesive waterproof backing.
• Need to overlap the wound by 2–3cm.
• Initially change each day, but as discharge decreases can leave for up to 7 days.

Table 12.25 Suitable dressings for different wound types

Wound type	Dressing property	Dressing type
Dry necrotic	Moisture retentive	Hydrocolloids
		Hydrogels
Slough-covered	Moisture retentive	Hydrocolloids
	Absorptive	Hydrogels
	Perhaps: absorbs odour, antimicrobial	
Clean exudating	Absorptive	Hydrocolloids
	Perhaps absorbs odour, antimicrobial	Foams
	Alginates	
	If exudates high:	
	knitted varicose	
	primary dressing	
Dry	Paraffin gauze	
Moisture retentive	Absorbent perforated plastic film or vapour-permeable adhesive film	
Low adherence		Thermal insulation

Allevyn®
- Plastic-net-covered polyurethane foam bonded to a vapour-permeable polyurethane film backing.
- The backing is water and bacteria proof.
- Can be left on a clean non-infected wound for 3–4 days.

Syprosorb® (discontinued)
- Layered absorbent polyurethane foam vapour-permeable dressing.
- Used for wounds with light to moderate exudates.
- Change dressing when exudate is within 1cm of dressing edge.

Cavi-Care®
- Conforming cavity dressing for deep uninfected wounds.

Allevyn cavity wound dressing®
- Foam chippings in a perforated film.

Types of dressing 2

Hydrocolloids

- Made from cellulose, gelatin, and pectins to absorb water and form a gel, providing a moist environment.
- Backing of vapour-permeable polyurethane film or foam.
- Some are available as a paste.
- Some have a wide adhesive border.
- Suitable for granulating wounds with a low to moderate exudate, including surgical wounds, pressure sores, leg ulcers, and minor burns.
- Promote rehydration and autolytic debridement of dry, sloughy, or necrotic wounds.
- Manage blisters.
- Impermeability to water allows bathing and showering with the dressing in place.
- Should be left in place for 4–5 days provided that there is no infection.

Contraindications

- Infected wounds.
- Patients who are hypersensitive to hydrocolloid or its constituents.

Problems

Adhesion can be difficult, with the sides of the dressing rolling. To avoid this:

- allow a 2cm overlap from the wound margin to the side of the dressing;
- cover the dressing with an adhesive retention sheet if movement is likely to dislodge it;
- warm the dressing with the hands, preserving asepsis, prior to use;
- ask the patient not to put weight on the area for 20min, to allow adhesion to be maximized.[1]

Hydrogels

- Made from copolymer starch.
- Capable of significant fluid retention.
- Two types, amorphous and sheet:
  - amorphous hydrogels do not have a firm structure—their viscosity reduces as moisture is absorbed (e.g. Intrasite Gel®);
  - sheet hydrogels retain their structure as fluid is absorbed (e.g. Geliperm®).
- Used for dry, sloughy, lightly exudating, granulating, or necrotic wounds.
- Can be used as a carrier for metronidazole for smelly fungating wounds.
- Apply a thick layer of gel followed by a secondary dressing when using an amorphous hydrogel.
- A secondary dressing is also required when using a sheet hydrogel.
- Secondary dressings:
  - perforated plastic film, followed by an absorbent pad if exudate is heavy;
  - a vapour-permeable film dressing if exudate is light.

• Dressings need to be changed every 3–4 days or daily when used with a dry wound.

Contraindications:
• Infected or heavily exudating wounds
• Allergic reaction to some preparations
• Not to be used for wounds that are infected with *Pseudomonas.*

Vapour-permeable films and membranes
• Vapour-permeable polyurethane film coated with a synthetic adhesive.
• Used for:
  • post-operative dressings;
  • decubitus ulcers;
  • stoma care;
  • to prevent skin breakdown.
• Used as secondary dressings over alginates and foams.
• Sometimes used to protect vulnerable skin from damage.
• Allow the passage of water vapour and oxygen, but not liquid water or micro-organisms.
• Provide a moist healing environment.

Contraindications
Not suitable for large wounds with heavy exudate, as exudates may cause the adhesive edges to wrinkle and allow risk of bacterial entry.

1. Bux, M. (1996). Selection and use of wound dressings. *Wound Care for Pharmacists.* Summer, 11–16.

Types of preparation

Emollients
Used to treat dry and scaling skin:
- soothe and hydrate skin;
- preparations with high water content produce a greater cooling effect on the skin (suitable for those suffering pruritus);
- a preparation with high oil content will help those with severely dry skin by sealing the skin and preventing further water loss;
- should be applied in the direction of hair growth.

Creams
Oil-in-water emulsions have two actions:
- water is lost from the cream by evaporation and absorption by the skin which it cools;
- the water loss from the emulsion combined with the mechanical action of applying the mixture releases the oils onto the surface of the skin, preventing further water loss;
- an example is aqueous cream which is a light emollient.

Ointments
Greasy preparations, commonly using a base of soft paraffin or a combination of soft, liquid, and hard paraffin:
- do not normally contain water;
- more occlusive than creams;
- effective for chronic dry lesions;
- an example is emulsifying ointment.

Contraindications
Sensitivity to hydrous wool fat (lanolin) should be suspected if a reaction occurs.

Both aqueous cream and emulsifying ointment can be used as soap substitutes.

Corticosteroids
Hormones found in the cortex of the adrenal glands:
- mineralocorticoids control the balance between water and the mineral content of the body;
- glucocorticoids help maintain the normal blood glucose to assist the body in times of stress and injury;
- large amounts of corticosteroids suppress the autoimmune system—this anti-inflammatory effect is the reason for their use;
- they act by inhibiting the enzymes that stimulate the formation of prostaglandin and leukotriene to suppress the allergic/immune and inflammatory responses.

Adverse effects

Mild and moderately potent topical corticosteroids are rarely associated with adverse effects. Systemic absorption is increased if:

- they are applied over a wide area;
- the skin is damaged;
- they are covered by an occlusive dressing;

If the treatment is long term, systemic, and high dose, the following can occur:

- Hyperglycaemia
- Protein catabolism, leading to loss of bone mass, muscle atrophy, and thin skin
- Lipolysis, which can lead to Cushing's syndrome: 'moon face', or 'buffalo hump'
- Lessening of resistance to infection
- Poor wound healing
- Oedema
- Increased BP
- Sodium and water retention
- Hypokalaemia
- Hirsutism
- Allergic reactions
- Increased gastric acidity.

Always start on the least potent preparation (Table 12.26) and work up.

Further reading

Berliner, E., Ozbilgin, B., and Zarin, D.A. (2003). A systematic review of pneumatic compression for treatment of chronic venous insufficiency and venous ulcers. *Journal of Vascular Surgery*, **37**, 539–44.

Briggs, M. and Nelson, E.A. (2003). *Topical agents or dressings for pain in venous leg ulcers (Cochrane Review)*. www.thecochranelibrary.com

Enoch, S., Grey, J.E., and Harding, K.G. (2006). ABC of wound healing: non-surgical and drug treatments. *British Medical Journal*, **332**, 900–3.

Rajendran, S., Rigby, A.J., and Anand, S.C. (2007). Venous leg ulcer treatment and practice–Part 3. The use of compression therapy systems. *Journal of Wound Care*, **16**, 107–9.

Table 12.26 Preparation potency of corticosteroids

Potency	Preparation
Mildly potent	Hydrocortisone
Moderately potent	Alclometasone
	Clobetasone
	Fluocortolone
	Fludroxycortide
Potent	Beclometasone
	Betamethasone
	Diflucortolone
	Flucinonide
	Fluocinolone
	Fluticasone
	Mometasone
	Triamcinolone
Very potent	Clobetasol

Substance misuse and dependency

Substance misuse

Definition
Substance misuse is the harmful use of any substance, such as alcohol, prescribed medications (e.g. diazepam), illicit drugs (e.g. heroin, cannabis, cocaine), and other substances (e.g. glue, lighter fluid, magic mushrooms).[1]

Controlled drugs
These are preparations that are subject to the Misuse of Drugs Act 2005 which categorizes drugs as class A, B, or C. The drugs are termed controlled substances, with class A being the most dangerous.

Offences under the Misuse of Drugs Act 2005
- Unlawful possession of a controlled substance.
- Possession of a controlled substance with intent to supply it:
  - supplying or offering to supply a controlled drug is an offence even if no charge is made for the drug.
- Allowing premises you occupy or manage to be used unlawfully for the purpose of producing or supplying controlled drugs.

Classification of drugs under the Misuse of Drugs Act 2005
Class A drugs
- Ecstasy
- LSD
- Heroin
- Cocaine
- Crack
- Magic mushrooms (whether prepared or fresh)
- Methylamphetamine (crystal meth)
- Any Class B drug prepared for injection e.g. amphetamine
- Methadone.

Penalties for possession: up to 7 years in prison or an unlimited fine or both.

Penalties for dealing: up to life in prison or an unlimited fine or both.

Class B drugs
- Cannabis
- Amphetamines
- Methylphenidate
- Pholcodine.

Penalties for possession: up to 5 years in prison or an unlimited fine or both.

Penalties for dealing: up to 14 years in prison or an unlimited fine or both.

Class C drugs
- Tranquillizers
- Some painkillers, GHB (gamma-hydroxybutyrate)
- Ketamine.

Penalties for possession: up to 2 years in prison or an unlimited fine or both.

Penalties for dealing: up to 14 years in prison or an unlimited fine or both.

A full list of controlled substances can be found at: http://drugs.homeoffice. gov.uk/drugs-laws/misuse-of-drugs-act/ (accessed 13 September 2009).

Common drugs and substances of abuse and dependence

- Cocaine
- Diamorphine (heroin)
- Morphine
- Synthetic opioids
- Amphetamines
- Flunitrazepam
- Benzodiazepines (e.g. temazepam)
- Barbiturates
- Cannabis
- Lysergide (LSD)
- 34-methylenedioxymetamphetamine (MDMA, ecstasy)
- Solvents and glue
- Petrol
- Antifreeze
- Alcohol
- Nicotine.

NB: nurse independent and supplementary prescribers and health professional prescribers are unable to prescribe diamorphine for drug addictions. The Nursing and Midwifery Council have produced guidance regarding the prescribing of the above:
🖳 www.nmc-uk.org/aDisplayDocument.aspx?DocumentID=7166

1. Castledine G. and Close A. (2009) *Oxford Handbook of Adult Nursing*. Oxford University Press, Oxford.

Background

The 2008–2009 drug strategy aims to reduce the harm that drugs cause to society, to communities, and to individuals and their families, and comprises the following four strands of work.

- Protecting communities by:
  - tackling drug supply;
  - tackling drug-related crime;
  - preventing antisocial behaviour.
- Preventing harm to children, young people, and families affected by drug misuse.
- Delivering new approaches to drug treatment and social re-integration.
- Public information campaigns, communications, and community engagement.

The Information Centre Statistics on Drug Misuse: England 2007

🖳 http://www.ic.nhs.uk/webfiles/publications/drugmisuse07/Drugs%20mis useEnland%202007%20with%20links%20and%20buttons.pdf (accessed 13 September 2009)

Main findings regarding drug abuse by adults aged 16–59 years living in England or Wales

- In 2005–2006, 10.5% of adults had used one or more illicit drug in the previous year.
- The use of any Class A drug had increased from 2.7% in 1998 to 3.4% in 2005–2006, mainly due to a rise in the use of cocaine powder.
- 13.7% of men compared with 7.4% of women had taken drugs in the preceding year.
- Drug use by adults aged 16–24 years fell in 2006 from 31.8% (1998) to 25.2%, but Class A drug use remained stable.

The government's 10-year strategy for reducing drug misuse (Tackling Drugs to Build a Better Britain) seeks to move the emphasis from reactive rehabilitation to prevention. To help with this a drug prevention resource pack has been available since 2003.

Further to this, in 2005 a briefing on nurse prescribing in substance misuse was published by the National Treatment Agency for Substance Misuse (🖳 www.dh.gov.uk).

Nicotine replacement therapy as an aid to smoking cessation

Effects of tobacco smoke

Tobacco smoke contains over 300 chemical compounds, including irritants such as tars, nicotine, and carbon monoxide, which are responsible for causing both short- and long-term effects.

Long-term effects
- Coronary heart disease
- Peripheral vascular disease (PVD)
- Cerebrovascular disease
- Lung cancer
- Peptic ulceration
- Chronic obstructive pulmonary disease (COPD)
- Low birthweight at term for babies of mothers who smoked during their pregnancy.

Short-term effects
- Emotional dependence on nicotine.
- Decreased removal of secretions from the lung as the cilia lining the bronchi are less active.
- The oxygen-carrying capacity of the blood is reduced as there is an increase in carboxyhaemoglobin.
- Loss of appetite.

Nicotine

This agonist acts on receptors in the CNS to cause neuronal excitement, resulting in:
- tolerance;
- physical dependence;
- psychological dependence (cravings).

Nicotine is highly addictive. Withdrawal symptoms include:
- the need to smoke tobacco;
- depression;
- irritability;
- insomnia;
- difficulty in concentration;
- restlessness;
- increased appetite, resulting in weight gain.

Smoking cessation interventions have proved to be a cost-effective way of preserving health and reducing ill-health caused by smoking tobacco.

Nicotine replacement therapy is useful as an aid to smoking cessation in those who smoke more than 10 cigarettes a day and its efficacy is enhanced if it is combined with behavioural support.

📖 Prescribing for public health, p. 205.

Alcohol misuse

The misuse of alcohol is the most common form of substance misuse. The WHO International Statistical Classification of Diseases and Related Health Problems, 10th revision (ICD-10)[1] categorizes alcohol-use disorders according to the level of alcohol consumption as follows.

Hazardous drinking
- Drinking above safe levels—8 units daily for men and 6 units for women.
- No significant alcohol-related problems to date.
- Binge drinking is defined as drinking over twice the recommended safe levels in a day.

Harmful drinking
- Drinking over the safe levels.
- Evidence of alcohol-related problems (Table 12.27).

Alcohol dependence
Alcohol dependence is defined in ICD-10 as:
> a cluster of physiological, behavioural, and cognitive phenomena in which the use of alcohol takes on a much higher priority for a given individual than other behaviors.[1]

A central characteristic is the desire to drink alcohol, and a return to drinking after a period of abstinence.[2]

Alcohol dependence
A definite diagnosis of dependence on alcohol is usually made only if three or more of the ICD-10 criteria for alcohol dependence have been noted over the preceding year:
- a strong desire or sense of compulsion to drink alcohol;
- difficulty in controlling drinking in terms of its:
  - onset;
  - termination;
  - level of use.
- a physiological withdrawal state (e.g. tremor, sweating, rapid heart rate, anxiety, insomnia, or less commonly seizures, disorientation, hallucinations) when drinking has ceased or reduced, or drinking to relieve or avoid such a withdrawal state;
- evidence of tolerance (i.e. increased amounts of alcohol are required in order to achieve effects originally produced by smaller amounts);
- progressive neglect of alternative pleasures or interests because of drinking, and increased amounts of time necessary to obtain or take alcohol, or to recover from its effects;
- persisting with alcohol use despite awareness of overtly harmful consequences.

1. WHO (1992) *The ICD-10 classification of mental and behavioural disorders. Clinical descriptions and diagnostic guidelines.* World Health Organization, Geneva.
2. SIGN (2003) *The management of harmful drinking and alcohol dependence in primary care.* Scottish Intercollegiate Guidelines Network. 🖳 www.sign.ac.uk (accessed 4 February 2009).

Table 12.27 Complications of alcohol abuse

Complication	Finding
Alcohol-related mortality[1]	22 000 premature deaths per year
Liver damage[2]	Fatty liver: 90% of persistent heavy drinkers, asymptomatic Alcoholic hepatitis: 40% of heavy drinkers, often the precursor to cirrhosis Cirrhosis: 8–30% of heavy drinkers*
Cardiovascular disease[3]	Excessive alcohol consumption ↑ risk of: raised blood pressure (binge drinking may be particularly implicated) haemorrhagic stroke coronary heart disease cardiomyopathy arrhythmias
Cancer[4]	Alcohol causes ↑ risk of squamous carcinoma of: oropharynx larynx oesophagus. Heavy alcohol consumption is associated with carcinoma of: liver stomach colon rectum lung pancreas breast
Other medical complications[5]	Gout Gastrointestinal haemorrhage Pancreatitis Neurological problems (e.g. seizures, neuropathy, acute confusional states, subdural haematoma) Falls (in elderly people) Wernicke's encephalopathy and Korsakoff's psychosis Impotence/fertility problems Risk of trauma when intoxicated.

*Heavy drinking is defined as a minimum of 20 units daily for 5 years

1. Information Centre (2006). *Statistics on alcohol: England 2006.* Information Centre, London.
2. Raistrick, D., Hodgson, R., and Ritson, B. (1999). *Tackling alcohol together.* Free Association Books, London.
3. British Heart Foundation (2006). *Coronary heart disease statistics,* Chapter 7. www.heartstart.org (accessed 9 September 2009).
4. WHO/FAO (2003). *Joint WHO/FAO Expert Consultation on Diet, Nutrition and the Prevention of Chronic Diseases,* pp. 95–104. WHO, Geneva.
5. SIGN (2003). *The management of harmful drinking and alcohol dependence in primary care.* Scottish Intercollegiate Guidelines Network.

Prescribing for the urinary system

Brief description of the urinary system

Structure of the urinary system (Fig. 12.9)

The urinary system comprises:
- kidneys (usually two);
- paired ureters;
- bladder;
- urethra.

Urine drains from the kidneys at a rate of about 1mL/min.

Kidneys
- Each kidney is the size of a fist and is supplied with blood via the renal arteries and veins.
- The kidney consists of three regions:
  - pelvis (transferring waste products from the medulla to the ureters);
  - cortex (the outer covering);
  - medulla.
- There are about 225km of fine blood vessels in each kidney.
- The filtration of blood to remove waste products takes place in glomeruli which contain Bowman's capsules and glomerular capillaries and are located in the medulla region of the kidney.
- In addition to glomerular filtration to remove waste products, the kidneys also play a role in:
  - control of blood pressure;
  - maintenance of the acid–base balance of the blood;
  - hormone production;
  - synthesis of vitamin D.

Ureters

The two ureters carry urine from the pelvis of the kidneys to the bladder.

Bladder
- The bladder is a hollow muscular organ with three orifices in its wall (openings to the two ureters and the urethra). It acts as a reservoir for urine (up to 600mL between voidings) and expels urine at micturition.
- Bladder control and voiding involve the automonic (sympathetic and parasympathetic) and somatic nervous systems.
- The bladder is supported by the pelvic floor and two muscle groups.
- The bladder wall consists of four layers:
  - the peritoneum, covering the surface of the bladder;
  - the detrusor muscle;
  - the submucosa;
  - the mucosa.
- The parasympathetic nerves control voiding by stimulating:
  - the detrusor muscle to contract;
  - the internal urethral sphincter to relax.

A child's bladder capacity can be calculated using:

bladder capacity (mL) = (age in years × 30) + 30.

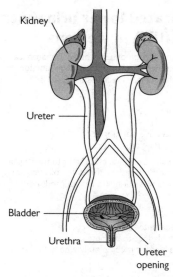

Fig. 12.9 Diagram of the urinary system. Reproduced from Glasper, E.A., McEwing, G., and Richardson, J. (2006). *Oxford Handbook of Children's and Young People's Nursing*, by kind permission of Oxford University Press.

Urethra

This forms a conduit to take urine from the bladder to the meatus (opening). In females it is about 4cm long and has an external sphincter. In males it is about 20cm long with both an external and internal sphincter.

📖 Prescribing for sexual health, pp. 381–398.

Functions of the urinary system

- Excretion: removal of waste products from body fluids.
- Elimination: removal of waste products to outside the body.

The vital functions of the urinary system are performed by the kidneys. However, problems with any of the conduction systems have an effect on renal function.

Uncomplicated lower urinary tract infection (UTI) in women

The patient has an infection of her otherwise anatomically and physiologically normal urinary tract, with normal renal function and no associated illness to impair the defence mechanisms.

Risk factors

- Sexual intercourse
- Family history of UTI
- Use of a contraceptive diaphragm
- More common during pregnancy.

As women have a short urethra, close to both the vagina and the rectum, there is little protection against the entry of micro-organisms into the bladder. Normal changes during pregnancy predispose to infection.

Prevention

- Adequate fluid intake.
- Empty the bladder after sexual intercourse.
- Don't allow the bladder to become overfull.
- Ensure that the bladder is completely emptied when passing urine.

Causes

- *Escherichia coli* is the causative organism in 70% of cases.
- The remaining 30% of cases are caused by Proteus mirabilis, Klebsiella pneumonia, and Staphylococcus saprophyticus.

Assessment

Patient's history and clinical signs.

Signs and symptoms

- Positive dipstick for:
  - pus in the urine (leucocyte esterase test);
  - bacteria that alter nitrate in the urine to nitrite (nitrate reductase test).
- Lower abdominal discomfort.
- Burning pain on passing urine.
- Frequency.
- Urgency.
- Cloudy or foul-smelling urine.
- Confusion (especially in the older woman).
- Dysuria.
- Haematuria.

Treatment

- Encourage patients to drink 3L of fluid per day.
- Give sodium bicarbonate or potassium citrate to make the urine more alkaline and reduce the burning sensation on voiding.
- Cranberry products.[1,2]

- Oral antibiotics may be prescribed, e.g. cefalexin or trimethoprim (see current BNF for full list).
- Avoid trimethoprim in pregnancy.
- Treat all UTIs during pregnancy and confirm cessation of the infection by urine sample culture.
- Mild analgesia or hot pads for localized pain relief.

1. Avorn, J. Monane, H., Gurwitz, J.H., et al. (1994). Reduction of bacteriuria and pyuria after ingestion of cranberry juice. *JAMA*, **271**, 751–4.
2. Eichhorts, A.M., Janken, J.K., and Mullen, T.M. (1997). The therapeutic value of cranberries in treating and preventing urinary tract infections. *Online Journal of Knowledge Synthesis in Nursing*, **4**, 7–17.

Problems with catheter patency

- Patients with indwelling catheters are prone to patency problems such as:
  - blockage;
  - catheter encrustation;
  - inflammatory reactions;
  - trauma;
  - bladder infections;
  - pain and discomfort.
- 50% of patients have blockages secondary to encrustation.
- *Proteus*, *Klebsiella*, and *Pseudomonas* bacteria specifically facilitate the process of encrustation by providing urease enzymes that release ammonia and hydrogen ions from the urine, increasing its alkalinity.
- Micro-organisms also collect on the surface of the catheter, producing a biofilm that produces a glycocalyx (a thick coat of polysaccharides).

Risk factors
After 14 days, silicone-coated, Teflon®-coated, and latex catheters are more likely to become encrusted than all-silicone catheters.[1]

Prevention
- Hydrogel-coated and all-silicone catheters appear to be resistant to encrustation for up to 18 weeks.
- Hydrogel-coated catheters are more resistant to biofilm than silicone-coated ones.
- It is possible to predict the length of time that a catheter will last for individual patients by observing patterns of catheter life for each patient, thus preventing blockages by replacing catheters in time.
- Reducing urine alkalinity by consumption of cranberry juice may prolong catheter patency and prevent infection.
- Hydrogel-coated, all-silicone, and silicone catheters require changing every 3 months to avoid blockage.
- Latex catheters require changing every 6 weeks.

Treatment
Blocked catheters require changing (often painful for the patient) or washing out.

Washout
- Warm catheter patency solutions to body temperature.
- Performed washout using aseptic technique.
- Encourage patients to maintain adequate fluid intake to keep urine dilute.
- Suggest that patients try cranberry products.

1. Winn, C. (1998). Complications with urinary catheters. *Professional Nurse*, **13**, S7–10.

Urinary incontinence

Definition
An involuntary or inappropriate loss of urine which can be demonstrated objectively.[1] It can be classified into six categories, although they are not mutually exclusive.

Urge incontinence
This is caused by instability of the detrusor muscle, or hyper-reflexia, which causes the bladder to contract at times other than intended urination. The bladder may not empty completely and a residual volume greater than 100mL is common. The cause is unknown but it may be due to obstruction or neurological disease.

Overflow incontinence
The bladder overfills and urine leaks into the ureter. Symptoms include voiding small amounts of urine, hesitancy, poor flow, or post-micturition dribble. This condition may follow hysterectomy or be caused by faecal impaction, unwanted effects of a drug regime, or prostatic hyperplasia.

Stress incontinence
An involuntary urine leak when abdominal pressure increases during physical activity, e.g. exercise or coughing. It is usually caused by muscular damage to the bladder outlet because of weakness of the pelvic floor musculature. It is often precipitated by childbirth or post-menopausal oestrogen deficiency, or is a complication following prostatic surgery.

Neuropathic bladder disorder
Caused by injury or disease of neuronal control which results in dysfunction of the lower urinary tract. Often associated with open or closed spina bifida, spinal chord tumour, trauma, and transverse myelitis.

Post-micturition dribble
Slight incontinence following micturition in males as the bulbo spongiosum muscle fails to evacuate the distal bulb of the urethra.

Functional incontinence
Despite a healthy and normal urinary tract, inappropriate voiding occurs because of environmental factors such as inaccessible toilets or impaired mobility.

Nocturnal enuresis
Involuntary leakage of urine occurring during sleep.

Nocturia
One or more voids at night, each of which is preceded and followed by sleep.

Assessment

- Full symptom and medical history including for women:
  - gynaecological;
  - obstetric.
- And for men and women:
  - surgical;
  - neurological.
- Holistic assessment.
- Baseline clinical assessment including mid-stream urine (MSU).
- Measurement of a post-void residual.
- Discussion of the patient's perception of the problem.
- Completion of a three-day bladder diary.

Physical examination;

- Abdominal
- Vaginal.

Following a complete assessment, an accurate diagnosis can be made and appropriate treatment decided, guided by local formularies and patient choice.[2]

1. National Prescribing Centre (1999). *Nurse prescribing resource pack—urinary incontinence.* NPC, London.
2. NICE (2006). *Urinary incontinence: the management of urinary incontinence in women. Clinical guideline 40.* 🖳 www.nice.org.uk (accessed 2 February 2010).

Overactive bladder

Definition

Urinary urgency with or without urge incontinence, usually with frequency and nocturia.[1] Prevalence in the general population is 14–16%.[2]

Prescribing for an overactive bladder

In 2008, 2.85 million prescriptions were written for anticholinergic drugs (also known as antimuscarinics).[3] These inhibit acetylcholine from binding at the muscarinic receptors in the detrusor muscle of the bladder. This reduces the involuntary contractions of the detrusor muscle whilst maintaining normal voiding.

Side effects of anticholinergics[4]

- Dry mouth
- Constipation
- Blurred vision
- Dry eyes
- Drowsiness
- Difficulty in voiding
- Skin reactions.

Drugs that cause urinary incontinence

- Parasympathomimetics (e.g. distigmine bromide, bethanechol chloride) stimulate contraction of the detrusor muscle.
- Alpha-blockers (e.g. alfuzosin, doxazosin, prazosin, and tamsulosin) cause relaxation of the striated muscle of the urethral sphincter.
- Diuretics, alcohol, and caffeine may worsen frequency, urgency, and urinary incontinence.

Resources

Continent Products Directory, Continence Foundation, 307 Hatton Square, 16 Baldwin Gardens, London EC19 7RJ. ⌨ http://www.continence-foundation.org.uk/products/ (accessed 3 February 2010).

PromoCon 2001 (Promoting Continence through Product Awareness), Disabled Living, Redbank House, 4 St Chad's Street, Cheetham, Manchester M8 8QA. ☏ Product helpline: 0161 834 2001.

MDA. ⌨ www.medical-devices.gov.uk (accessed 3 February 2010).

Local continence advisor telephone number

1. Abrams, P., Cardozo, I., Fall, M. *et al.* (2002). The standardisation of terminology of lower urinary tract function: report from the Standardisation Sub-committee of the International Continence Society. *Neurourology and Urodynamics*, **21**, 167–78.
2. Irwin, D., Milsom, I., and Hunskaar, S. (2006). Population based survey of urinary incontinence, overactive bladder and other lower urinary tract symptoms in five countries: results of the EPIC study. *European Urology*, **50**, 1306–14.
3. Roesner, M. and Wagg, A. (2008). Greater evidence of action of urinary incontinence is needed. *Guidelines in Practice*, **11**, 27–32.
4. *British National Formulary* (latest edn). British Medical Association and Royal Pharmaceutical Society of Great Britain, London.

Prescribing for sexual health

Brief overview of the female reproductive system

Structure and function

Ovaries (female gonads)

The ovaries are suspended, by the mesovarium, suspensory and ovarian ligaments, either side of the pelvis within the peritoneal cavity.

Ovaries produce oestrogen (Table 12.24), a hormone that stimulates the production and maturation of follicles which ripen to produce ova. This process is called oogenesis and occurs every 28 days between puberty and menopause.

Follicle stimulating hormone (FSH) and luteinizing hormone (LH), secreted by the hypothalamus, situated in the anterior lobe of the pituitary gland, control the menstrual cycle. This cycle facilitates the release of a mature ovum each month and prepares the lining of the uterus to receive and implant the fertilized ovum.

Fallopian or ovarian tubes

These muscular tubes, approximately 12 cm in length, are the conduit for the ripened ova between the ovary and uterus.

The widest part of the tube is proximate to the ovary and is called the infundibulum. This has a number of finger-like projections, called fimbriae, which waft fluid from the peritoneal cavity into the tube. The lining of the tube contains cilia, and the combination of strong muscular contractions and beating of the cilia enables the ova to be transported along the tube to the uterus.

The tube also provides an environment full of nutrients for both the sperm (spermatozoa) and fertilized egg.

Uterus

This hollow, pear-shaped organ is situated leaning forward within the pelvis behind the bladder. It consists of the body, or corpus, and the cervix. It is supported and stabilized by a broad ligament, other suspensory ligaments, skeletal muscles, and the fascia of the pelvic floor.

The body (corpus)

The fundus of the body is situated at its junction with the Fallopian tubes. This part is comprised of muscle and myometrium which is lined with endometrium (glandular tissue). Part of this endometrial tissue is shed during menstruation. During pregnancy the endometrium deals with the physiological needs of the developing fetus.

The cervix

At the lower end of the uterus, this structure, which points towards the spine, extends into the vagina and forms a curved surface enclosing a central opening called the cervical os. The cervix consists of mainly connective tissue with a little muscle. Cervical glands are situated within the epithelial lining of the cervix.

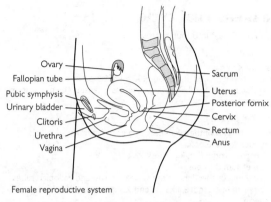

Female reproductive system

Fig. 12.10 Brief overview of the female reproductive system. Reproduced from Glasper, EA, McEwing, G, and Richardson, J. (2006) *Oxford Handbook of Children's and Young People's Nursing*, by kind permission of Oxford University Press.

The vagina

Comprising bundles of smooth muscles, this tube passes through the pelvic floor and perineum. When pelvic and peritoneal muscles contract, a sphincter is formed around the opening to the vagina. Nutrients, for the flora of bacteria in the vagina, and lubricating secretions are provided by cervical glands. These maintain an acidic environment which can affect the motility of spermatozoa.

The external genitalia

Contained within the vulva, the labia minora and majora and the clitoris comprise the female external genitalia. Surrounding the vaginal opening is an area rich in sebaceous, sweat and mucus-secreting glands. Anterior to the vulva and the pubic symphysis is a bulging area of adipose deposit, the mons pubis.

Prescribing for public health, p. 205.

The menstrual cycle

This can be divided into four phases:

Menstruaton

- Lasts for 4–6 days.
- Endometrium is shed and about 400 ml of blood is lost.
- Secretion of FSH and LH begin to increase, causing the maturation of several ovarian follicles.

Follicular phase

- On about day 6 of the cycle only one of the stimulated follicles continues to develop.
- Oestrogen production increases.
- Endometrium thickens.
- Cervical mucus throughout the vagina, uterus, and Fallopian tubes becomes thinner, more alkaline and viscous, aiding the passage of sperm.

Ovulatory phase

- Increased oestrogen stimulates the growth of the follicle.
- During mid-cycle there is a further increase in oestrogen production followed by a surge of LH from the pituitary gland.
- 34–38 h after this surge the follicle bursts.

Luteal phase

- The cells of the ruptured follicle multiply and become the corpus luteum.
- The yellowish corpus luteum produces progesterone (Table 12.24) and moderate amounts of oestrogen.
- During the next 7 days high levels of progesterone are secreted to prepare the body for pregnancy.
- Increasing the vascularization of the endometrium.
- Endometrial glands enlarge and secrete fluids containing glucose, amino acids, and mucus.
- Cervical mucus thickens.
- If fertilization does not occur, the corpus luteum degenerates after 7 days.
- Production of oestrogen and progesterone is reduced over the 12 days following ovulation.
- Endometrial lining is shed.
- Oestrogen and progesterone are further reduced.
- FSH and LH begin a new cycle.

Fertilization

- Only one sperm normally fertilizes the ovum.
- The ovum travels to the uterus and implants in the endometrium.

Table 12.24 Main activities of oestrogen, progesterone, and progestogen

Hormone	Activity
Oestrogen	Development of sex hormone in women
	Breast development
	Fat distribution
	Hair distribution
	During menstrual cycle:
	Growth of endometrium
	Movement of fimbriae and contraction of uterine tube walls to enable passage of ovum
	Increase in sexual drive
	Thinning of cervical mucus
	Increased suppleness of vagina enabling it to expand during pregnancy, labour, and intercourse
	Water retention
	Stimulation of bone and muscle growth
	Stimulation of hepatic production of sex hormone binding globulin, HDL[a] and blood clotting factors
Progesterone	Continued preparation of the uterus for pregnancy
	In combination with prolactin, stimulates the breasts to produce milk
	Thickening of cervical mucus
Progestogen	Derived from testosterone; can stimulate excess hair growth and acne
	Increase in appetite and weight gain
	Reduction of sex drive
	Increased risk of CVD by the reduction of HDL and an increase in LDL levels
	Reduction in sex hormone binding globulin
Sex hormone binding globulin	Reduces male characteristics
	Affects circulating testosterone and progestogens

[a]HDLs are complexes of lipid and protein which transport cholesterol away from peripheral tissue to the liver where they are stored or excreted in the bile.

Brief overview of the male reproductive system

Structure and function

The penis

When in flaccid state it is a soft cylinder of spongy tissue. Only ½ the length of the penis is visible outside the body.

The penis allows urine to be voided and the expulsion of spermatozoa during sexual intercourse or stimulation.

The penis has three main sections:

The root

This section attaches the penis to the underside of the pelvis.

The body

The tubular part of the penis, which comprises three cylindrical columns of erectile tissue, two corpora cavernosum and the corpus spongiosum.

The corpora cavernosa lie adjacent to each other and contain most of the erectile tissue of the penis. Within these structures are small spaces, the lacunar spaces, which are surrounded by smooth muscle. A tough fibrous coat, the tunica albicans, encases each of the corpora cavernoss.

The corpus spongiosum protects and surrounds the urethra on the underside of the penis. The tissue of the corpus spongiosum is erectile and the whole length expands during an erection. At the distal end the corpus spongiosum widens to form the glans or head of the penis.

The glans or head

This refers to the expanded distal end of the penis, which is surrounded by the prepuce or foreskin and contains the external urethral meatus.

The urethra

This has two functions, both to allow the voiding of urine from the bladder and to act as a channel for semen during ejaculation. A sphincter between the bladder and urethra contracts during ejaculation, preventing urine entering the urethra and sperm entering the bladder at this time.

The testicles (testes)

Two testicles are contained separately within the scrotum, a thin sack of skin and involuntary muscle, which hang on the outside of the body. This enables the testicles to be kept cool; in cold weather the involuntary muscle contracts and draws the scrotum nearer to the body to prevent overcooling. This muscular contraction also occurs in states of fear, anger, and sexual arousal.

The testicles produce and store spermatozoa and supply testosterone. This hormone is responsible for the production of male features such as facial hair, a deep voice, and the ability to have an erection.

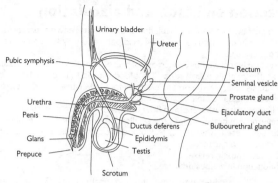

Fig. 12.11 Brief overview of the male reproductive system. Reproduced from Glasper, EA, McEwing, G, and Richardson, J. (2006) *Oxford Handbook of Children's and Young People's Nursing*, by kind permission of Oxford University Press.

The prostate

This is a walnut-sized gland which produces prostatic fluid, a rich source of prostaglandin E, and accounts for 20% of semen volume.

📖 Prescribing for problems within the endocrine system, pp. 267–284.

Erection emission and ejaculation

It is important to note that ejaculation and erection are two separate functions. A man can ejaculate from a flaccid penis and may have an erection without ejaculation.

Erection is achieved by an increase of pressure in a low-pressure system. When the penis is flaccid it has less blood supplied (1/8th to 1/10th the erect penis volume), the pressure is therefore lower than when it is erect.

Erection has three important components:

1. High-pressure arterial blood flow through the centre of each corpus cavernosum branching into the smaller arteries within the erectile tissue. These tiny arterioles leak blood into the lacunar spaces, causing the penis to expand.
2. Smooth muscle relaxation.
3. Reduction in venous drainage.

(1) and (2) are under autonomic and hormonal control; (3) occurs as a result of (1) and (2).

During sexual arousal the brain sends messages via parasympathetic nerves within the spinal cord, which cause smooth muscles to relax, arterial walls to dilate, and blood flow to increase.

During sexual activity sperm are propelled from the penis in two stages, emission and ejaculation:

• emission involves contraction of the smooth muscle of the vas deferens, seminal vesicles, and prostate gland, expelling semen into the urethra;
• ejaculation is achieved by contraction of the striated muscle at the base of the penis which enables semen to be expelled from the penis.

During heterosexual intercourse, sperm reach the uterine tubes within hours of intercourse and ejaculation, although they are viable for up to 7 days. During this period they become more able to adhere to the ovum, which improves the facilitation of fertilization.

Contraception

Contraception is an integral part of sexual health and should be considered during consultations. The consultation should include a full medical history and a sexual, reproductive, and previous contraceptive history to identify additional risks and factors which may influence choice and effective use of any method. Consent issues in young people are covered by the Fraser Guidance (see p.101). A list of available training in contraception and sexual health can be obtained from: www.guna.org.uk. The document *Sexual Health Competencies* is published by the RCN.[1]

Contraceptive prescribing in the UK should be evidence guided. UK policy and guidance comes from a number of sources including:
• NICE Guidance on Long Acting Reversible Contraception (LARC);[2]
• MEDFASH Recommended Standards for Sexual Health Services;[3]
• National Strategy for Sexual Health;[4]

and from The Faculty of Sexual and Reproductive HealthCare (FSRH) Clinical Effectiveness Unit in the form of:
• evidence based guidance documents on all currently available methods of contraception;
• UK Selected Practice Recommendations[5] (adapted from the WHO Selected Practice Recommendations[6]); and, in particular;
• UK Medical Eligibility Criteria (UKMEC)[7](adapted from the WHO Medical Eligibility Criteria[8]).

The UKMEC[7] give 4 categories of eligibility for use of contraception:
1. no restriction to use
2. benefits usually outweigh risks
3. risks usually outweigh benefits
4. unacceptable risk.

Use of a method with category 3 requires expert clinical judgement and/or referral to a specialist provider.

All FSRH publications and guidance are available from 🖳 http://www.ffphrc.org.uk/

Comprehensive information and individual method leaflets for patients are available from 🖳 www.fpa.org.uk.

With thanks to Shelley Mehigan, Clinical Nurse Specialist in Contraception, Sexual Health Service, Berkshire East PCT.

Combined hormonal contraception (CHC)

Combined hormonal contraception contains the synthetic hormones oestrogen and progestogen.

Action of CHC

- The main action is prevention of ovulation.
- Cervical mucus remains viscous and is no longer stretchy, impairing the transport and penetration of sperm.
- Alters the endometrium to make it less receptive to implantation.
- Interferes with motility within the fallopian tubes.

There are several different types of CHC:

- *monophasic pills*: each tablet contains a fixed amount of oestrogen and progestogen. Tablets are taken orally usually for 21 consecutive days followed by 7 days with no tablets, during which withdrawal bleeding occurs;
- *phased pills*: these contain varying amounts of hormones depending on the stage of the cycle;
- *everyday pills*: these may be monophasic or phased and consist of active pills and inactive pills. They are taken for each of the 28 days. As some of the pills are inactive, it is essential to take them in the correct order;
- *patches*: patches applied weekly for 3 weeks followed by a 7-day break;
- *vaginal ring*: A ring is inserted into the vagina for 3 weeks, removed for 7 days and then a new ring is inserted.

UKMEC category 3/4[7]include:

- Past history of, or current: thrombosis; ischaemic arterial disease; stroke; breast cancer; liver disease.
- Known or suspected thrombophilia.
- Migraine with aura.
- Smoker aged 35 or over—or stopped less than a year ago.
- BMI >35.
- Multiple risks for arterial disease (age, BMI, smoker, migraine, hypertension).
- Hypertension >140 systolic, >90 diastolic.
- Breastfeeding.

Advantages of CHCs

- Reliable and reversible.
- Convenient and easy to use, not related to intercourse.
- Bleeding is predictable and regular and may be lighter and less painful.
- Can reduce premenstrual signs and symptoms including a reduction in acne in some women.
- Reduces the risk of benign breast disease, endometriosis, ectopic pregnancy, and ovarian cysts.
- Reduces endometrial and ovarian cancer.
- Reduces risk of pelvic inflammatory disease (PID).

Disadvantages of CHCs

- Cannot be taken by women with contraindications or risk factors for venous or arterial disease.
- Need to be taken correctly and consistently (pills daily; patches weekly, ring monthly)—requires adequate teaching of the method by the prescriber.
- Risk of thromboembolism, heart disease, increase in BP, jaundice, gallstones, liver cancer.
- Risk of failure if taking interacting medication or if severe diarrhoea and vomiting with COC.
- Possible link with cancer of the breast and cervix.
- May need to be discontinued prior to some planned surgery.
- Do not protect against sexually transmitted infection (STI).
- Side effects in some women including headaches, acne, breast tenderness and bloating.
- Patches may be visible.

Progestogen-only pill (POP)

POPs contain the synthetic hormone progestogen. The older POPs containing norethisterone, etynodiol diacetate, or levonorgestrel do not prevent ovulation consistently. Cerazette® which contains desogestrel, prevents ovulation 98% of the time. This may, therefore, be more suitable for younger women who may be more fertile, or for those for whom prevention of pregnancy is paramount. POPs are suitable for women who have contraindications to CHC or who choose them as a preferred method.

Action of POPs

- Possible prevention of ovulation—this is the main mode of action of Cerazette®.
- Thickening of cervical mucus, impeding the transit of sperm.
- Thinning of endometrial lining of the uterus, which prevents implantation.
- Interference with motility within the fallopian tubes.

Advantages of POPs

- Can be taken by women who have contraindications to or risks for CHC, including those who smoke, are breast feeding, or have migraine with aura.
- No increased risk of cardiovascular disease (CVD), venous thrombolism or hypertension.
- Can be continued prior to surgery.
- Are suitable for women who are breast feeding.
- May reduce dysmenorrhoea and premenstrual signs.

Disadvantages of POPs

- Older versions may be less effective.
- Need to be taken correctly and consistently—requires adequate teaching of the method by the prescriber.
- Older POPs needs to be taken within 3 hours of the time of day that the previous day's pill was taken (12 hrs for Cerazette®).
- Periods may become irregular or disappear completely.
- Can cause development of functional ovarian cysts.
- Possible Increased risk of ectopic pregnancy.

Injected progestogens

Long acting reversible contraception (LARC). Depo-Provera® and Noristerat® similar to the POP but main action is to prevent ovulation. They are given by IM injection every 12 (Depo-Provera®) or 8 (Noristerat®) weeks. Periods usually stop completely with Depo-Provera®.

Advantages of injectables
In addition to those for POP:
• Very effective, lasts for 12 or 8 weeks, reduced risk of endometrial cancer, particularly good for women with problem periods or premenstrual symptoms.

Disadvantages of injectables
Possibility of disrupted or irregular bleeding in a few women particularly at start, weight gain, delayed return to fertility, cannot be removed, theoretical connection with osteoporosis in some women (unconfirmed). MHRA advises review after 2 years with Depo-Provera®.

Implanted progestogens (Nexplanon®)

Long acting reversible contraception (LARC). Similar to the POP but main action is to prevent ovulation. Single rod inserted subdermally in the inner aspect of the upper arm. Must only be fitted or removed by those who have had specific training (RCN)[9]. Protection lasts for up to 3 years.

Advantages of implants
In addition to those for POP:
• very effective, lasts for 3 years, quickly reversible on removal, no follow-up unless problems.

Disadvantages of implants
• Disrupted or irregular bleeding which may continue for 3 years, though some women will have amenorrhoea; minor surgery to remove (removal may be difficult if not inserted correctly), can cause development of functional ovarian cysts, possible increased risk of ectopic pregnancy if method fails.

Intra-uterine devices (IUDs)

Long acting reversible contraception (LARC): Fitted into the uterus and consist of a plastic carrier with copper wire and/or copper bands. Must only be fitted or removed by those who have had specific training (RCN).[10]

Mode of action
• Main effect is by the copper ions to prevent fertilization.
• Foreign body reaction disrupts the endometrium and prevents implantation.

Advantages of IUDs
Very effective for up to 10 years depending on device; if fitted over the age of 40 may remain in place until after the menopause.

Disadvantages of IUDs
Periods may be longer, heavier and more painful; increased risk of pelvic infection for women at risk of sexually transmitted infection (STI); rarely can be expelled or perforate; apparent increased risk of ectopic pregnancy with older IUDs with less than 300mm^2 copper as less effective at preventing extra-uterine pregnancies.

Intra-uterine system (IUS/Mirena®)
Long acting reversible contraception (LARC): Fitted into the uterus and consists of a silastic T shaped device with a capsule containing levonorgestrel. Must only be fitted or removed by those who have had specific training (RCN).[10] Also licensed for use for the treatment of menorrhagia.

Mode of action
Similar to the POP—main action is to prevent implantation, rarely prevents ovulation.

Advantages of IUS
Same as POP but with the addition of significant reduction of bleeding—many older women end up with amenorrhoea.

Disadvantages of IUS
Irregular bleeding pattern particularly at start.

Emergency contraception
2 oral preparations or a copper-containing IUD.

Oral preparations
1. Levonelle® 1500—POM; Levonelle® One Step—Pharmacy product
Contains levonorgestrel—licensed for emergency contraception up to 72 hours after unprotected sexual intercourse (UPSI) or contraceptive failure.

Mode of action
Depends on when taken in menstrual cycle. May prevent or delay ovulation, alters endometrium, affects ovum transport and alters normal corpus luteal function.
• Can be taken up to 72 hours (3 days) after a single episode of unprotected intercourse.
• Less effective than an IUD.
• Efficacy deteriorates with time.
• Can be given more than once in a cycle.

2. ellaOne®[11]

Contains ulipristal acetate—is a selective progesterone receptor modulator licensed for emergency contraception up to 120 hours after UPSI or contraceptive failure.

- New product.
- Primary mechanism of action is inhibition or delay of ovulation.
- Licensed for use up to 120 hours.
- Potential interaction with progestogen containing products so additional contraception required until next bleed.
- Ulipristal is contraindicated in pregnancy or suspected pregnancy, as well as in those with a hypersensitivity to any of the excipients. In the absence of specific studies to monitor safety, ulipristal is not recommended in those with severe hepatic impairment, nor is it recommended in women with severe asthma insufficiently.

Controlled by oral glucocorticoids. As it is not known whether ulipristal is excreted in breast milk, breastfeeding women are advised not to breast-feed for 36 hours after treatment.

IUD

- A copper IUD can be inserted up to 120 hours (5 days) after unprotected sex.
- If more than 5 days since unprotected intercourse (or multiple episodes) the device will still be effective if inserted up to 5 days after the earliest calculated day when ovulation could have occurred.

Spermicides

- These need to be used in conjunction with barrier methods as their failure rate is high if used alone.
- They contain an active ingredient, which destroys the sperm membrane and alters the pH of the vaginal environment, and need to be introduced into the vagina before intercourse.
- Available as cream, pessaries, or foams.

Female barrier methods of contraception

These provide a barrier between the egg and sperm.

Diaphragm

- A dome-shaped device made of latex or silicone, which is positioned in the vagina to cover the cervix.
- If used correctly, with a spermicidal preparation, it can be up to 96% effective.
- Available with flat, coil or arcing springs in various sizes which need to be fitted by a trained clinician.

Cervical cap

The cap is smaller than the diaphragm and is made of silicone. It covers the cervix and is held in place by suction to the vaginal or cervical wall and is between 92 and 96% effective if used correctly with a spermicide.

Female condom/Femidom

A one-size, loose fitting, lubricated sheath made of polyurethane inserted into the vagina.

Male barrier methods of contraception

The condom or sheath

These cover the erect penis, retain the sperm at ejaculation, and prevent its entering the vagina. They should be used with a spermicide and are available in a number of styles, sizes, and finishes.

Further reading

Belfield, T. (1999). *FPA Contraceptive Handbook: A Guide for Family Planning and Other Health Professionals*, 3rd edition. Family Planning Association, London.

Belfield, T., Carter, Y., Matthews, P. (2006). *The Handbook of Sexual Health in Primary Care*, 2nd revised edition. Family Planning Association, London.

1. RCN (2004). *Sexual Health Competences: an integrated career and competency framework for sexual and reproductive health nursing*. RCN, London.
2. National Institute for Health and Clinical Excellence (2005). *Long-acting reversible contra-ception: the effective and appropriate use of long-acting reversible contraception*. 🖳 www.nice.org.uk.
3. DH/Medical Foundation for AIDS and Sexual Health (2005). *Recommended standards for sexual health services*. DH, London.
4. DH. (2001). *National Strategy for Sexual Health and HIV*. DH, London.
5. Faculty of Family Planning and Reproductive Health Care (2002). *UK Selected Practice Recom-mendations for Contraceptive Use*. www.ffprhc.org.uk.
6. World Health Organization (2005). *Selected Practice Recommendations for Contraceptive Use*. Second Ed. WHO, Geneva.
7. Faculty of Sexual and Reproductive HealthCare, Clinical Effectiveness Unit (2009). *UK Medical Eligibility Criteria for Contraceptive Use*. www.fsrh.org.
8. World Health Organization. (2009). *Medical Eligibility Criteria for Contraceptive Use*. Fourth Ed. WHO, Geneva.
9. RCN (2008). *Inserting and removing subdermal contraceptive implants. Accreditation and training guidance for nurses*. RCN, London. http://www.rcn.org.uk/__data/assets/pdf_file/0004/199381/002_240.pdf.
10. RCN (2008). *Intrauterine techniques. RCN accreditation and training guidance for nurses and mid-wives*. RCN, London. http://www.rcn.org.uk/__data/assets/pdf_file/0007/199357/003_179.pdf.

Common conditions

Bacterial vaginosis

Bacterial infection of the vagina; only 50% of women with this infection report symptoms.

Cause

- The most common cause is an alteration in the normal flora of the vagina, from a predominance of *Lactobacillus* to a high concentration of anaerobic bacteria.
- It has been identified that the incidence of bacterial vaginosis is increased in women using IUDs and those taking oral contraceptives.
- Other risk factors include new or multiple sexual partners, sexual debut at a young age, and douching.[1]

Treatment

- Clindamycin cream 2% (Dalacin® cream).
- Metronidazole vaginal gel 0.75% (Zidoval® vaginal gel).
- Metronidazole PO.

Vulvovaginal candidiasis (thrush)

Cause

This inflammation is usually caused by a yeast, *Candida albicans*.

Signs and symptoms

Vulval itching and soreness; vaginal discharge; pain during intercourse.

Treatment: all partners

GI in BNF for imidazole preparations, which are formulated as pessaries, capsules, or intravaginal creams.

📖 Prescribing for the prevention and treatment of infections, pp. 309–16.

Dysmenorrhoea

Lower abdominal or pelvic pain experienced during menstruation.

Treatment

To control the pain with minimal side effects (📖 Prescribing for pain, pp. 317–30). NSAIDs have been used beneficially (e.g. mefenamic acid).

Balanitis

An inflammation of the glans penis.

Cause

Usually caused by bacterial or fungal infections and often associated with phimosis, an inability to retract the foreskin.

Signs and symptoms

Redness, itch, discharge

Treatment

As vulvovaginal candidiasis, with imidazoles or antifungals such as nystatin.

---

1. BASHH CEG Group. (1999). *National Guidelines on the management of bacterial vaginosis.* BASHH CEG Group, London. 🖳 www.agum.org.uk.

Prescribing for palliative care

Prescribing for palliative care

Definition

The Gold Standard Framework[1] aims to improve palliative care delivery. Symptom management is one of the seven key tasks of the framework. Prescribing for people who require palliative care involves active total care and suppression of symptoms for those whose disease is not responsive to curative treatments. In addition to control of pain and other symptoms, it involves a holistic approach, embracing social, psychological, and spiritual dimensions. Palliation aims to relieve symptoms and offer support to the patient and their family and/or carers, thus optimizing the patient's quality of life. Care is provided by a multidisciplinary team and may be delivered in the patient's home, at a day hospice, or at an inpatient hospice.

Palliative care may be required by patients who have:
- cancer;
- a debilitating progressive illness, such as heart failure;
- multiple sclerosis;
- motor neuron disease;
- HIV/AIDS.

In March 2004 NICE issued general guidelines aimed at improving and supporting palliative care services for adults with cancer to facilitate the implementation of the NHS Cancer Plan for England[2] and the NHS Plan for Wales (Improving Health in Wales).[3] The key aims are as follows.
- *People who are affected by cancer should be involved in developing cancer services.*
- *There should be good communication, and people affected by cancer should be involved in decision making.*
- *Information should be available free of charge.*
- *People affected by cancer should be offered a range of physical, emotional, spiritual and social support.*
- *There should be services to help people living with the after-effects of cancer manage these for themselves.*
- *People with advanced cancer should have access to a range of services to improve their quality of life.*
- *There should be support for people dying from cancer.*
- *The needs of family and other carers of people with cancer should be met.*
- *There should be a trained workforce to provide services.*[4]

In 2009 NICE issued specific guidance on caring for people with advanced breast cancer.[5]

Treatment

The number of drugs should be limited to as few as possible, as taking oral medication can be an effort. The treatment goal of any new medication needs to be monitored.

Prescribing by members of a multi-disciplinary team requires liaison between the professionals involved. Communication and record-keeping are key to ensuring that all medications prescribed are compatible with

each other and with the possible multipathology of the patient. The seven principles of safe prescribing need to be considered along with the following (📖 Seven principles of safe prescribing, p. 94).
• Size, shape, and taste of medication.
• Avoidance of inconvenient doses or dose intervals.
• The risk of adverse effects and drug interactions.
• Reinforce regimens with written advice. To avoid confusion for the patient and their family the medication regimen and the purpose of the drug should be written down.

Oral medications are usually satisfactory provided that the patient is not suffering from:
• nausea;
• dysphagia;
• vomiting;
• intestinal obstruction;
• coma.

Rectal, transdermal, and parenteral routes offer different options.

NB: it is imperative to be aware of differing potencies when switching between different opioids and/or different routes of administration.

Negotiating a contract

As with all prescribing, it is important to reach a concordant agreement with your patient (📖 Concordance, p. 84; 📖 The prescribing pyramid, p. 94). In addition to the recognition and treatment of symptoms identified through assessment and examination, it is important to consider:
• patient preference and concordance;
• patient perception of severity of symptoms;
• quality of life issues;
• value for money considerations;
• the roles of other members of the multidisciplinary team.

📖 Concordance, p. 84.
📖 Ensuring an effective consultation, p. 190.

Further reading

WHO Europe (2004). *Palliative care: the solid facts*. WHO, Milan. 🖥 www.euro.who.int
WHO Europe (2004). *Better palliative care for older people*. WHO, Milan. 🖥 www.euro.who.int

1. *The Gold Standard Framework for community palliative care*.
🖥 http://www.goldstandardsframework.nhs.uk/
2. Department of Health (2001). *The NHS Cancer Plan*.
🖥 www.doh.gov.uk/cancer/cancerplan.htm
3. National Assembly for Wales (2001). Improving health in Wales: a plan for the NHS and its partners. 🖥 www.wales.gov.uk/healthplanonline/health_plan/content/nhsplan-e.pdf
4. NICE (2004). Guidelines and updates. 🖥 www.nice.org.uk/csgsp (accessed 3 December 2010)
5. NICE (2009). Guidelines and updates. 🖥 http://guidance.nice.org.uk/CG81 (accessed 4 February 2011)

Management of anxiety

Approximately 25% of people who are terminally ill suffer alterations in mood such as anxiety or depression.[1]

Definition of depression

A universally unpleasant emotion than can be acute/transient or chronic/persistent.[1]

Possible causes of anxiety

- Situational
- Organic
- Psychiatric
- Drug-induced (Table 12.29)
- Spiritual.

Signs of anxiety and depression

- Poor concentration
- Indecisiveness
- Insomnia
- Irritability
- Sweating
- Tremor
- Panic attacks
- Apprehension
- Worry
- Inability to relax
- Difficulty in falling asleep and unrefreshing sleep
- Nightmares.

Symptoms of anxiety and depression

- Muscular aches and fatigue
- Restlessness
- Trembling
- Jumpiness
- Tension headaches
- Shortness of breath
- Palpitations
- Dizziness
- Sweating
- Dry mouth
- Nausea
- Diarrhoea
- Urinary frequency.

Treatment

Benzodiazepine.

---

1. Lloyd-Williams, M., Dennis, M., and Taylor, F. (2004). A prospective study to determine the association between physical symptoms and depression in patients with advanced cancer. *Palliative Medicine*, **18**, 558–63.

Management of pain in palliative care

It is imperative to assess each pain that a person has as there may be more than one type. Use a validated and structured pain assessment tool in your discussion and, where possible, record the nature and severity of the pain(s) as perceived by the patient. Failing that, ask those who are taking care of them. The choice of analgesic will depend on the severity and cause of the pain.

Prescribe analgesia in a stepwise approach moving to the next step when the maximal dose of the analgesic is reached as shown in the WHO analgesic ladder (Fig. 12.12). See also Table 12.29.

📖 Prescribing for pain, pp. 317–330.

Opioids

- If non-opioids prove insufficient for mild to moderate pain control, opioids such as codeine and dextropropoxyphene may be given alone or in combination with non-opioids.
- Tramadol may be useful for moderate pain.
- Morphine is the most useful opiate if the above are failing to control pain (Fig. 12.12).
- Morphine often causes nausea and vomiting in adults and may need to be given with an anti-emetic.
- Other unwanted effects of morphine use include drowsiness and constipation.
- Larger doses may cause respiratory depression and hypotension.
- Consideration of possible dependence is not a deterrent for use of morphine in terminal illness.
- Patients are often prescribed morphine tablets in slow-release formulation for pain control in palliative care.
- Alongside this they may be prescibed non-slow-release morphine to take when their pain is not controlled by the slow-release formulation. This is sometimes called a 'rescue dose'.
- The active life of non-slow-release morphine is ~4hr and it can be administered up to six times daily.
- A rescue dose may be needed ~30min before activity which causes pain (e.g. wound re-dressing).

Strong opioids

e.g.
Morphine,
Diamorphine,
Fentanyl,
Methadone,
Hydromorphone,
Oxycodone,
± Adjuvant*

Weak opioids

e.g.
Codeine,
Dihydroodeine,
Dextropropoxy-
phene,
Tramadol,
± Adjuvant*

Non-opioid
analgesics
e.g. NSAIDs
paracetamol

Fig. 12.12 WHO analgesic ladder (reproduced with permission).[1]

*Adjuvant analgesics are drugs that have a primary indication which is not pain but can potentiate or enhance the effect of opioids, can treat the symptoms of the pain, or can help balance the doses to minimize the dose-related unwanted effects of opioids.

Table 12.29 Drugs that may affect renal and hepatic function

Area	Drug name	Symptom control
Renal	Aspirin	Pain
	Baclofen	Muscle spasm
	Cimetidine	Gastric hyperacidity
	Domperidone	Nausea and vomiting
	Famotidine	Gastric hyperacidity
	Ibuprofen	Mild to moderate pain
	Metoclopramide	Nausea and vomiting
	Ranitidine	Gastric hyperacidity
Hepatic	Aspirin	Mild to moderate pain
	Cimetidine	Gastric hyperacidity
	Cyclizine	Nausea and vomiting
	Dantrolene	Muscle spasm
	Diclofenac	Pain (NSAID external use)
	Ibuprofen	Pain (NSAID)
	Ketoprofen	Pain (NSAID external use)
	Metoclopramide	Nausea and vomiting
	Metronidazole	Fungating wounds
	Miconazole	Oral candidiasis (local)
	Paracetamol	Pain
	Ranitidine	Gastric hyperacidity

Adapted from BNF 44.[2]

Breakthrough pain

The formula for calculating the morphine dose for breakthrough pain is:

breakthrough dose = (total daily dose of slow-release morphine)/6

Further information

- Changing patients from oral morphine to diamorphine via a syringe driver: see table in BNF 'Prescribing in palliative care').
- Changing from oral morphine to fentanyl patch (slow-release dose over 3 days): see BNF 7.2 and 'Prescribing in palliative care'.

Further reading

Davis, A. (ed.) (2006). *Cancer-related breakthrough pain.* Oxford University Press, Oxford.
National Patient Safety Agency (2008). *Reducing dosing errors with opioid medicines. Rapid Response Report.* ☐ www.npsa.nhs.uk
SIGN (2008) Control of pain in adults with cancer: a national clinical guideline. ☐ www.sign.ac.uk

1. World Health Organization (1986). *Cancer pain relief.* WHO, Geneva.
2. *British National Formulary 44* (2002). British Medical Association and Royal Pharmaceutical Association of Great Britain, London.

Management of further palliative care related conditions (A–Z)

Constipation

Possible causes

- Stress
- Diet
- Lack of exercise
- Reduced fluid intake
- Side-effect medication
- Underlying disease process.

Treatment

See 📖 Constipation, p. 304.

People taking opioid analgesics should take both a stimulant laxative and a softening laxative.[1] Bulk-forming laxatives are less useful for palliative care constipation because:

- they are unpalatable;
- they need to be taken with a minimum of 200–300mL of water;
- they can cause intestinal obstruction if taken with too little water.

Normal advice regarding increasing fluids, dietary fibre, and exercise may be inappropriate for palliative care patients.

Cough

This may be a symptom of an underlying pathology (e.g. asthma or post-nasal drip) and prescribing must follow assessment of the causes.

- If the cough is productive help in expectoration may be required, e.g. physiotherapy or antibiotics if an infection is causative.
- A persistent dry cough may need to be suppressed with an opioid although there are unwanted effects such as sputum retention and ventilatory failure which may contraindicate its use.

Practical aspects regarding the comfort of the patient should be taken into consideration:

- position;
- avoiding smoke or fume inhalation;
- use of a humidifier if the air in the room is very dry.

Diarrhoea

Possible causes

- Excessive use of laxatives, antibiotics, antacids
- Infection
- Fistula
- Anxiety
- Irritable bowel
- Neurological dysfunction
- Autonomic insufficiency.

Dry mouth
Establish the cause: it could be dehydration, infection, anxiety, or an unwanted effect of a medication, and resolve where possible.

Excessive respiratory secretions
The BNF has recommended the use of hyoscine hydrobromide although it can cause agitation. It notes that hyoscine butylbromide has fewer unwanted side effects but is less effective in controlling these secretions.

Fungating wounds
Wound care products containing charcoal may be useful when dressing these often malodorous wounds. See Table 12.25 in 📖 Types of dressing 1, p. 355.

Gastric hyperactivity
It should be noted that H2-receptor antagonists, which are useful for this symptom, do not protect against ulceration caused by the NSAIDs commonly prescribed for pain relief in patients requiring palliative care.

Muscle spasm
Possible causes
- Drug induced
- Meningeal metaseses
- Bone metastases
- Nerve compression
- Peripheral neuropathy
- Polymyostis
- Spinal degeneration.

Treatment
- Try simple measures:
  - heat pad;
  - massage;
  - relaxation.
- Consider transcutaneous electric nerve stimulation (TENS) over the trigger point if the pain is myofascial.
- If the trigger points are multiple or the muscle spasm is widespread, a muscle relaxant (e.g. diazepam) should be considered.

Nausea and vomiting

Care consists of the management of symptoms. Therefore it is important to remember that oral antiemetics will not be absorbed if there is gastric stasis.

Possible causes
- Chemoreceptor trigger zone:
  - biochemical abnormality;
  - hypercalcaemia;
  - liver failure;
  - renal failure;
  - sepsis;
  - drugs (e.g. opioids, antibiotics).
- Via vestibular system:
  - drugs (e.g. aspirin).
- Via cortical centres:
  - psychological factors (e.g. anxiety);
  - sites, smells, tastes;
  - conditioned vomiting;
  - raised intracranial pressure.

Treatment
- Dietary measures:
  - liquid and soft foods, selected by the patient;
  - small meals, eaten slowly.
- Environmental measures:
  - avoidance of noxious or suggestive smells and odours;
  - use of relaxation techniques;
  - use of antiemetics selected depending on presumed causative mechanism (e.g. metoclopramide—commence adequate dose before vomiting starts if possible).

Oral candidiasis

60% of patients with cancer have oral problems: either dry mouth or Candida. 📖 Prescribing for gastrointestinal problems, pp. 285–308.

Restlessness, agitation, and confusion

Possible causes in people requiring palliative care:
- Cognitive impairment
- Drug reaction.

Treatment
Phenothiazines such as levomepromazine and antipsychotic (neuroleptic) preparations.

Further information

For further information beyond the scope of this handbook:
- www.macmillan.org.uk
- www.cancerresearchuk.org/aboutcancer.
- National Cancer Institute. www.cancer.gov/cancerinfo/pdq/supportivecare
- National Council for Hospice and Specialist Palliative Care Services (NCHSPCS). www.hospice-spec-council.org.uk/

Cancer helplines

Cancer BACUP ☎ 0808001234
CancerHelp UK www.cancerhelp.org.uk

1. Twycross, R. and Wilcock, A. (eds) (2007). *Palliative care formulary* (3rd edn). palliativedrugs.com

Disposal of medicines following death

Following the enquiry into the ease with which Dr Shipman obtained controlled drugs with which he killed many of his patients, the Department of Health amended legislation regarding the management of controlled drugs in the UK. The Misuse of Drugs Regulations 2001 has been amended and the Controlled Drugs (Supervision of Management and Use) Regulations 2006 came into effect on 1 January 2007.

📖 Controlled drugs (CDs), p. 98.

At the time of going to press all drugs, once dispensed, are the patient's property and pass to their family on their death. This poses a problem as it is illegal to possess controlled drugs that have not been prescribed for you.

After the death of a family member relatives should be encouraged to return any unused medications to the pharmacy. If this is not possible, a community nurse, with the owners' permission and witnessed by another member of the health-care professional team, may destroy any unused controlled drugs.

Further reading

Department of Health (2007). *Safer management of controlled drugs: early action*. TSO, London.

McNicol, E., Strassels, S.A., Goudas, L., et al. (2007) *NSAIDS or paracetamol, alone or combined with opioids, for cancer pain (Cochrane Review)*. Cochrane Library, Issue 2. Wiley, Chichester.

Complementary and alternative medicines and over-the-counter drugs

Complementary and alternative medicine (CAM)

The Department of Health Steering Group Report[1] recommended that complentary health practitioners come under the regulation of a single professional body that is likely to be the Health Professions Council (HPC).

Professional body guidance

The Nursing and Midwifery Council (NMC) Professional Code of Conduct states:

> You must ensure that the use of complementary or alternative therapies is safe and in the best interests of those in your care.[2]

Standard 23 of the Standards for Medicines Management states:

> Registrants must have successfully undertaken training and be competent to practise the administration of complementary and alternative therapies.[3]

The Nursing and Midwifery Council have published guidelines relating to complementary therapies and homeopathy.[4] All registered health-care practitioners are advised that when practising complementary therapies and homeopathy, they are fully accountable and must satisfy themselves that they are competent to do so. They must respect the wishes of patients who are using these treatments. This guidance is to be used in conjunction with the NMC Standards for Medicines Management[3] and the NMC Standards of Proficiency for Nurse and Midwife Prescribers.[5]

What is CAM?

- The treatment of disease using methods other than recognized/conventional medicine.
- Use of homeopathic, herbal, aromatherapy, and (OTC) vitamin supplements to treat conditions.

Problems

- Often not adequately clinically trialled.
- Might not have a product licence.
- Poor manufacturing process.
- Adulteration to include toxic substances and conventional drugs.
- Misidentification of herbs.
- Substitution of herbs.
- Varying strengths of preparations.
- Incomplete labelling.
- Incorrect dosage and instructions.
- Patients may see treatments/medications as 'natural' and not inform their health professional that they are taking them.
- Information not readily available in 'conventional' textbooks.

When prescribing

- Always ask the patient what else they are taking, including OTC medication and herbal medicines.
- Consider potential drug interactions.[6,7]

History[8]

- At least 5000 years old.
- Interest in CAM has grown over past two decades.
- Over 31 million visits to CAM practitioners in 1998.
- One in five Britons seeks complementary or alternative therapy.
- Perceived to be 'safe'.
- Research is lagging behind.
- Health-care professionals are assumed to know about CAM.

Recommendations of House of Lords Select Committee 2000

- Tougher regulation.
- More rigorous testing.
- Greater supervision of practice.
- Only those with a statutory regulation or powerful self-regulation should be available on NHS.
- Only by referral from GP.

Further reading

Department of Health (2007). *Trust, assurance and safety—the regulation of health professionals in the 21st century*. TSO, London.
Department of Health (2009). *Joint consultation on the report to ministers from the Department of Health Steering Group on the statutory regulation of practitioners of acupuncture, herbal medicine, traditional Chinese medicine and other traditional medicine systems practised in the UK*. TSO, London.

1. Department of Health (2009). *Joint consultation on the report to ministers from the Department of Health Steering Group on the statutory regulation of practitioners of acupuncture, herbal medicine, traditional Chinese medicine and other traditional medicine systems practised in the UK*. TSO, London.
2. Nursing and Midwifery Council (2008). *The code: standards of conduct, performance and ethics for nurses and midwives*. NMC, London.
3. Nursing and Midwifery Council (2008). *Standards for medicines management*. NMC, London.
4. Nursing and Midwifery Council (2008) *Complementary therapies and homeopathy advice sheet.* ⊠ http://www.nmc-uk.org/aArticle.aspx?ArticleID=3056 (accessed 25 October 2009).
5. Nursing and Midwifery Council (2006) *Standards of proficiency for nurse and midwife prescribers*. NMC, London.
6. *British National Formulary* (latest edn). British Medical Association and the Royal Pharmaceutical Society of Great Britain, London.
7. Stockley, I.H. (2009) *Drug interactions* (8th edn). Pharamceutical Press, London.
8. Thomas, K, Nicholl J.P., and Coleman, P. (2001). Use and expenditure on complementary therapies in England: a population based survey. *Complementary Therapies in Medicine*, **9**, 2–11.

Homeopathic and herbal medicines

Homeopathy

- Homeopathy: from *homeos* (similar) and *pathos* (disease).
- Like cures like—the mild effects of the remedy mimic the symptoms of the disease.
- The greater the dilution, the greater the therapeutic effect (serial dilution)—hardly any or no trace of active ingredient.
- Manufacture controlled by the Medicines Act 1968.
- Medical claims cannot be made for remedies; however, leaflets can be displayed near the product.
- Medical homeopaths are medically qualified and regulated by the GMC.
- Non-medical homeopaths are regulated by different bodies (Fellowship of Homeopaths etc.).

Effects on patients

- Limited evidence with regard to ADRs.
- Little evidence with regard to drug interactions.

Herbalism

Regulated by National Institute of Medical Herbalists 1864 (professional body). 🖥 http://www.nimh.org.uk/ (accessed 22 October 2009).
  Phytotherapy is the science of herbalism.

Herbal medicines (Table 13.1)

- Plant-derived medicines at pharmacological doses where effects can be measured.
- Symptom-based approach to diagnosis.

In 2008 the Medicines and Health Care Products Regulatory Agency (MHRA) produced the document *Public health risk with herbal medicines: an overview*, warning the public and professionals of the dangers associated with taking herbal medicines. The document can be accessed at 🖥 http://www.mhra.gov.uk/Safetyinformation/Generalsafetyinformatio-nandadvice/Product-specificinformationandadvice/Herbalmedicines/index.htm

Regulation of herbal medicines

- Licensed:
  - marketing authorization (product licence) issued by MHRA;
  - have to meet safety, quality, and efficacy standards similarly to conventional drugs.
- Unlicensed:
  - exempt from licensing requirements (Section 12 of Medicines Act 1968).

Section 12 Medicines Act 1968

- Section 12 (1): a person can make, sell, and supply herbal remedies as part of business provided that the remedy is manufactured on the premises and supplied as a consequence of consultation between the patient and the herbalist.

Table 13.1 Commonly used herbal medicines

Drug	Indications	Side effects	Interactions	Cautions/contraindications
Gluco-samine	Relief of joint pain	Mild GI symptoms, rash, drowsiness, headache, insomnia		Diabetes may alter glucose sensitivity. Caution in breastfeeding. Contraindicated if allergic to shellfish
Saw palmetto	Urogenital conditions: benign prostatic hyperplasia	Dizziness and GI disturbance Rare side effects: mild pruritus, headache and hypertension. Erectile dysfunction (similar to placebo effect in studies)	Hormonal therapies (contraception and HRT)	Cautions: pregnancy and breastfeeding. Hormone-dependent cancers
Valerian	Insomnia	Headache, drowsiness (sedation), GI symptoms Rarely: nervous excitability, cardiac disturbances on sudden withdrawal (not confirmed in trials) Can cause dependency		Pregnancy and breastfeeding Before driving or operating heavy machinery Not to be taken if known hyper-sensitivity
St John's wort	Mild depression		Liver enzyme inducer for anti-epileptics, theophylline, combined hormonal contraceptive, SSRIs, warfarin	Avoid during pregnancy, breast-feeding Avoid when taking anti-epileptics, theophylline, combined hormonal contraceptive, SSRIs, or warfarin

(Continued)

Table 13.1 (*Contd.*)

Drug	Indications	Side effects	Interactions	Cautions/contraindications
Echinacea	Prevention of upper respiratory tract infections	Nausea, dizziness, shortness of breath, burning and numbing sensation in tongue, dermatitis, hepatitis, pruritus, hepatotoxicity	Other hepatotoxic drugs, e.g. anabolic steroids, amiodarone, ketoconazole, and methotrexate may also decrease the effect of immuno-suppressants	Cautions: asthma, atopy, allergy or hypersensitivity to sunflowers, liver dysfunction, TB, diabetes, HIV, systemic lupus, and other autoimmune diseases

- Section 12(2): allows manufacture and supply where:
  - process of manufacture consists of drying, crushing or comminuting;
  - remedy sold without any written recommendation as to its use;
  - remedy sold under a designation which only specifies the plant and the process and does not apply any other name to the remedy.

📖 The legal differences between prescribing, administering, and dispensing, p. 18.

Safety of homeopathic and herbal medicines

Safety should be considered for the following reasons:
- lack of data;
- 'natural' does not always mean safe (e.g. digitalis);
- remember herbal remedies are medicines;
- report adverse reactions to a doctor or pharmacist;
- may interact with other medicines.

Alert
- Patients taking drugs with a narrow therapeutic index (e.g. warfarin) or a drug therapy which is considered critical (e.g. insulin) should avoid complementary medicines.
- Women who are pregnant or breastfeeding should avoid complementary medicines.
- Kava-kava is now withdrawn from the market because of Yellow Card reporting of severe hepatotoxicity.
- Some Chinese medicines contain harmful excipients.
- 📖 Basic principles of pharmacology, pp. 53–64.

Reporting
- Report to the MHRA using the Yellow Card scheme.
- Important for all drugs, especially those that are less well known.
- 📖 Drug effects, p. 66

Further reading
Zollman, C. and Vickers, A. (1999). ABC of complementary medicine. What is complementary medicine? *BMJ*, **319**, 693–6. 🖥 http://www.mcs.gov.uk/ourwork/licensingmeds/herbalsafety
UKMI complementary medicines summaries, December 2002. 🖥 www.ukmi.nhs.uk

Other complementary therapies

Chiropractic

A form of health care which focuses on correcting spinal problems and the function of the nervous system without the use of drugs or surgery.
- Professional or representative association: British Chiropractic Association
- Contact e-mail: enquiries@chiropractic-uk.co.uk

Osteopathy

A system of health care which focuses on balancing the musculoskeletal system to prevent and treat disease.
- Professional or representative association: British Osteopathic Association
- Website: 🖳 www.osteopathy.org

Acupuncture

Based on the ancient Chinese technique of inserting thin needles at specific points in the body. Used to control pain and other symptoms.
- Professional or representative association: British Acupuncture Council
- Website: 🖳 www.acupuncture.org.uk

Reflexology

Based on the ancient Chinese technique of restoring energy flow through the body by the application of pressure point massage (mainly the feet, but can be the hands or ears).
- Professional or representative association: British Reflexology Association
- Website: 🖳 www.britreflex.co.uk

Aromatherapy

Uses essential oils (either extracts or essences often in conjunction with massage) to prevent or to treat disease.
- Professional or representative association: British Council of Practising Aromatherapists
- Email: info@bcapa.org
- Professional or representative association: Aromatherapy Organisations Council
- Website: 🖳 www.aromatherapycouncil.co.uk

Healing

Can be defined as natural or spiritual. The use of either hands-on or no-touch techniques to restore the energy flow through the body to support the body's own healing mechanisms.

- Professional or representative association: National Federation of Spiritual Healers (The Healing Trust)
- Website: 🖥 www.nfsh.org.uk

Naturopathy

The use of natural agents to support the internal balance of the body, promoting health and well-being.

- Professional or representative association: The British Naturopathic Association
- Website: 🖥 www.naturopaths.org.uk

Over-the-counter (OTC) drugs

Background
The NHS Plan[1] placed emphasis on encouraging a growth in self-care by extending the range of medicines available over the counter. To facilitate this, many items which were formerly prescription-only medicines (POMs) have been classified as pharmacy (P) or general sales list (GSL).

It is acknowledged that this increase in the number of medications available OTC will not necessarily reduce the prescribing burden of either doctors or NMPs. It is unlikely that patients with enduring conditions who do not currently pay for their prescriptions will elect to purchase them OTC.[1]

It is important to note that OTC licenses may not mirror POM licenses. For example, hydrocortisone 1% cream sold OTC may not be used on the face. Before advising OTC purchase, always be sure that the licence permits the use required.

Responsibilities
- Prescribers are equally accountable whether they recommend an OTC drug or prescribe a product, and it is important to bear in mind the Nursing and Midwifery Council standards on prescribing.[3]
- NMPs need to be vigilant when taking a medication history to ensure that patients tell them about all products they are taking, including OTCs and home remedies.
- It may be helpful to set up local guidelines to ensure good communication between community pharmacists, GPs, and non-medical prescribers to ensure the best use of OTC products for the benefit of patients.[4]

Possible problems
Several problems are engendered by the move to extended availability of OTC products.
- Many patients may take OTC products and fail to inform their GP, leading to potential drug interactions.
- Direct advertising to the general public, which is permitted for OTC products, may increase demand for the product as a prescribed item.

- Direct advertising may also lead to products being taken which are not required, or which are contraindicated by other medication being taken, either prescribed or OTC.
- Ethical issues of equity and fairness arise if a decision is made to recommend a product as an OTC to one patient whilst deciding to prescribe for another, even if the decision to prescribe is based on evidence that the patient would choose not to purchase the item even if it is essential.

📖 Prescribing for GI problems, pp. 285–308; 📖 Ethics, p. 138; 📖 Cost-effective prescribing, p. 438.

1. Department of Health (2000). *The NHS Plan: a plan for investment, a plan for reform.* TSO, London.
2. Bellingham, C. (2002). To switch or not? Pharmacists' opinions. *Pharmaceutical Journal*, **268**,
3. Nursing and Midwifery Council (2006). *Standards of proficiency for nurse and midwife prescribers.* NMC, London.
4. Nursing and Midwifery Council (2008). *The code: standards of conduct, performance and ethics for nurses and midwives.* NMC, London.

Section 4

Accountability

Audit

Audit

Audit is a systematic and official examination of a record, process, structure, environment, or account to evaluate performance.[1]

Clinical audit

The National Institute for Health and Clinical Excellence (NICE), the Commission for Health Improvement (CHI, functions now taken over by the Healthcare Commission), the Royal College of Nursing (RCN), and the University of Leicester give the following definition of clinical audit.

Clinical audit is a quality improvement process that seeks to improve patient care and outcomes through systematic review of care against explicit criteria and the implementation of change. Aspects of the structure, processes, and outcomes of care are selected and systematically evaluated against explicit criteria. Where indicated, changes are implemented at an individual, team, or service level and further monitoring is used to confirm improvement in healthcare delivery.[2]

Audit policy driver timeline

Audit requirements have been driven by government policy and professional bodies.

2000

- The NHS Plan[3] proposed that it should be mandatory for doctors to take part in clinical audit and that this should be extended to facilitate the involvement of:
  - nurses and midwives;
  - therapists;
  - other NHS staff.
- Audit Scotland, a statutory body was set up under the Public Finance and Accountability (Scotland) Act.

2001

- Improving Health in Wales[4] introduced annual appraisals that address the results of audit. The General Medical Council (GMC) advised all doctors that they '*must take part in regular and systematic medical and clinical audit*'.[5]
- The UK Central Council for Nursing, Midwifery and Health Visiting (UKCC) states that initiatives, such as clinical audit, are '*the business of every registered practitioner*'.[6]
- The Report of the Public Inquiry into Children's Heart Surgery at the Bristol Royal Infirmary 1984–1995 makes the following recommendations:
  The process of clinical audit, which is now widely practised within trusts, should be at the core of a system of local monitoring of performance. Clinical audit must be fully supported by trusts. They should ensure that healthcare professionals have access to the necessary time, facilities, advice, and expertise in order to conduct audit effectively.[7]

2004
- Public Audit (Wales) Act 2004
- First Audit Scotland Report on the NHS (🖳 www.audit-scotland.gov.uk).

2005
- The Wales Audit Office was created by amalgamating the office of the Audit Commission in Wales with that of the National Audit Office in Wales, under the Auditor General for Wales.
- The Chief Medical Officer's report *Good doctors, safer patients* called for clinical audit to enable to reach its potential as a rich source of information to support service improvement.[8]

2007
- The White Paper *Trust, assurance and safety* set out the mechanisms put in place to take the work of audit forward.[9]

2008
- The HealthCare Quality Improvement Partnership, an amalgamation of the Academy of Medical Royal Colleges, the Royal College of Nursing and the Long Term Conditions Alliance, created to host the National Clinical Audit and Patients' Outcomes Programme (NCAPOP).
- Launch of *Clinical Audit Today*, a UK online clinical audit journal (🖳 http://www.clinicalauditsupport.com)

2009
- An Audit Scotland report outlines changes in NHS spending and the management of capital.[10]

2010
- The National Archives—http://webarchive.nationalarchives.gov.uk contains details of the Enhanced Recovery Partnership programme.

1. Marquis, B.L. and Huston, C.J. (2006). *Leadership roles and management functions in nursing* (5th edn). Lippincott Williams & Wilkins, Philadelphia, PA.
2. NICE, CHI, RCN, and University of Leicester (2002). *Principles for best practice in clinical audit.* Radcliffe Medical Press, Abingdon.
3. Department of Health (2000). *NHS Plan: a plan for investment, a plan for reform.* TSO, London.
4. Minister for Health and Social Services (2001). *Improving health in Wales: a plan for the NHS and its partners.* National Assembly for Wales, Cardiff.
5. General Medical Council (2001). *Good medical practice.* GMC, London.
6. UK Central Council for Nursing (2001). *Professional self-regulation and clinical governance.* UKCCN, London.
7. Department of Health (2001). *Learning from Bristol: the Department of Health's response to the Report of the Public Inquiry into Children's Heart Surgery at the Bristol Royal Infirmary 1984–1995.* Command paper CM 5207. TSO, London.
8. 🖳 www.dh.gov.uk/en/Publicationsandstatistics/DH_4137232 (accessed 23 September 2009).
9. 🖳 www.dh.gov.uk/en/Publicationsandstatistics/DH_065946 (accessed 23 September 2009).
10. 🖳 www.audit-scotland.gov.uk (accessed 23 September 2009).

The relationship of clinical audit to clinical governance

NICE notes that clinical audit is at the heart of clinical governance as it provides the processes for evaluation of the quality of care delivered to patients, highlighting best practice and areas for improvement. NICE and the Healthcare Commission endorsed the publication *Principles for best practice in clinical audit*.[1] This booklet and the accompanying CD draw on a systematic review of audit literature and detail the audit process including:
- methods;
- tools;
- techniques;
- activities.

The document contains information regarding each stage of the audit process:
- preparing for audit;
- selecting audit criteria;
- measuring levels of performance;
- making and sustaining improvements in care.

---

1. NICE, CHI, RCN, and University of Leicester (2002). *Principles for best practice in clinical audit*. Radcliffe Medical Press, Abingdon.

Characteristics of a clinical audit

Table 14.1 Main characteristics of a clinical audit

Characteristic	Application
Topic area	Is it:
	relevant to the local situation?
	relevant to patient care?
Purpose	Does it:
	evaluate care delivery?
	monitor?
	deliver better patient care?
	make effective use of resources?
Timescale	Short for quick results and feedback
	Longer for a more in-depth study
Method	Measurement against implicit or explicit standards
	Opportunistic: makes use of existing data (e.g. patient's notes for a retrospective study)
Feedback and dissemination	Local (other professions, managers, purchasers, etc.)
	National/international (conferences, professional bodies, etc.)
Mechanisms of feedback and dissemination	Internal reports
	Audit meetings
	Publications

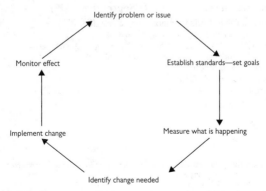

Fig. 14.1 Clinical audit cycle. Adapted from Humphries, J. and Green, J. (2002). *Nurse prescribing* (2nd edn). Palgrave, Basingstoke.

Differences between audit and research

Both activities contribute to improving the effectiveness of clinical care. The main differences are shown in Table 14.2.[1]

Table 14.2 Main differences between audit and research

Research	Audit
Defines or helps to define what makes good practice.	Measures if good practice—defined by research and/or expert opinion—is being followed every day with every patient
Advances knowledge of good practice	Helps to improve the actual quality of care being given to patients at a local level

Considerations when preparing a clinical audit proposal

- What do you want the audit to be about?
- What do you want to achieve?
- How can the audit contribute to quality of care?
- How will you measure practice?
- How will you collect data?
- How will you get support for the audit?
- Who will support you?
- Discuss any financial assistance/funding available with the clinical effectiveness or audit department of your trust.
- Arrange for audit to be included in your department/directorate service plan for the next year.

(Adapted from NHS[2].)

Useful resources (accessed 23 September 2009)

- National Clinical Audit Support Programme (NCASP) www.nhsia.nhs.uk/phsmi/pages/ncasp.asp
- NHS Quality Improvement Scotland www.crag.scot.nhs.uk
- Clinical Standards Board for Scotland (CSBS) www.nhshealthqulity.org
- Health of Wales (HOWIS) www.wales.nhs.uk
- Northern Ireland Audit office www.niauditoffice.gov.uk

1. Bowling, A. (2003). *Research methods in health: investigating health and health services* (2nd edn). Open University Press, Buckingham.
2. NHS Executive (2000). *Achieving effective practice. a clinical effectiveness and research information pack for nurses, midwives and health visitors. No. 6: Preparing a proposal for clinical audit.* TSO, London.

Approaches to audit 1

Prescription analysis and cost tabulation (PACT)
as an audit tool

Since the introduction of computerized prescribing information in 1998 at
the then Prescription Pricing Authority (PPA) it has been possible to make
prescription analysis and costing reports available to trusts and individual
prescribers.

The analysis of primary care prescribing in England was improved by
the introduction of Prescribing Analysis and Cost (PACT) data in 1991 by
the Prescription Pricing Division (PPD) of the Business Services Authority
(PPDBSA). PACT data (ePACT) are an important starting point for
understanding prescribing trends and activity.

ePACT offers a service for pharmaceutical and prescribing advisors and
is available for:
• primary care trusts (PCTs);
• strategic health authorities (SHAs);
• agencies acting on behalf of groups of other organizations.

It allows real-time online analysis of the previous 60 months prescribing
data held on the NHS Prescription Services Prescribing Database. Data
are updated on a monthly basis (6 weeks after the month in which the
prescription was dispensed) and can be selected according to:
• reporting period (i.e. month/quarter/year);
• prescribing organization (e.g. practice, PCT);
• BNF classification;
• controlled drugs tag.

The data available include:
• budgets and expenditure forecasts;
• costs and volumes of prescribing;
• prescribing totals by prescribers at all BNF levels;
• prescribing from non-medical prescribers;
• the working environment of nurses and supplementary prescribers
  (i.e. community or practice);
• patient list sizes;
• Low Income Scheme Index scores for practices;
• average daily quantities and defined daily doses;
• prescribing on behalf of PCT/practice;
• dispensing contractor name and address.

Data can be displayed in tabular and graphical formats. Variations in prescribing practice can be analysed in detail, trends can be identified, and
comparisons made.

National Patient Safety Agency (NPSA) (www.npsa.nhs.uk)

This agency, founded in 2001, promotes patient safety and has already issued medication alerts which require action by the NHS on many topics. Examples include the use of:

- potassium chloride;
- methotrexate;
- diamorphine and morphine;
- Repevax® and Revaxis®;
- anticoagulant medicines;
- liquid medicines administered via oral and other enteral routes;
- injectable medicines;
- epidural injections and infusions;
- paediatric intravenous infusions.

The abolition of NPSA was announced in 2010—the safety functions have been transferred to the National Commissioning Board.

Approaches to audit 2

The National Prescribing Centre (www.npc.co.uk)
The National Prescribing Centre is a health service organization formed in April 1996 by the Department of Health. It aims to support both individuals and the NHS in general to deliver medicines:
• rationally;
• that are evidence based;
• safely;
• cost effectively.

This is achieved through:
• evidenced-based therapeutic support:
  • MeReC;
  • New Medicines Scheme;
  • NPCi.
• medicines management support;
• prescriber support;
• non-medical prescribing programmes;
• supporting policy into practice.
The NPC offers support and teaching material. In addition, it has published a glossary of terms which cover prescribing rationales. For example, prescribed items may be ascribed to:
• the patient (this is 1 for 1);
• the prescribing unit (weighted depending on patient type), e.g. a surgery with a predominance of older patients is expected to prescribe more items per head than a surgery where the catchment area is a university and the predominance will be younger patients who, it is expected, will be healthier and require fewer prescriptions).
Local and national cost comparisons are facilitated by an attempt to create an average and remove demographic discrepancies by the creation of prescribing units (PUs) and ASTRO-PUs:
• ASTRO-PU—adjusted for age, sex, temporary resident originated prescribing unit;
• STAR-PU—adjusted for specific therapeutic group, age/sex-related prescribing units.

This glossary can be accessed at: ⌨ http://www.npc.co.uk/policy/prescribing/prescribingTerms/bodybup.htm (accessed 23 September 2009).
All the time of going to press the NPC is to become a part of NICE in April 2011.

NHS Business Services Authority (NHSBSA) (www.nhsbsa.nhs.uk)

The NHSBSA provides prescribing data and indications of prescribing trends. For example, in June 2007 the NHSBSA database, which records those registered to prescribe, included:
- 7472 nurse independent prescribers and 22,569 prescribing community practitioners;
- 411 pharmacist prescribers;
- 13 physiotherapists;
- 6 podiatrists.

The PPD received its first prescription from a podiatrist in June 2007.

Scottish Medicines Consortium (SMC) (ww.scottishmedicines.org.uk)

In Scotland the Scottish Medicines Consortium (SMC) provides advice to NHS Boards and Area Drug and Therapeutics Committees (ADTCs) regarding the status of:
- all newly licensed medicines;
- all new formulations of existing medicines;
- all new indications for established products (licensed from January 2002).

Cost-effective prescribing

The NHSBSA (see above) reported that in the period June 2006–June 2007 there was an overall rise in prescribing cost of 3.1% and in prescription numbers of 4.6%.[1] Specific rises were as follows.

- Nurses prescribed 8.1 million items—71.1% rise in prescription numbers.
- Pharmacists prescribed 46,927 items—163% rise in prescription numbers.

These increases have considerable cost implications for the NHS. Therefore it is the responsibility of the prescriber always to consider the cost of any items prescribed as it is essential to optimize the total NHS budget and avoid wasting resources.

- Consider recommending an OTC product which often costs the patient less than a prescription and costs the NHS nothing.
- Where possible prescribe a drug by the generic name:
  - except for dressings or appliances where bioavailability problems are so important that the patient should always receive the same brand (see current edition of the BNF).

Information regarding the relative costs of prescribable items can be obtained from the Drug Tariff at: 🖳 http://www.nhsbsa.nhs.uk/924.aspx.

📖 Over-the counter (OTC) drugs, p. 422; 📖 Safe prescribing, p. 88.

The aim is to facilitate the implementation of national targets and guidelines and to calculate the cost of such implementation.

Prescribing Support Unit (PSU) (www.ic.nhs.uk/services/prescribing-support-unit-psu)

The NHS Information Centre hosts the PSU which plays an important role in improving the cost-effectiveness of prescribed drugs in the UK by:

- supporting policy initiatives concerned with primary care;
- producing regular reports and standard tables based on prescription activity data;
- providing informed advice;
- analysing the national drugs bill.

The PSU hosts and manages Prescription Cost Analysis (PCA), the national prescribing information database, which is used for answering questions regarding all aspects of the primary care drugs bill from;

- Parliament;
- the public and private sectors.

The data used to populate the PCA database are provided by the Prescription Pricing Division (PPD) of the Business Services Authority (BSA). The PSU is also responsible for:

- annual publication of information on the number and type of pharmacies in the country;
- advising on prescribing issues and policy;
- analysis of prescribing data.

The PSU gives advice on prescribing issues and policy to:
- the Department of Health;
- the National Institute for Health and Clinical Excellence;
- the Audit Commission;
- the Healthcare Commission.

UK Medicines Information (UKMi) (🖳 www.ukmi.nhs.uk)
UKMi is an NHS pharmacy-based service. It aims to provide evidence of therapeutic use of medicines to support:
- safety;
- effectiveness;
- efficiency.
  The UKMi service is provided by a network of:
- 260 local medicines information centres (based in the pharmacy departments of most hospital trusts);
- 16 regional centres;
- national centres (Northern Ireland and Wales).

The Prescribing Outlook series
This is published on the UKMi website and is targeted at NHS budget holders and prescribing planners to enable them to assess the impact of new drugs both at a therapeutic and economic level.
- **Prescribing Outlook A** is produced in collaboration with the NPC and National Horizon Scanning Centre (NHSC) and includes:
  - information on drugs that have a planned launch date in the following 12–18 months;
  - drugs already on the market but with new indications;
  - brief clinical and therapeutic data;
  - information on predicted launch dates;
  - potential target population;
  - estimated impact on service delivery;
  - cost implications.
- **Prescribing Outlook B** contains information on existing and forthcoming:
  - NICE guidance;
  - NSFs;
  - GMS contracts;
  - other national targets that may have budgetary implications over the following 12–18 months.
The aim is to facilitate the implementation of national targets and guidelines and to calculate the cost of such implementation.
- **Prescribing Outlook C** is an Excel spreadsheet based on the content of Prescribing Outlooks A and B which allows crude calculations of potential costs of prescribing changes for a local population.

Further reading
🖳 www.dh.gov.uk/PublicationsAndStatistics

1. 🖳 www.nhsbsa.nhs.uk/PrescriptionServices/Documents/Volume_and_cost_year_to_ June_2007.pdf (accessed 23 September 2009).

Evidence-based prescribing

What is evidence-based prescribing (EBP)?

Evidence-based prescribing involves the application of rigorous methodology to support the assessment of all available evidence to facilitate a safe, effective, and cost-effective prescribing decision in order to deliver the best treatment and care available. In order to further best practice it is important to disseminate the findings of audit and research. Evidence of your prescribing practice can be referred to in your appraisal, and key knowledge and skills which you need to acquire can be identified to further your career and to advance best practice.

The benefits of EBP
- Improves clinical practice.
- Improves outcome for patients.
- Highlights the use of less effective prescribing practices.

Evidence-based prescribing decisions provided by quantitative methods must be based on rigorous considerations about the efficacy of the treatment and its clinical effectiveness.

Points to consider when evaluating quantitative evidence
- What is the best available evidence?
- How will it affect/change existing evidence-based practice?
- What will the health outcomes for the patient be?
- Clinical and cost effectiveness.
- Disseminating information.

Good sources of quantitative evidence
- BNF.
- Bulletins (MeReC, Bandolier, etc.).
- National Prescribing Centre.
- Journals (e.g. *Clinical Evidence*).
- Medicines Compendium (🖳 www.medicines.org.uk).
- Association of the British Pharmaceutical Industry (ABPI).
- National Institute of Health and Clinical Excellence (NICE).

Sources of quantitative data
- Systematic reviews and databases (e.g. Cochrane Database, Centre for Reviews and Dissemination).
- Local prescribing support services/harmaceutical advisor.
- PACT/EPACT (local and national prescribing audit).
- Drug bulletins/information service.
- National Prescribing Centre (NPC).
- Locally provided education/training.
- Locally/regionally developed guidelines/information/research/case studies.
- Support networks.
- Committee for Safety on Medicines (CSM).
- National Health Service Executive.

Examples of guidelines and protocols
- Jointly developed locally between nurses, GPs, pharmacists, and allied health professional prescribers (e.g. local formularies based on national evidence and best practice).
- PRODIGY for primary care evidence.
- NICE technical appraisals.

Best practice

Best practice is:
- up to date;
- benchmarked against comparative sources where available;
- in line with local and national guidelines.

Good practice suggested by analysis of prescribing practices (audit):
- breakdown of data by therapeutic area;
- review of PACT data (recommended quarterly);
- Prescription Pricing Authority (PPA) reviews provide potential for savings by prescribing generic medicines;
- benchmarking against other areas and other prescribers.

PACT data

In primary care PACT data can be used to:
- review prescribing habits;
- monitor adherence to prescribing policies;
- compare performance between prescribers;
- monitor expenditure and cost-effectiveness.

Prescribing data are monitored locally in secondary care.

Local and national formulary development and maintenance

- Provides rational evidence-based policies.
- Considers cost in context of appropriate care.
- Needs regular updating and maintenance.

Sources supporting clinical appraisal skills

- Critical Appraisal Skills Programme.
- Centre for Evidence Based Medicine.
- Centre for Evidence Based Nursing.
- National Prescribing Centre.
- Nurse Prescriber website.
- Patient medication records.

Inductive and deductive reasoning

Analysis of evidence is based on:
- deductive reasoning (if A and B are true, then C will follow);
- inductive reasoning (based on likelihood of probability rather than certainty);
- arguments from authority (based on accurately reported reasoning from a respected authority).

Evaluating the evidence

When evaluating the evidence from drug companies ask the following questions.

- How biased are the claims about evidence?
- How do you know the level of bias or accurate reporting?
- Would you prescribe any of these products?
- Why should you prescribe this drug?
- Why shouldn't you prescribe this drug?
- How did you come to your decision?
- How did the evidence rank in the hierarchy of evidence?
- Who sponsored the trials?
- What is the methodology?
- How many subjects were in the cohort (pre- and post-marketing)?
- How old were the subjects?

Methods of researching evidence are ranked according to their quality and credibility (Table 15.1).[1]

Table 15.1 The hierarchy of quantitative evidence in relation to prescribing

No. 1	Systematic reviews	Published and unpublished research is collated and each piece is assessed by an independent reviewer The results are then combined and findings discussed
No. 2	Randomized control trials (RCTs) Used to assess relative effects of a treatment	Compares group 1 who are being treated with the new drug with group 2 who are identical in every way except that they are not being treated (control group). Participants are randomly chosen for each group. Can be 3 groups: 1 on the new treatment, 1 on standard treatment, and 1 on placebo
Cohort studies	Observational studies of patients who are being treated with a new drug	Subjects may be followed up over a long time period
Case–control studies	A group of patients who, for example, are taking the drug in question are studied for their medical histories which are compared with those of other patients within the group to look for similarities and emerging patterns	Faster production of results than cohort studies but not as reliable
Cross-sectional surveys	Used to measure the frequency of risk factors in patients who, for example, are taking a drug within a defined population and a particular time	Statistical inferencing
Case reports and case studies	Descriptions of medical histories of single patients are compared with case histories of patients who have similar case reports. This can be useful when searching for rare side effects	Not valid statistically because of lack of a comparative control group

Adapted from Jones, C. (2002). Research methods. *Pharmaceutical Journal*, **28**, 839–42.

1. Granby, T. (2005). Evidence based prescribing. *Nurse Prescriber*, **2** (21 February 2005). Cited in: www.nurse-prescriber.co.uk/Articles/Evidence-based_Px.htm

Qualitative evidence

Remember that it is also of the utmost importance to consider evidence relating to participants lived experiences (qualitative evidence) as these reflect quality-of-life issues which may affect concordance.

When reading a paper

Consider the potential risk and benefits to the patient in relation to the following.

- The absolute risk to the patient: How does taking the new drug reduce the patient's risk of dying?
- The absolute risk reduction: By what percentage as measured against the control group (those who have not taken the drug) can taking the new drug reduce the patient's risk of dying?
- The relative risk: What are the chances of the patients dying from the condition which is being treated if they do not have the drug in relation to the population in general?
- Relative risk reduction: how much is the risk of dying from the condition which is being treated reduced in the group who are taking the drug compared with the percentage risk of dying as a result of the condition for members of the control group (those who have been selected for the trial but who have not taken the drug)?
- Numbers needed to treat: How many patients will need to be treated before the effects of the new drug become evident?
- Odds ratio: How effective is the drug compared with its not being effective? The number of times that a treatment is effective is divided by the number of times that it is not effective (any number greater than 1 indicates a good odds ratio).

Qualitative studies may also reveal factors which influence patient's decisions regarding their concordance with treatments prescribed. For example, despite the evidence to support the efficacy of the practice of many-layered bandaging to promote leg ulcer healing, it has been shown that patients dislike this treatment so much that they remove their bandages.[1]

Further reading

Kendall, S. (1997). What do we mean by evidence? Implications for primary health care nursing. *Journal of Interprofessional Care*, 11, 23–34.

1. Rycroft-Malone, J., Seers, K., Titchen, A., Kitson, A., Harvey, G., and McCormack, B. (2004). What counts as evidence in evidence based practice? *Journal of Advanced Nursing*, **47**, 81–90.

Managing the role

Clinical governance and clinical supervision

In addition to the criminal and civil legal system, all health professionals, including those regulated by the Health Professions Council, are subject to professional codes of conduct developed with their professional bodies. These professional accountabilities exist regardless of the work setting. 📖 Nursing and Midwifery Council and Health Professions Council codes, p. 20.

Clinical governance provides part of the regulatory requirements for all services delivered by the NHS, including services regulated by the Care Quality Commission (CQC) who monitor the delivery of all health and adult social care in England.

Clinical supervision is a component of clinical governance and exists to provide clinical staff with support and opportunities for professional development. It is anticipated that, through these measures, the quality and performance of clinical practice will be maintained and high standards of patient and staff safety will be delivered.

In general the expansion of prescribing to professions working in both the NHS and the private sector requires consideration of clinical supervision and governance arrangements.

Definiotion of clinical supervision

[A] term used to describe a formal process of professional support and learning which enables practitioners to develop knowledge and competence, assume responsibility for their own practice and enhance consumer protection and safety of care in complex situations.

Central to the process of learning and to the expansion of scope of practice clinical supervision should be seen as a means of encouraging self assessment and analytical and reflective skills.[1]

Aims of clinical supervision

- Development of professional expertise.
- Development of quality care.
- A safeguard for standards of practice.
- Issues from clinical supervision will feed into the more strategic clinical governance arena.

Components

- Educational: development of the skills, attitudes, understanding, and abilities of an individual practitioner.
- Restorative: provision of an emotionally supportive environment to allow and help practioners to explore their feeling regarding their therapeutic work with patients and clients.
- Managerial: provision of an opportunity for quality control and a consideration of the organizational responsibilities of the individual.

Action for the clinical supervisor

- Confirm a common belief and purpose for clinical supervision, possibly through use of a contract (see below).

- Commit energy and time to the role of supervisor.
- Listen to the individual and be led by their agenda and style for learning.
- Identify how a practitioner can learn from both the positive and negative influences of practice.
- Be confident and explore new ideas, providing support as well as challenge.
- Promise respect, mutual trust, confidentiality, and sensitivity.

Example of the components of a clinical supervision contract

The contract must be clear and agreed by all and contain the following.
- Statement of the purpose of supervision (see above).
- Focus of supervision, i.e. reflection by the supervisees.
- An explicit statement of the responsibilities of the supervisor/ supervisee or group.
- Venue, time, frequency, and length of each session.
- Respect for confidentiality.
- How could best practice identified in other areas be modified to suit local conditions?
- Note taking, i.e. type of notes and an agreement that secretarial support will include typing the notes of meetings.
- Valuation of each session.
- Dates set to review points that require action.
- Signatures of the parties and date.

NB: it is important to include a mutually agreed plan of action regarding what to do if a breach of the code of conduct is identified.
📖 Nursing and Midwifery Council and Health Professions Council codes, p. 20

Remember

- Clinical supervisions meetings are not a confessional.
- Ensure time for support and identification of developmental needs.
- Clinical supervision can only be as useful as the participants want it to be.
- Group work may be helpful for reflection on practice.

Clinical supervision at the local level results in clinical effectiveness for the organization and patient, which in turn leads into the more strategic arena of clinical governance. 📖 Reflective practice, p. 130.

Further reading

Butterworth, T., Carson, J., White, E., et al. (1997). *It is good to talk: an evaluation study of clinical supervision in 23 sites in England and Scotland*. University of Manchester.
Driscoll, J. (2004). *Practising clinical supervision: a reflective approach*. Balliére Tindall, London.
RCN (2000). *Realising clinical effectiveness and clinical governance through clinical supervision*. Radcliffe Medical Press, Abingdon.
RCN (2002). Lesson cards: 'invaluable assistance' to clinical governance. *Quality Improvement Network News*, Winter 2002-03.
Scottish Department of Health (1997). Designed to care. 🖥 www.scotland.gov.uk/Publications. (accessed 2 February 2010).

Clinical governance (CG)

The Department of Health defines clinical governance as the system through which NHS organizations are accountable and through which they demonstrate their continuous improvement in quality.

Definition

- CG is a framework which helps all prescribers to continuously improve quality and safeguard standards of care.[1]
- CG places quality at the centre of NHS reforms, and through the Care Standards Act (2000)[2] and the Care Quality Commission applies it across the independent sector.

Aims of CG

- Improve the quality of information for both patients and staff.
- Promote collaboration, partnership and team working.
- Reduce variations in practice.
- Implement EBP, including the use of audit and practice development.

Key principles for CG[1]

- Focus on improving the quality of care.
- Apply to all health care regardless of the venue for delivery.
- Public and patient involvement is essential.
- Demands partnership between all professional groups and patients.
- Health professionals have a key role to play in the implementation of CG.
- An enabling culture is needed which celebrates success and learns from mistakes.

CG resources

- Patients' forums: details available from local councils.
- ▢ www.dpp.org: the Disease Prevention Panel (DPP) is a charity, partly funded by the Department of Health, producing unbiased user-tested health information.
- Clinical Governance Support Team (CGST): ▢ www.cgsupport.org
- Changing Workforce Programme: ▢ www.modern.nhs.uk
- NHS performance indicators (only 2002): ▢ www.doh.gov.uk/ nhsperformanceindicators
- Sources of social statistics, health services, and public health: ▢ http:// www.parliament.uk/commons/lib/research/briefings/SNSG-03843.pdf (accessed 22 September 2009)
- Education for Health: ▢ www.educationforhealth.org.uk (accessed 22 September 2009). Education for Health aims to provide a consistent, comprehensive, and innovative approach to professional health training across the fields of cardiovascular disease and respiratory health.
- ▢ http://www.dh.gov.uk/en/Publichealth/Patientsafety/ Clinicalgovernance/DH_114 (accessed 22 September 2009).

See also Table 16.1.

Table 16.1 Clinical governance—underpinning policy and support

Country	Policy/legislation	Support
England	*The new NHS: modern, dependable*[3]	Clinical Governance Support team – established 1999 Contact: ▢ www.cgsupport.org
Northern Ireland	*Best practice–best care* Incorporated in: Health and Personal Social Services (Quality and Improvement and Regulation) Order 2003	Clinical and Social Care Governance Support Team Contact: ▢ www.dhsspsni. gov.uk
Scotland	*Designed to care* *Partnership for care*	NHS Quality improvement Scotland ▢ http://www.nhshealthquality. org/nhsqis/CCC
Wales	*Putting patients first*	Clinical Governance Support and Development Unit ▢ http://www.wales.nhs.uk/ publications/ whitepaper98_e.pdf

All web sites given in this table were accessed on 22 September 2009

Further reading

RCN (2002). Lesson cards: 'invaluable assistance' to clinical governance. *Quality Improvement Network News*, Winter 2002-03.

1. RCN (1998). Cited in *Clinical governance: an RCN resource guide*. RCN, London 2003.
▢ www.rcn.org.uk
2. Department of Health (2000). *Care Standards Act*. TSO, London.
3. Department of Health (1997). *The new NHS: modern, dependable*. TSO, London.

Continuous professional development (CPD)

Taking an example from nursing, in order to maintain registration the NMC stipulates that nurses and midwives must comply with the PREP. The PREP handbook states that:

> the PREP standard enables you to demonstrate to the people in your care, your colleagues and yourself that you are keeping up to date and developing your practice.[1]

In order to maintain their registration, nurse and midwife prescribers must have satisfied the PREP requirements by undertaking CPD:

- 450hr of study;
- at least 35hr of learning relevant to their practice.

Other health professional bodies have similar rulings.

📖 Working as a prescriber, p. 168.

---

1. NMC. *Guidance for continuing professional development for nurse and midwife prescribers.* 🖥 http://www.nmc-uk.org/aDisplayDocument.aspx?documentID=4488 (accessed 3 February 2010).

Change management

Davidhizar[1] suggests there are three main drivers for change in contemporary health care:
- technology;
- information availability;
- growing populations.

The shortage of doctors and a decrease in junior doctors' hours are additional components of the catalyst that brought about non-medical prescribing.

Marquis and Houston[2] outline feelings of loss, stress, achievement, and pride as normal reactions to change, and cite the need of a change agent to make the process successful.

Change agent

Definition

A person skilled in the theory and implementation of planned change, who possesses well-developed leadership and management skills.

Change theory was identified in the mid 1900s by Lewin,[3] who described three phases through which the process must go before a planned change becomes part of a system.
- *Unfreezing:* the change agent persuades those opposing the change of its necessity.
- *Movement:* the change agent has to ensure that the driving forces for the change exceed the restraining forces of the system. If possible, change should be approached gradually to enable those involved to be fully assimilated in the change.
- *Refreezing:* to ensure that the change becomes integrated into the normal working patterns, the change agent needs to support the adaptive efforts of those adopting the change.

Change strategies

Because many change agents within non-medical prescribing do not have a hierarchical power base and are attempting to influence their peers and fellow professionals, a normative–re-educative strategy which uses group process may well be appropriate.
- The change agent assumes that because humans are social animals, they are more influenced by others than by facts.
- Skill with interpersonal relationships enables the change agent to focus on non-cognitive determinants of behaviour, such as roles, relationships, attitudes, and feelings.

Change resisters

Silber[4] suggests that a person's ability to cope with change rests on:

- their flexibility to events;
- their evaluation of the immediate situation;
- the anticipated consequences of the change;
- what is in it for them—what they have to lose or gain.

1. Davidhizar, R. (1996). Surviving organizational change. *Health Care Supervisor*, **14**, 19–24.
2. Marquis, B.L. and Houston, C. (2000). *Leadership roles and management functions in nursing* (3rd edn). Lippincott Williams & Wilkins, Philadelphia, PA.
3. Lewin, K. (1951). *Field theory in social sciences*. Harper & Row, New York.
4. Silber, M.B. (1993). The 'C's' in excellence: choice and change. *Nursing Management*, **24**, 60–2.

Responsibilities

Nurses have the responsibility to keep their knowledge current, and some useful resources for doing this are presented in this section.

Information sources

Where to get up-to-date information

National guidelines

The National Institute for Health and Clinical Excellence (NICE) provides up-to-date technology appraisals. These are nationally recognized guidelines which adhere to the best clinical evidence base and account for best practice and cost effective prescribing. Technology appraisals are updated every 5 years.

Nationally recognized guidelines are also produced by:

- British Thoracic Society (BTS): 🖥 www.brit.thoracic.org.uk
- British Hypertensive Society (BHS): 🖥 www.bhs.org.uk
- Diabetes UK (DUK): 🖥 www.diabetes.org.uk
- British Heart Foundation (BHF): 🖥 www.bhf.org.uk
- Scottish Intercollegiate Guidelines Network (SIGN): 🖥 www.sign.ac.uk

Prodigy (🖥 www.prodigy.nhs.uk) has evolved to form the NHS Clinical Knowledge Summaries (CKS) (🖥 www.cks.nhs.uk) which provide a nationally recognized knowledge source for non-medical prescribers in primary and secondary care.

Local guidelines

Guidelines exist to help direct the prescriber to the best, safest, and most effective evidence-based prescribing. Guidelines do not seek to impose, and, in supplementary prescribing (in agreement with the doctor) independent prescriber, and patient, can be tailored to meet the needs of the individual. However, whenever possible, it is best practice for the non-medical prescriber working for the NHS to follow the guidelines as indicated both nationally and, if working in the NHS, within the local NHS formulary.

Locally produced NHS formularies provide evidence-based guidelines, formularies, and protocols for prescribing medications and appliances and also recommend safe and cost-effective prescribing for locally accepted practice.

PACT data

PACT and SPA (Scottish Prescribing Analysis) are available as audit reports of practitioners' prescribing on a quarterly (three-monthly) basis. These data provide a comparison between local and national prescribing patterns and can be broken down to indicate individual prescribing patterns.

📖 Reflective practice, p. 130.

The Drug Tariff

The Drug Tariff is produced monthly as a joint compilation between the Department of Health and the Prescription Pricing Authority,[1] now known as the NHS Business Services Authority.

The following useful information is contained in the Drug Tariff.

- The basic price of named drugs, appliances, and chemical reagents.
- Endorsements including pack sizes.
- Whether the prescription is in pharmacopoeial or generic form.

- Brand name and name of the manufacturer or wholesaler from whom the drug was purchased.
- Quantity supplied (if at variance with quantity ordered).
- Pharmacists' professional payments fees.
- Commonly used pack sizes.
- Advice on domicillary oxygen service.
- Advice to care homes.
- Borderline substances.
- The Dental Prescribing Formulary.
- The District Nurse and Health Visitor Prescribers' Formulary.
- The Nurse Prescribers' Extended Formulary.
- Drugs and other substances not to be prescribed under the NHS pharmaceutical services (blacklisted drugs).
- Drugs to be prescribed in certain circumstances under the NHS pharmaceutical services.

1. Department of Health (2005). *Drug Tariff* (latest edn). TSO, London. ⬚ http://www.drugtariff.com/ (accessed 26 June 2010).

Regional Medicines Information Services

Regional Medicines Information Services, also known as UK Medicines Information Services (UKMi), provides NHS pharmacist and technical advice for all health-care professionals.

All medicines information activities can be accessed on the UKMi website at 🖥 www.ukmi.nhs.uk Links are available to other related sites, such as UKMi central and Druginofzone, providing region specific information.

This service provides prescribing information and advice regarding the following.
- Pregnancy
- Breastfeeding
- Alternative medicines
- Complementary therapies
- News and email alerts
- Bulletins
- Product updates and information
- Purchasing and Supplies Agency (PASA):
  - alerts and drug shortages;
  - patent expiry;
  - changes to product characteristics summaries.
- Information on new drugs:
  - information on drugs tracked through clinical development phases 2 and 3;
  - evaluated appraisals on drugs likely to make an impact on NHS prescribing;
  - service and financial framework (SAFF) planning.
- Support for evidence-based practice:
  - FAQs database;
  - critical appraisal trials (CATs);
  - toolkits for the National Service Frameworks (NSFs);
  - available evaluations for complementary medicines;
  - one-stop reference shop.
- Training:
  - UKMi workbook providing tutorials facilitating user access to information on particular aspects of prescribing;
  - MiCAL—a CD which includes details of critical appraisal literature searching and information sources;
  - packages for regional pharmacy training programmes.
- Shared-care guidelines
- Details of prescribing committee decisions and project information
- Support for national organizations:
  - NHS Direct;
  - walk-in centres;
  - National Electronic Library for Health (NeHL).
- National Patient Safety Agency
- Some are part of the National Poisons Information Service

- Local medicines information support:
  - enquiry answering service for all health professionals;
  - local bulletins;
  - clinical pharmacy, clinical governance and medicines management support;
  - educational support.

Advice and support

Advisory Committee on Borderline Substances
NICE
🖥 www.nice.org.uk

Action on Smoking and Health
ASH
🖥 www.ash.org

Age Concern
General enquiries: 0208-765-7200
Information line: 0800-009966
🖥 www.ageconcern.co.uk

Alcohol Concern
Email: contact@alcoholconcern.org.uk
🖥 www.alcoholconcern.org.uk

Allergy UK
Telephone: 0208-303-8525
🖥 www.allergyfoundation.com

Alzheimer's Society
Telephone: 0845-300-0326
Email: enquiries@alzheimers.org.uk
🖥 www.alzeheimers.org.uk

Anaphylaxis Campaign
Telephone: 01252-542029
Email: Info@anaphylaxis.org.uk
🖥 www.anaphylaxis.org.uk

Asthma UK
Telephone: 0845-701-0203 (Mon–Fri 9am–5pm)
🖥 www.asthma.org.uk

Blood Pressure Association
🖥 www.bpassoc.org.uk

British Association of Dermatologists
🖥 www.bad.org.uk

British Cardiac Society
🖥 www.bcs.com

British Dermatological Nursing Group
🖥 www.bdng.org.uk

British Heart Foundation
Telephone Heart Information Line: 0845-070-8070
🖥 www.bhf.org.uk

British Herbal Medicines Association (BHMA)
⌨ www.trusthomeopathy.org

British Kidney Patient Association (BKPA)
Telephone: 0142-047-2021/2 (9am–5pm)
⌨ www.britishkidney-pa.co.uk

British Lung Foundation
Email: enquiries@blf-uk.org
⌨ www.lunguk.org/support-groups.asp

British Menopause Society
⌨ www.the–bms.org

British Pain Society
Email info@britishpainsociety.org
⌨ www.britishpainsociety.org

British Pregnancy Advisory Service (BPAS)
Actionline: 0845-730-4030
⌨ www.bpas.org

British Thoracic Society
Email: bts@brit-thoracic.org.uk
⌨ www.brit-thoracic.org.uk

British Thyroid Foundation
⌨ www.btf-thyroid.org

British Vascular Foundation
Email: bvf@care4free.net
⌨ www.bvf.org.uk

Colon Cancer Concern
Infoline: 0870-506-050 (Mon–Fri. 10am–4pm)
Email: info@coloncancer.org.uk
⌨ www.coloncancer.org.uk

Colostomy Association
Freephone helpline: 0800-587-6744
⌨ www.colostomyassociation.org.uk

Continence Foundation
Helpline: 0845-345-0165 (Mon- Fri. 9.30am–1pm)
Email: continence-help@dialpipex.com
⌨ www.continence-foundation.org.uk

Carers Line
Telephone: 0808-808-7777 (Mon–Fri. 10am–12noon and 2pm–4pm)

Depression Alliance
⌨ www.depressionalliance.org

Diabetes UK
Careline: 0845-120-2960 (Mon–Fri 9am–5pm) (low-call rate)
Email: info@diabetes.org.uk
🖳 www.diabetes.org.uk

Disability Information Trust
🖳 www.abilityonline.org.uk/disability.information.trust.htm

Disabled Living Foundation
Telephone: 0845-130-9177 (low-call rate)
Text phone: 020-7432-8009 (Mon–Fri 10.00am–1pm)
🖳 www.dlf.org.uk

Family Heart Association
Email: md@familyheart.org
🖳 www.familyheart.org

Ileostomy and Internal Pouch Support Group (IA)
Freephone: 0800-018-4724
Email: info@the-ia.org.uk
🖳 www.the-ia.org.uk

Impotence Association
Helpline: 0870-774-3571
Email: info@sda.uk.net
🖳 www.sda.uk.net

Irritable Bowel Syndrome (IBS) Network
Telephone: 01543 492192 (Mon–Fri. 6am–8pm, Sat 10am–12 noon)
Email: info@ibsnetwork.org.uk
🖳 www.ibsnetwork.org.uk

Long-Term Medical Conditions Alliance (LMCA)
Email: info@lmca.org.uk
🖳 www.lmca.org.uk

Marie Stopes International
Telephone-One Call
Abortion, emergency contraception: 0845-300-8090
Vasectomy, female sterilization: 0845-300-0212
Health screening: 0845-300-0460
Email: info@mariestopes.org.uk
🖳 www.mariestopes.org.uk

Menopause Amarant Trust
Helpline telephone: 01293-413 000 (Mon–Fri 11.00am–6pm)
🖳 www.amarantmenopausetrust.org.uk

National Eczema Society
Helpline: 0870-241-3604 (Mon–Fri 8am–8pm)
🖳 www.eczema.org

National Fertility Association (ISSUE)
Helpline: 01922-722-888
Email: info@issue.c.uk
🖳 www.infertilitynetworkuk.com

National Osteoporosis Society (NOS)
Helpline: 0845-450-0230
Email: info@nos.org.uk
🖳 www.nos.org.uk

National Prescribing Centre
Telephone: 0151-794-8134
🖳 www.npc.co.uk

National Respiratory Training Centre
Health professional helpline: 01926-493-63
Email: enquiries@nrts.org.uk
🖳 www.nrts.org.uk

Necrobiosis Support Network
Telephone: 020-7878-2308

NHS Stop Smoking Helpline
Telephone: 0800-169-0169

Nurses Hypotension Association
Email: secretary@nha.uk.net
🖳 www.nha.uk.net

Nursing and Midwifery Council (NMC)
Telephone: 020-7637-7181
🖳 www.nmc.uk.org

Paracetamol Information Centre
Email gb@butlers.u-net.com
🖳 www.pharmweb.net/paracetamol.htm

Psoriasis Association
Telephone: 0845-676-0076 (Mon–Thurs 9.15am–4.45pm; Fri. 9.15am–4.30pm)
🖳 www.psoriasis-association.org.uk

Royal College of Nursing (RCN)
Information and advice for members telephone: 0845-772-6100
🖳 www.rcn.org.uk

Samaritans
Telephone: 08457-909090 (charged at local rates)
Email Jo@samaritans.org
🖳 www.samaritans.org

Smoking Cessation Action in Primary care (SCAPE)
30 Orange Street
London WC2H 71Z

Urostomy Association
Telephone: 01245-224-294 (10am–12am)

Women's Health Concern
Email (counselling and advice): counseling@womens-health-concern.org
🖳 www.womens-health-concern.org

Wound Care Society
🖳 www.woundcaresociety.org

Additional prescribing information available in the BNF

The Community Practitioners' Formulary/British National Formulary (CPF/BNF) contains invaluable information for the prescriber, both in the notes on drugs and preparations and in the various appendices.

UK health departments distribute BNFs to NHS hospitals and prescribing doctors and nurses. It is available free online to NHS staff at ⌨ www.bnf.org

Requests for extra copies and details of changes for mailing can be made by contacting the NHS Response line: 08701-555-455.

Pharmaid

Even BNFs which are 6–12 months old are of use for those working in developing countries. The Commonwealth Pharmaceutical Association has a scheme, Pharmaid, which despatches older BNFs, in the month of November, to areas where they may be of use.

Please contact ⌨ www.pharmaid.com or check the health-related press for details of this scheme.

Additional prescribing information available within appendices of the BNF

- Drug interactions.
- Liver disease.
- Renal impairment.
- Pregnancy and breastfeeding.
- Intravenous additives.
- Borderline substances.
- Wound management products and elastic hosiery.
- Cautionary and advisory labels for dispensing.
- Basic net prices (see Drug Tariff, published monthly, for information; OTCs are at retail price which includes VAT).
- Changes to the names of drugs in accordance with the EEC directive 92/27/EEC. This states that where the British Approved Name (BAN) is different from the Recommended International Non-proprietary name (rINN), the BAN must be changed to the rINN.
- Index of manufacturers and their contact details.
- Index of 'special order' manufacturers.
- A table of approximate conversions:
  - pounds (lb) and stones to kilograms (kg);
  - fluid ounces (fl oz) to millilitres (mL);
  - imperial to metric length;
  - mass;
  - volume;
  - other units.

- A table for ideal body weight, height, and surface area for children aged newborn to 12 years, and for adults (male and female).
- Contact details for:
  - Driver and Vehicle Licensing Authority (DVLA);
  - information on medications prohibited for sportsmen and women;
  - Poisons Information Services;
  - information on travel immunization requirements;
  - patient information lines;
  - medicines information services.

Working outside the UK

Working outside the UK

This is a developing area and all workers in health care who would like to work abroad should approach their professional bodies, the Nursing and Midwifery council and the Health Professional Council, for specific information regarding:

- recognition of their general and prescribing qualifications outside the UK;
- working and prescribing outside the UK.

The point of contact for information regarding work permits, scope of practice, and visas is the relevant embassy or high commission.

The requirements, registration, permits, and recognition of qualifications vary from country to country within the European Union (EU) and from state to state within other countries. Therefore it is advisable to check the specifics with the embassy or high commission of the country/countries in which you wish to work.

At the present time the Royal College of Nursing (RCN) offers guidance to their members regarding working in:

- Australia
- Bahamas
- Bahrain
- Barbados
- Bermuda
- British Virgin Islands
- Brunei
- Canada
- Cayman Islands
- Cyprus
- European Union (EU)
- European Economic Area (EEA)
- Gambia
- Ghana
- Gibraltar
- Hong Kong
- Jordan
- Kenya
- Malaysia
- Malta
- Mauritius
- New Zealand
- Nigeria
- Papua New Guinea
- Saudi Arabia
- Seychelles
- Singapore
- South Africa
- Switzerland
- Turkey
- United Arab Emirates
- USA

- Zambia
- Zimbabwe.

General advice and examples regarding working in
- USA
- EU
- Australia;

are given in the remainder of this chapter.

United States of America

Health care in the USA

In addition to the two public health-care programmes Medicare and Medicaid, both created in 1965, individuals rely on private health insurers to provide their health-care.

- **Medicare** is the federal government's health programme primarily serving Americans who are aged over 65.
- **Medicaid** is a joint federal–state programme designed primarily to finance health care for the poor.
  Both provide care for the disabled.

Together, Medicare and Medicaid cover more than 80 million Americans. Medicare beneficiaries and Medicaid recipients are entitled to outpatient medical care from physicians and hospital care from the same medical professionals who provide health-care to individuals with private health insurance.

For further information on gaining an employment visa and other useful immigration checks visit:

- US State Department website ▦ www.state.gov (accessed 2 February 2010).
- National Immigration Services ▦ www.myvisa.com (accessed 2 February 2010).

NB: this information is current and there may be changes to the US system whilst the book is being printed.

Working as a nurse in the USA

- In order to practice as a registered nurse in the USA you will need both a licence to practice there and a work permit.
- Salaries, conditions, and the cost of living vary from state to state and there are no national agreements.
- A car may be essential to enable you to work in some areas as hospitals are built on the outer fringes of cities.
- Annual leave entitlement may be as little as 2–4 weeks.
- Check that your employment package includes health insurance.

In the USA there is only one category of first-level nurse; the Registered Nurse (RN). The RN qualification is the equivalent to the UK's Registered General Nurse (RGN). Only a RGN is eligible to apply for nurse registration in the USA.

Requirements

There are three main requirements for gaining employment.

- Sitting and passing the Commission on Graduates of Foreign Nursing Schools (CGFNS) examination.
- Once you have passed your CGFNS examination you are eligible to take the NCLEX-RN® examination in a chosen state. Joining a recruitment agency which sponsors nurses to fly to the USA is a good way of sitting and gaining this qualification.

- Only New York and Florida do not require you to pass your CGFNS before you take the state NCLEX-RN® examination.

NB: Each state has its own board of nursing and different eligibility criteria for foreign nurses.

Visa/work permit

- Prospective employers have to prove that they have made every effort to recruit a person who already has the right to work and reside in the USA before they can employ foreign nurses.
- Unless you are a US citizen by marriage or birth you must have the correct visa to enter the USA.
- If you work on a visitor's visa you run the risk of being deported.

European Union

One of the effects of the EU is to allow greater freedom of movement for individuals between EU countries and those which have signed the European Economic Area (EEA) agreement. There has been some harmonization to enable movement between EU member countries and a good source of information is: 🖳 http://www.dfes.gov.uk/europeopen/uktoeu

For example, within the field of pharmacy, the Approved European Pharmacy Qualifications Order of Council 2007 No. 564 states that the UK government policy intention behind the mutual recognition of professional qualifications is to ensure that:
• people have free movement rights around the EU;
• those who have acquired a professional qualification in one member state (in this case in the field of pharmacy) are able to move to another member state and practise in that state on the basis of the qualification that they have already acquired.

With some professions, including pharmacy, this has also led to the harmonization of minimum training conditions throughout the EU.

Additional details can be obtained from the Professional Regulation Branch at the Department of Health (telephone: 0113-254-5789; email: stephen.arthur@dh.gsi.gov.uk)

At the time of going to press the EU comprises: Austria, Belgium, Bulgaria, Cyprus, Czech Republic, Denmark, Estonia, Finland, France, Germany, Greece, Hungary, Republic of Ireland, Italy, Latvia, Liechtenstein, Lithuania, Luxembourg, Malta, Netherlands, Poland, Portugal, Romania, Slovakia, Slovenia, Spain, Sweden, and the UK.

The EEA covers the EU countries plus Iceland, Liechtenstein, and Norway.

Information on living, working, studying, or travelling in other EU countries can be obtained from 🖳 www.europa.eu.int/eures (accessed 2 February 2010) or Freephone 00800-4080-4080.

Embassies may be able provide general advice on employment and residence in the host country. A list of embassies can be obtained from the Foreign and Commonwealth Office website 🖳 www.fco.gov.uk (accessed 2 February 2010).

The qualifications in the following professions are automatically recognized in other EU countries:
• midwife;
• pharmacist;
• doctor;
• nurse;
• dentist;
• veterinary surgeon.

The main obstacle to employment is language. Prospects of employment are generally poor if you do not have a good command of the language of the country. Some 'British' and 'American' hospitals in Europe welcome applications for employment from UK-trained personnel, but the working language of these hospitals is the language of the country.

Recognition of nursing qualifications

Mutual recognition of first-level registered general nurses' and midwives' qualifications apply to all of the EU and EEA member countries. Although Switzerland is not a member of the EU or EEA there is mutual recognition of nursing qualifications.

Registered general/adult branch nurses and midwives moving between EU and EEA countries are able to register their qualifications. First, you must verify your qualifications and training with the Nursing and Midwifery Council (NMC). Application forms can be obtained from the NMC registration dept and a NMC fact sheet can be downloaded from ▣ www.nmc-uk.org.

Nurses on other parts of the NMC register:
- child health;
- learning disability;
- mental health nurses;

may be able to take advantage of the General Systems Provisions of EU Directive 2005/36/EC to obtain recognition of their UK nursing qualifications in another EU/EEA country.

NB: Not all EU/EEA countries have the same variety of basic nursing qualifications as the UK, and some other EU/EEA countries have nurse training leading to basic qualifications that have no equivalent in the UK.

RCN members can obtain additional information on nursing abroad at ▣ www.rcn.org.uk or ▣ international.office@rcn.org.uk (both accessed 2 February 2010).

For independent information and a chance to contact nurses who have already experienced working abroad try ▣ www.21stcenturynurse.com (accessed 2 February 2010).

Nurses who keep up their registration will not require a Return to Practice (RTP) course on return to working for the NHS in the UK.

Australia

Administratively Australia is divided into six states and two territories, each with their own legislation. It is a requirement to have the appropriate work visa and, for example, a nurse or midwife will need to be registered by the board of the state or territory in which they intend to work.
The Department of Immigration and Citizenship lists the following regional offices for information regarding visas and registration:

New South Wales
Parramatta Office
  9 Wentworth Street, Parramatta, NSW 2150
  Fax: (02)8861-4422

Sydney Office
  Ground Floor, 26 Lee Street, Sydney NSW 2000
  Fax: (02)8862 6096

Tasmania
Hobart Office
  Level 13, 188 Collins Street, Hobart, TAS 7000
  Fax (03)6223-8247

Australian Capital Territory
Canberra Regional Office
  3 Lonsdale Street, Braddon, ACT 2612
  Fax: (02)6248-0479

Victoria
Melbourne Office
  CBD Office, Ground Floor, Casselden Place, 2 Lonsdale Street, Melbourne, VIC 3000
  Fax: (03)9235-3300

Dandenong Office
  51 Princes Highway, Dandenong, VIC 3175
  Fax: (03)8762-2625

South Australia
Adelaide Office
  Level 3, 55 Currie Street, Adelaide, SA 5000
  Fax: (08)8237-6699

Northern Territory
Darwin Office
  Pella House, 40 Cavenagh Street, Darwin NT 0800
  Fax: (08)8981-6245

Queensland
Brisbane Office
  299 Adelaide Street, Brisbane, QLD 4000
  Fax: (07)3136-7347
Gold Coast Office
  Level 1, 72 Nerang Street, Southport, QLD 4215
  Fax: (07)5591-5402

Cairns Office
Level 2, GHD Building, 95 Spence Street, Cairns, QLD 4870
Fax: (07)4051-0198

Thursday Island Office
Commonwealth Centre, Hastings Street, PO Box 299, Thursday Island,
Fax: (08)9___ ___ ___ton Street, West Perth, WA

Working as a nurse in Australia

To practice as a registered nurse in Australia you need to follow the procedure outlined below.

- Be registered as a nurse the board of the state/territory in which you wish to practice.
- You will also need to have ready applied for and received the relevant visa/work permit entitling you to work.
- Each state or territory has own legislation and arrangements regarding nurses from overseas.
- If you are not registered you cannot work. One of the easiest and cheapest states in which to register is New South Wales (NSW).

Registration

- The Australian Nursing Council Incorporated (ANCI) Assessment is a requirement before initial registration is possible.
- Application forms and detailed information are available on their website.
- Once registered in one state it is relatively easy to transfer your registration to another state.

Visas and work permits for all health-care professionals

Categories

If you are a citizen of the UK, Republic of Ireland, Canada, or the Netherlands, and/or if you are aged between 18 and 25 years or between 26 and 30 years at the time of application and can show that your entry to Australia will be of benefit to both yourself and Australia, you are eligible for a working holiday visa (WHV).

Obtaining a working holiday visa

- You need to apply to the Australian High Commission before you leave.
- It is illegal to enter Australia without your WHV.
- This type of visa allows you to work for up to 3 months with one employer and for a total of 12 months.

If you do not fall into the categories listed above you will need a work permit (WP).

Obtaining a work permit

● First, you need to be offered a position or be sponsored ... to work.

● A WP allows you to work for over 3 months and ...

Useful contact addresses

● Australian High Commission, ... : canberra@
  4LA . ⌨ http://www.australia.o... (... February 2010).

● Royal College of Nursing Aus...
  Australia. Tel: +61-6282-...
  ...na.org.au; ⌨ www...

Information ... and application forms obtained from the Department of Immigration and Multicultural and Indigenous Affairs (DIMIA) website:
⌨ www.imm...gov.au (accessed 2 Feb... 010)
⌨ http://www...anc.org.au/registration... (accessed 2 February 2010).

Index